T0290472

Scleroderma: Best Approaches to Patient Care

Editor

TRACY M. FRECH

RHEUMATIC DISEASE CLINICS OF NORTH AMERICA

www.rheumatic.theclinics.com

Consulting Editor
MICHAEL H. WEISMAN

May 2023 • Volume 49 • Number 2

ELSEVIER

1600 John F. Kennedy Boulevard • Suite 1800 • Philadelphia, Pennsylvania, 19103-2899
http://www.theclinics.com

RHEUMATIC DISEASE CLINICS OF NORTH AMERICA Volume 49, Number 2
May 2023 ISSN 0889-857X, ISBN 13: 978-0-323-96079-3

Editor: Joanna Gascoine
Developmental Editor: Karen Justine S. Dino

Rheumatic Disease Clinics of North America (ISSN 0889-857X) is published quarterly by Elsevier Inc., 360 Park Avenue South, New York, NY 10010-1710. Months of issue are February, May, August, and November. Business and editorial offices: 1600 John F. Kennedy Boulevard, Suite 1800, Philadelphia, PA 19103-2899. Periodicals postage paid at New York, NY and additional mailing offices. Subscription prices are USD 377.00 per year for US individuals, USD 865.00 per year for US institutions, USD 100.00 per year for US students and residents, USD 444.00 per year for Canadian individuals, USD 1081.00 per year for Canadian institutions, USD 100.00 per year for Canadian students/residents, USD 484.00 per year for international individuals, USD 1081.00 per year for international institutions, and USD 230.00 per year for foreign students/residents. To receive student/ resident rate, orders must be accompanied by name of affiliated institution, date of term, and the *signature* of program/residency coordinator on institution letterhead. Orders will be billed at individual rate until proof of status received. Foreign air speed delivery is included in all *Clinics* subscription prices. All prices are subject to change without notice. **POSTMASTER:** Send address changes to *Rheumatic Disease Clinics of North America,* Elsevier Health Sciences Division, Subscription Customer Service, 3251 Riverport Lane, Maryland Heights, MO 63043. **Customer Service: 1-800-654-2452 (US and Canada). From outside of the US and Canada: 314-447- 8871. Fax: 314-447-8029. For print support, e-mail: JournalsCustomerService-usa@elsevier.com. For on-line support, e-mail: JournalsOnlineSupport-usa@elsevier.com.**

Reprints. For copies of 100 or more of articles in this publication, please contact the Commercial Reprints Department, Elsevier Inc., 360 Park Avenue South, New York, New York, 10010-1710; Tel.: +1-212-633- 3874, Fax: +1-212-633-3820, and E-mail: reprints@elsevier.com.

Rheumatic Disease Clinics of North America is covered in *MEDLINE/PubMed (Index Medicus), Current Contents/Clinical Medicine, Science Citation Index, ISI/BIOMED,* and *EMBASE/Excerpta Medica.*

Contributors

CONSULTING EDITOR

MICHAEL H. WEISMAN, MD
Adjunct Professor of Medicine, Stanford University, Distinguished Professor of Medicine Emeritus, David Geffen School of Medicine at UCLA, Professor of Medicine Emeritus, Cedars-Sinai Medical Center, Los Angeles, California, USA

EDITOR

TRACY M. FRECH, MD, MS
Division of Rheumatology and Immunology, Department of Internal Medicine, Vanderbilt University Medical Center, Division of Rheumatology, Tennessee Valley Healthcare System, Veterans Affair Medical Center, Nashville, Tennessee, USA

AUTHORS

VINEET AGRAWAL, MD, PhD
Division of Cardiovascular Medicine, Vanderbilt University Medical Center, Nashville, Tennessee, USA

SHERVIN ASSASSI, MD, MS
Professor and Director, Division of Rheumatology, The University of Texas Health Science Center at Houston, Houston, Texas, USA

MURRAY BARRON, MD
Division of Rheumatology, Montreal, Quebec, Canada

COSIMO BRUNI, MD, PhD
Post-Doc Researcher, Department of Rheumatology, University Hospital Zurich, University of Zurich, Zurich, Switzerland; Division of Rheumatology, Department of Experimental Medicine, Careggi University Hospital - University of Florence, Florence, Italy

EVAN BUSMAN
Healthcare Patient Advocate, Atlanta, Georgia, USA

LEONARDO MARTIN CALDERON, MD
Department of Medicine, Schulich School of Medicine and Dentistry, University of Western Ontario, London, Ontario, Canada

CORRADO CAMPOCHIARO, MD
Senior Lecturer, Consultant in Rheumatology and Clinical Immunology, Unit of Immunology, Rheumatology, Allergy and Rare Diseases (UnIRAR), IRCCS San Raffaele Hospital, Vita-Salute San Raffaele University, Milan, Italy

FLAVIA V. CASTELINO, MD
Division of Rheumatology, Massachusetts General Hospital, Boston, Massachusetts, USA

HUMZA A. CHAUDHRY, BS
New Orleans Scleroderma and Sarcoidosis Patient Care and Research Center, Tulane University School of Medicine, New Orleans, Louisiana, USA

ERIN CHEW, MD
Division of Rheumatology and Immunology, Vanderbilt University Medical Center, Nashville, Tennessee, USA

ANGELA CHRISTENSEN, MD
Doctors Hospital, Renaissance, Texas, USA

LORINDA CHUNG, MD, MS
Departments of Medicine and Dermatology, Division of Immunology and Rheumatology, Stanford University School of Medicine, Palo Alto VA Healthcare System, Palo Alto, California, USA

MAURIZIO CUTOLO, MD
Professor of Rheumatology and Internal Medicine, Director, Laboratory of Experimental Rheumatology and Academic Division of Clinical Rheumatology, Director of the Postgraduate School of Rheumatology, Deputy-Chair of the European Rare Connective Tissue Disease Network ReCONNET-ERN, Deputy Chair, Department of Internal Medicine and Medical Specialties, University of Genova, IRCCS San Martino Polyclinic Hospital, Genova, Italy

JESKA K. DE VRIES-BOUWSTRA, MD, PhD
Rheumatologist, Assistant Professor, Head of the Leiden Clinic for Systemic Sclerosis, Department of Rheumatology, Leiden University Hospital, Leiden, the Netherlands

CHRISTOPHER P. DENTON, PhD, FRCP
Professor, Division of Medicine, Department of Inflammation, Centre for Rheumatology, University College London, London, United Kingdom

JÖRG H.W. DISTLER, MD
Department of Internal Medicine 3 - Rheumatology and Immunology, Friedrich–Alexander University Erlangen–Nuremberg (fau) and University Hospital Erlangen, Erlangen, Germany

ROBYN T. DOMSIC, MD, MPH
Division of Rheumatology and Clinical Immunology, University of Pittsburgh School of Medicine, Pittsburgh, Pennsylvania, USA

KIM FLIGELSTONE
Patient Research Partner, Scleroderma & Raynaud Society, UK (SRUK), Federation of European Scleroderma Associations, United Kingdom

IVAN FOELDVARI, MD
Head of the Hamburg Centre for Pediatric and Adolescence Rheumatology, Centre for Treatment of Scleroderma and Uveitis in Childhood and Adolescence, Teaching Unit of the Asklepios Campus of the Semmelweis Medical School, Budapest, Hungary; An der Schön Klinik Hamburg Eilbek, Hamburg, Germany

TRACY M. FRECH, MD, MS
Division of Rheumatology and Immunology, Department of Internal Medicine, Vanderbilt University Medical Center, Division of Rheumatology, Tennessee Valley Healthcare System, Veterans Affair Medical Center, Nashville, Tennessee, USA

JESSICA K. GORDON, MD, MSc
Department of Rheumatology, Hospital for Special Surgery, New York, New York, USA

FAYE N. HANT, DO, MSCR
Professor of Medicine, Director of the Rheumatology Fellowship Program, Division of Rheumatology and Immunology, Department of Medicine, Medical University of South Carolina, Charleston, South Carolina, USA

ARIANE L. HERRICK, MD, FRCP
Division of Musculoskeletal and Dermatological Sciences, The University of Manchester, Northern Care Alliance NHS Foundation Trust, Manchester Academic Health Science Centre, Manchester, United Kingdom

ANNA-MARIA HOFFMANN-VOLD, MD, PhD
Senior Consultant and Senior Researcher, Head of the Inflammatory and Fibrotic Rheumatic Disease Research Area, Department of Rheumatology, Oslo University Hospital - Rikshospitalet, Oslo, Norway

VIVIEN M. HSU, MD
RWJ–Scleroderma Program, Rutgers Robert Wood Johnson Medical School, New Brunswick, New Jersey, USA

MARIE HUDSON, MD, MPH, FRCPC
Central Manchester NHS Foundation Trust, Department of Medicine, McGill University, Division of Rheumatology, Lady Davis Institute for Medical Research, Jewish General Hospital, Montreal, Quebec, Canada

MICHAEL HUGHES, BSc (Hons), MBBS, MSc, MRCP (UK) (Rheumatology), PhD
Department of Rheumatology, Tameside and Glossop Integrated Care NHS Foundation Trust, Ashton-under-Lyne, United Kingdom; Division of Musculoskeletal and Dermatological Sciences, The University of Manchester, Manchester, United Kingdom

KELLY JENSEN, MD, MPH
New Orleans Scleroderma and Sarcoidosis Patient Care and Research Center, Tulane University School of Medicine, New Orleans, Louisiana, USA; University of Colorado School of Medicine, Denver, Colorado, USA

SINDHU R. JOHNSON, MD, PhD, FRCPC
Associate Professor of Medicine, Toronto Scleroderma Program, Division of Rheumatology, Department of Medicine, Mount Sinai Hospital, Toronto Western Hospital, Institute of Health Policy, Management and Evaluation, University of Toronto, Toronto, Ontario, Canada

CRISTIANE KAYSER, MD, PhD
Rheumatology Division, Escola Paulista de Medicina, Federal University of São Paulo (UNIFESP), São Paulo, São Paulo, Brazil

SAMARA M. KHALIQUE, MD
Department of Rheumatology, Virginia Tech Carilion Clinic School of Medicine, Roanoke, Virginia, USA

BENJAMIN D. KORMAN, MD
Division of Allergy, Immunology, and Rheumatology, University of Rochester Medical Center, Rochester, New York, USA

DANIEL J. LACHANT, DO
Division of Pulmonary and Critical Care Medicine, University of Rochester Medical Center, Rochester, New York, USA

NANCY LAZAR, MSW, LCSW
Direct Care Provider, Culver City, California, USA

EUN BONG LEE, MD, PhD
Professor, Division of Rheumatology, Seoul National University College of Medicine, Seoul, Republic of Korea

MARCO MATUCCI-CERINIC, MD, PhD
Professor, Division of Rheumatology and Scleroderma Unit, AOU Careggi, Florence, Department of Experimental and Clinical Medicine, University of Florence, Florence, Italy

ANNE MAWDSLEY
Raynaud's & Scleroderma Association–Care and Support, London, United Kingdom

ZSUZSANNA H. MCMAHAN, MD, MHS
Associate Professor, Division of Rheumatology, Johns Hopkins University, Baltimore, Maryland, USA

KATHLEEN MORRISROE, MBBS, FRACP, PhD
Department of Medicine, The University of Melbourne at St Vincent's Hospital (Melbourne), Department of Rheumatology, St Vincent's Hospital (Melbourne), Victoria, Australia

MAUREEN MURTAUGH, PhD, RDN
Department of Internal Medicine, Division of Epidemiology, University of Utah, Salt Lake City, Utah, USA

MANDANA NIKPOUR, MBBS, PhD
Professor, Department of Rheumatology, St Vincent's Hospital (Melbourne), Department of Medicine, The University of Melbourne at St Vincent's Hospital (Melbourne), Victoria, Australia

JOHN D. PAULING, BMedSci, BMBS, PhD, FRCP
Department of Rheumatology, North Bristol NHS Trust, Musculoskeletal Research Unit, Translational Health Sciences, Bristol Medical School, University of Bristol, Bristol, United Kingdom

JANET L. POOLE, PhD, OTR/L
Occupational Therapy Graduate Program, Department of Pediatrics, University of New Mexico, Albuquerque, New Mexico, USA

JANET E. POPE, MD
Department of Medicine, Schulich School of Medicine and Dentistry, University of Western Ontario, Division of Rheumatology, St. Joseph's Health Care, London, Ontario, Canada

ALANNAH QUINLIVAN, MBBS, BMeDSci
Doctor, Department of Rheumatology, St Vincent's Hospital (Melbourne), Department of Medicine, The University of Melbourne at St Vincent's Hospital (Melbourne), Victoria, Australia

GABRIELA RIEMEKASTEN, MD
Department of Rheumatology, University Medical Center Schleswig-Holstein, Campus Lübeck, Lübeck, Germany

TATIANA S. RODRiGUEZ-REYNA, MD, MSc
Clinical Researcher, Department of Immunology and Rheumatology, Instituto Nacional de Ciencias Médicas y Nutrición Salvador Zubirán, Mexico City, Mexico

ANNE-MARIE RUSSELL, PhD, APRN
Respiratory Institute, University of Exeter, Exeter, United Kingdom; Respiratory Medicine, Royal Devon University Healthcare NHS Foundation Trust, United Kingdom

LESLEY ANN SAKETKOO, MD, MPH
New Orleans Scleroderma and Sarcoidosis Patient Care and Research Center, University Medical Center – Comprehensive Pulmonary Hypertension Center and Interstitial Lung Disease Clinic Programs, Section of Pulmonary Medicine, Louisiana State University School of Medicine, Undergraduate Honors Department, Tulane University School of Medicine, New Orleans, Louisiana, USA

NORA SANDORFI, MD
Associate Professor of Medicine, University of Pennsylvania, Philadelphia, Pennsylvania, USA

AMI A. SHAH, MD, MS
Division of Rheumatology, Johns Hopkins School of Medicine, Johns Hopkins Scleroderma Center, Baltimore, Maryland, USA

VANESSA SMITH, MD
Professor of Medicine, Department of Internal Medicine, Ghent University, Department of Rheumatology, Ghent University Hospital, Unit for Molecular Immunology and Inflammation, VIB Inflammation Research Center (IRC), Ghent, Belgium; Member of ERN ReCONNET (Rare Connective Tissue Diseases)

VIRGINIA D. STEEN, MD
Division of Rheumatology, Department of Medicine, Georgetown University, Washington, DC, USA

ANTONIA VALENZUELA, MD, MS
Department of Rheumatology and Clinical Immunology, Pontificia Universidad Católica de Chile, Santiago, Chile

CECÍLIA VARJÚ, MD, PhD
Department of Rheumatology and Immunology, Medical School, University of Pécs, Pécs, Hungary

LUCAS VICTÓRIA DE OLIVEIRA MARTINS, MD, MSC
Rheumatology Division, Escola Paulista de Medicina, Federal University of São Paulo (Unifesp), São Paulo, São Paulo, Brazil

MADELON C. VONK, MD, PhD
Associate Professor, Systemic Sclerosis, Rheumatologist, Department of Rheumatology, Radboud University Nijmegen Medical Centre, Nijmegen, the Netherlands

SOPHIA C. WEINMANN, MD
Department of Medicine, Division of Rheumatology and Immunology, Duke University Hospital, Durham, North Carolina, USA

Contents

Systemic sclerosis (SSc) is a heterogeneous disease comprising of a wide spectrum of ages of onset, sex-based differences, ethnic variations, disease manifestations, differential serologic profiles, and variable response to therapy resulting in reduced health-related quality of life, disability, and survival. The ability to subset groups of patients with SSc can assist with refining the diagnosis, guide appropriate monitoring, inform aggressiveness of immunosuppression, and predict prognosis. The ability to subset patients with SSc has several important practical implications for patient care.

Systemic sclerosis (SSc) is a heterogenous systemic autoimmune disease of complex multi-organ manifestations with a disease-specific mortality of >50%. The patient journey is fraught with severe, diverse, and diffuse physical impairment, psychological burden, and diminishing health-related quality of life. SSc remains unfamiliar to many clinicians. Delayed/misdiagnosis, inadequate screening, and attention for common complications with potentially preventable disability/death contribute to patients feeling isolated and unsupported. We present actionable standards including screening, anticipatory guidance, and counseling in patient-centered SSc-care emphasizing psycho-social health as the central goal, whereas robust vigilance and efforts to improve biophysical health and survival are imperatives that support this goal.

As skin involvement is the hall mark of systemic sclerosis (SSc) and changes of skin involvement have shown to correlate with internal organ involvement, assessing the extend of skin involvement is key. Although the modified Rodnan skin score is a validated tool used to evaluate the skin in SSc, it has its drawbacks. Novel imagine methods are promising but should be further evaluated. As for molecule markers for skin

management practices are focused on the treatment of symptoms with little information available on how to use GI investigations in daily practice. This review demonstrates how to integrate the objective assessment of common lower GI symptoms into clinical care with the aim of guiding clinical decision making. Understanding the type of abnormal GI function that is affecting a patient and determining which parts of the gut are impacted can help clinicians to target therapy more precisely.

Joint involvement, including arthralgia, inflammatory arthritis, joint contractures and overlapping with rheumatoid arthritis, is a common manifestation and is associated with impared quality of life in systemic sclerosis (SSc). Few studies have evaluated the treatment of arthritis in SSc. Pharmacological approach includes low-dose corticosteroids, methotrexate, and hydroxychloroquine. Non-tumor necrosis factor biologics, especially rituximab and tocilizumab, may be a promising option for refractory cases.

Pulmonary hypertension (PH) is a leading cause of morbidity and mortality in systemic sclerosis (SSc). PH is a heterogenous condition and several different forms of PH are associated with SSc, including pulmonary arterial hypertension (PAH) resulting from a pulmonary arterial vasculopathy, PH due to interstitial lung disease, PH due to left heart disease, and PH due to thromboembolic disease. Extensive research has led to an improved understanding of the mediators involved in the pathogenesis of SSc-PH. Initial combination therapy is the preferred treatment approach for SSc-PAH and requires coordinated care with a multidisciplinary team including rheumatology, pulmonology, and cardiology.

Systemic sclerosis (SSc), also known as scleroderma, is a chronic autoimmune connective tissue disease and is associated with a significant economic burden resulting from health care utilization costs in addition to indirect costs attributable to SSc resulting from early retirement and lost productivity in those that remain in employment.

The optimal systemic sclerosis (SSc) care plan includes an occupational therapist and physical therapist as well as wound care experts and a registered dietitian if indicated. Screening instruments for functional and work disability, hand and mouth limitations, malnutrition, and dietary intake can identify the need for ancillary support services. Telemedicine can assist in developing effective ancillary treatment plans. Reimbursement for services may limit access for patients with SSc to expand their care team but a focus on prevention rather than management of damage is recognized as an important unmet need in SSc. In this review, the role of a comprehensive care team for SSc is discussed.

Each person who presents for scleroderma-focused care not only has their own psychosocial stressors in their day-to-day life but they also have scleroderma symptom-specific stressors as well as their own mental health reactions throughout their journey with this disease course. There are many actions patients can take to help and support themselves when they are faced with any of the mental health and social determinants of health stressors associated with this rare, chronic illness. Using the scleroderma specialty providers to inform, discuss, and address these areas with their patients can assist with more effective symptom and disease self-management.

Systemic sclerosis (SSc) is a rare multisystem autoimmune disease characterized by fibrosis, vasculopathy, and autoimmunity. There are multiple complications inherent to SSc and its management. One of these complications is increased infection risk, which can lead to decreased quality of life and increased morbidity and mortality. Patients with SSc have lower vaccination rates and decreased vaccine seroconversion secondary to immunosuppressive medications compared with the general population. The purpose of this review is to provide clinicians with an approach to vaccinations in SSc.

Systemic sclerosis (SSc) is a rare multisystem autoimmune disease characterized by fibrosis, vasculopathy, and autoimmunity. Lesser known complications inherent to SSc, such as malignancies and osteoporosis, can lead to decreased quality of life and increased morbidity and mortality. Patients with SSc have a greater risk of developing malignancies than the general population. In addition, they are more likely to be vitamin D deficient and are at great risk of osteoporosis-related fractures. However, these complications can be addressed through preventative measures. The purpose of this review is to provide clinicians with an approach to bone health and cancer screening in SSc.

Video content accompanies this article at http://www.rheumatic.
theclinics.com.

Rheumatology is rich in educational opportunities, learning about a variety
of diseases. Rheumatology subspecialty training is a time of unparalleled
learning, and within the curriculum of a training program, the connective
tissue diseases (CTDs) represent a unique challenge to the fellows. The
challenge therein lies in the multisystem presentations they are faced
with mastering. Scleroderma, as a rare and life-threatening CTD, remains
one of the most difficult conditions to manage and treat. In this article, the
authors focus on an approach to training the next generation of rheumatologists to take care of patients with scleroderma.

Emerging evidence shows that a complex interplay between cells and mediators and extracellular matrix factors may underlie the development and
persistence of fibrosis in systemic sclerosis. Similar processes may determine vasculopathy. This article reviews recent progress in understanding
how fibrosis becomes profibrotic and how the immune system, vascular,
and mesenchymal compartment affect disease development. Early phase
trials are informing about pathogenic mechanisms in vivo and reverse
translation for observational and randomized trials is allowing hypotheses
to be developed and tested. In addition to repurposing already available
drugs, these studies are paving the way for the next generation of targeted
therapeutics.

Systemic sclerosis (SSc) -related calcinosis can be a debilitating,
constantly painful, poorly understood vascular complication of calcium hydroxyapatite deposition in soft tissue structures that affects approximately
40% of both limited and diffuse cutaneous SSc subtypes. This publication
describes the iterative and multitiered international qualitative investigations that yielded remarkable insights into natural history, daily experience,
and complications of SSc-calcinosis providing pivotal information for
health management. Patient-driven question development and field
testing, according to Food and Drug Administration guidance, propelled
the development of a patient-reported outcome measure for SSc-
calcinosis, the Mawdsley Calcinosis Questionnaire.

Primary cardiac involvement in systemic sclerosis (SSc) is an important cause of morbidity and mortality. Abnormalities of cardiac structure and function can be detected on routine cardiopulmonary screening that is the standard of care for SSc monitoring. Cardiovascular magnetic resonance-extracellular volume (indicating diffuse fibrosis) and cardiac biomarkers may identify at-risk patients who would benefit from further evaluation including screening for atrial and ventricular arrhythmias with implantable loop recorders. The role of algorithm-based cardiac evaluation both before and after therapeutic initiation is one of the many unmet needs for SSc clinical care.

RHEUMATIC DISEASE CLINICS
OF NORTH AMERICA

SERIES OF RELATED INTEREST

Medical Clinics of North America
https://www.medical.theclinics.com/
Neurologic Clinics
https://www.neurologic.theclinics.com/
Dermatologic Clinics
https://www.derm.theclinics.com/
Physical Medicine and Rehabilitation Clinics of North America
https://www.pmr.theclinics.com/

THE CLINICS ARE AVAILABLE ONLINE!
Access your subscription at:
www.theclinics.com

Foreword

Scleroderma: Best Approaches to Patient Care

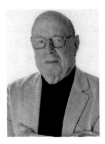

Michael H. Weisman, MD
Consulting Editor

This issue on systemic sclerosis is quite unlike anything that has come before, and the kudos have to go to Tracy Frech, who orchestrated the effort and selected the topics. For the very first time, we have a scholarly review of systemic sclerosis that is patient centered, comprehensive, and focused on clinical care that also addresses mental health, physical therapy, occupational therapy, and preventive care alongside organ system approaches. It has long been recognized that subsetting systemic sclerosis patients is critical for prognosis; now with modern tools and increased knowledge of therapeutic pathways, we can approach the patient based on much better knowledge of risk assessments. The new goals are to intervene early, and effectively. Tracy has given us the state-of-the-art approaches to the vascular complications of the disease, and the emphasis is always on collaboration with our colleagues in other specialties where their knowledge can be of critical importance. Perhaps it is useful to step back and realize the impact of this issue—with the tools at hand, we now can focus on therapeutics, and we have the possibility to train the next generation of

Rheum Dis Clin N Am 49 (2023) xvii–xviii
https://doi.org/10.1016/j.rdc.2023.02.001
0889-857X/23/© 2023 Elsevier Inc. All rights reserved.

rheumatologists to utilize the optimal ways to manage the systemic sclerosis patient. Tracy did a remarkable job here, and our specialty of Rheumatology is grateful for this issue.

Michael H. Weisman, MD
Adjunct Professor of Medicine
Stanford University
Distinguished Professor of Medicine Emeritus
David Geffen School of Medicine at UCLA, Professor of Medicine Emeritus
Cedars-Sinai Medical Center
10800 Wilshire Boulevard #404
Los Angeles, CA 90024, USA

E-mail address:
weisman@cshs.org

Preface

Best Approaches to the Care of Systemic Sclerosis Patients

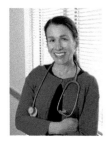

Tracy M. Frech, MD, MS
Editor

In this issue, the world's leading experts review the best approaches to patient care for patients with systemic sclerosis. Systemic sclerosis is an autoimmune disease with severe multiorgan system manifestations with heterogeneous rates of progression, which occurs in children and adults. This comprehensive series covers a thoughtful approach to assessing an individual patient and applying scientific principles of vasculopathy, fibrosis, and immune dysfunction to treatment decisions. Organ-specific manifestations and treatments, including skin, joint, heart, lung, and kidney, are reviewed by expert rheumatologists. A comprehensive care plan that involves professionals in mental health, occupational therapy, physical therapy, and wound care is highlighted as valuable in the care of the systemic sclerosis patient. The importance of education for trainees in a systemic sclerosis physical exam is discussed. The critical topic of involving patients as partners and registry-based discovery is reviewed. The only way to truly understand the burden of disease for patients with systemic sclerosis is with international partnerships and perspectives. This issue provides guidance for treating health care providers on best approaches to care of systemic sclerosis patients.

Tracy M. Frech, MD, MS
Division of Rheumatology and Immunology
Department of Internal Medicine
Vanderbilt University Medical Center
Tennessee Valley Healthcare System Veterans Affair Medical Center
1161 Medical Center Drive, 3113-B
Nashville, TN 37212, USA

E-mail address:
tracy.frech@vumc.edu

Rheum Dis Clin N Am 49 (2023) xix
https://doi.org/10.1016/j.rdc.2023.01.019
0889-857X/23/© 2023 Elsevier Inc. All rights reserved.

rheumatic.theclinics.com

Approach to Systemic Sclerosis Patient Assessment
How Does Patient Subsetting Help?

Sindhu R. Johnson, MD, PhD, FRCPC[a,b,*], Ivan Foeldvari, MD[c,d,*]

KEYWORDS

• Scleroderma • Systemic sclerosis • Classification criteria • Subsetting

KEY POINTS

• The ability to subset groups of patients with systemic sclerosis (SSc) can guide appropriate monitoring, inform treatment, predict outcomes, and inform prognosis.
• Extent of skin involvement is currently the strongest determinant of SSc subsets.
• SSc-specific antibodies, gene expression profiling, and nailfold capillary pattern are innovative means of further informing SSc subsets.

CLASSIFICATION OF SYSTEMIC SCLEROSIS

Classification and subclassification of systemic sclerosis (SSc) are important parts of both research and clinical practice.[1] SSc is a heterogeneous disease characterized by immune activation, vasculopathy, and fibrosis, affecting the skin and internal organs. Furthermore, there is variation in disease manifestations across ages (juvenile onset,[2] geriatric onset[3]), sexes,[4,5] and ethnicities.[6,7] SSc can result in diminished quality of life and early mortality.[8–10] The heterogeneity within SSc is problematic for the interpretation of research results and their application to patient care.[1] Heterogeneity among study patients can lead to imprecise estimates of treatment effect unrelated to the intervention itself.[1] Heterogeneity among study patients compromises comparison of results across studies.[1] The American College of Rheumatology (ACR) and the European League Against Rheumatism (EULAR) have recognized the need for classification criteria to identify more homogeneous groups of patients for inclusion into

[a] Toronto Scleroderma Program, Division of Rheumatology, Department of Medicine, Mount Sinai Hospital, Toronto Western Hospital, Ground Floor, East Wing, 399 Bathurst Street, Toronto, Ontario M5T 2S8, Canada; [b] Institute of Health Policy, Management and Evaluation, University of Toronto, Toronto, Ontario, Canada; [c] Centre for Treatment of Scleroderma and Uveitis in Childhood and Adolescence, Teaching Unit of the Asklepios Campus of the Semmelweis Medical School, Budapest, Hungary; [d] An der Schön Klinik Hamburg Eilbek, Dehnhaide 120, Hamburg 22081, Germany
* Corresponding authors.
E-mail addresses: Sindhu.Johnson@uhn.ca (S.R.J.); Foeldvari@t-online.de (I.F.)

Rheum Dis Clin N Am 49 (2023) 193–210
https://doi.org/10.1016/j.rdc.2023.01.001
0889-857X/23/© 2023 Elsevier Inc. All rights reserved.

research studies.[1,11,12] Classification is separate from diagnosis.[11] Over the last several decades, several iterations of classification criteria have been proposed.[1,13–15]

The ACR/EULAR classification criteria for SSc are currently the global standard for identifying patients into clinical trials and observational studies.[16–18] These classification criteria were developed in a multiphased international collaborative effort with a balanced use of data-driven and expert-based methods.[19–23] These classification criteria have excellent sensitivity of 91% and specificity of 92% compared with previous iterations of classification criteria.[17,24–27] They also have excellent sensitivity and specificity for early disease (less than 3 years disease duration). Furthermore, these excellent operating characteristics have been externally validated in other cohorts.[28–31] Every patient with juvenile SSc, who fulfills the pediatric classification criteria,[32] where cutaneous involvement of proximal the metacarpophalangeal (MCP) or metatarsophalangeal (MTP) joints is a major criteria, is sufficient to fulfill the ACR-EULAR classification criteria. The ACR/EULAR classification criteria were not formally validated for juvenile SSc. Further, the ACR/EULAR classification criteria for SSc do not substitute for diagnostic criteria.[18] The diagnosis of SSc remains within the judgment of the appropriately trained and experienced health care professional. In clinical practice, the inability to fulfill the classification criteria for SSc should not be used as justification to withhold appropriate therapy from a patient with SSc.

SUBSETS OF SYSTEMIC SCLEROSIS

Several methods of identifying subsets of patients with SSc are currently used based on extent of skin involvement, age of onset, disease duration, and presence of overlapping rheumatic diseases.

Limited Versus Diffuse Systemic Sclerosis

The criteria of Leroy and colleagues[33] are the most frequently cited subsetting system for SSc. This system categorizes SSc into diffuse cutaneous and limited cutaneous SSc.[33] Patients with limited SSc have skin involvement that is limited to distal to the knees and elbows but may include the face, neck, or upper chest. Diffuse SSc have skin thickening proximal to the elbows and knees and/or truncal involvement at any time in their disease course. **Table 1** compares the diffuse and limited subsets. Because of the ability to readily observe disease activity, rapidity of disease, and

Table 1 Limited and diffuse subset system	
Limited	**Diffuse**
Often experience symptoms of Raynaud phenomenon for years before cutaneous or internal organ manifestations	Usually develop Raynaud phenomenon within a year of onset of skin changes
Later onset of pulmonary arterial hypertension	Generally rapid progression with most patients peaking their skin thickness score within 2 y
Includes CREST syndrome, an acronym for calcinosis, Raynaud phenomenon, esophageal dysmotility, sclerodactyly, and telangiectasias	Can be accompanied by • Tendon friction rubs (a harbinger of active skin disease) • Finger and large joint contractures
Includes scleroderma sine scleroderma	More likely to develop • Severe interstitial lung disease • Scleroderma renal crisis • Myocardial involvement

poor outcomes, most SSc clinical trials focus on the evaluation of innovative therapies in the diffuse subset. As such, the limited subset has been called "unfairly neglected."[34]

This SSc subset system largely relies on extensive skin involvement. Extent of skin involvement has good discriminative validity with regard to dominant features (fibrotic vs vascular pathic), internal organ damage, and outcomes.[15] This system of subsetting is valuable for identifying patients with early SSc who may have a poor prognosis and will require close monitoring. The diffuse subset with rapidly progressive disease requires treatment that is more aggressive. However, in later stages of the disease, patients initially classified as rapid progressors may still have high disease severity due to the accumulated damage but low disease activity as a result of treatment or spontaneous remission. Furthermore, some patients with SSc develop visceral disease late in the disease course. Thus, the limited/diffuse system loses its predicted value in more advanced disease. In pediatric disease the differences are even less pronounced.[2]

Very Early Systemic Sclerosis

The very early diagnosis of SSc (VEDOSS) project of the European League Against Rheumatism Scleroderma Trials and Research group lists features that may precede characteristic skin thickening and internal organ involvement and facilitate earlier diagnosis.[35,36] A patient with Raynaud phenomenon and/or puffy fingers who are positive for antinuclear antibodies are considered to fulfill the VEDOSS criteria if they also have abnormal capillaroscopy and positive anticentromere antibodies (ACA) or positive anti-Scl-70 antibodies. Although RNA polymerase III antibodies were not captured in the preliminary dataset,[37] for practical purposes, this SSc-specific antibody is often included for VEDOSS characterization. Nationwide registries with VEDOSS subsetting and follow-up studies may give us valuable insights into the SSc natural history and main prognostic factors.[38]

Overlap Syndromes

SSc can overlap with other systemic autoimmune rheumatic diseases, mostly systemic lupus erythematosus (so-called lupoderma), rheumatoid arthritis, myositis, Sjogren syndrome, mixed connective tissue disease, and rarely vasculitis.[39,40] In the setting of juvenile SSc, overlap mostly occurs with juvenile dermatomyositiss.[2] In patients with juvenile dermatomyositis, calcinosis cutis usually occurs within 2 to 3 years from disease onset, which is faster than it occurs with other systemic autoimmune rheumatic diseases, where calcinosis cutis tends to occur at 8 years.[41] In juvenile dermatomyositis, anti-NXP-2 and anti-PM/Scl antibodies are associated with an increased risk of calcinosis.[42] In juvenile dermatomyositis, calcinotic lesions usually resorb over several years.[43] In contrast, in SSc-associated calcinosis, few lesions improve, whereas most of them either remain stable or progress at 1 year.[44]

The EULAR/ACR classification criteria for SSc can be applied to individuals with an overlap syndrome. Treatment is determined by which disease the manifestation is most likely to be attributed to. For example, if the symmetrical, inflammatory arthritis affecting the small joints of the hands is rheumatoid factor and/or anti-CCP positive, one may consider treatment with a tumor necrosis factor inhibitor, which is otherwise not generally effective in the setting of SSc.

JUVENILE-ONSET SYSTEMIC SCLEROSIS

Juvenile-onset SSc is classified according to the Pediatric Rheumatology European Society–American College of Rheumatology (PRES-ACR) classification criteria.[32] This classification consists of one major criteria, the scleroderma-specific skin induration proximal to the MCP or MTP joints, and at least 2 minor criteria, the SSc-specific organ involvement and antibody profile. The PRES-ACR criteria were never validated prospectively. In the juvenile scleroderma inception cohort we presented during an ACR meeting,[45] every patient who fulfills the PRES-ACR criteria automatically has 9 points of the adult ACR-EULAR classification criteria, which is sufficient to classify the patients as patients with SSc. Therefore, since 2014, the ACR-EULAR classification criteria are used as inclusion criteria for the juvenile scleroderma inception cohort,[46] which is the largest cohort of juvenile systemic scleroderma of the world.

REFINING SYSTEMIC SCLEROSIS SUBSETS

With advances in knowledge, our expectations for SSc subsetting have changed.[47] There have been calls for subsetting patients with SSc using a combination of multi-system involvement, genetic markers, autoantibody profiling, nailfold capillaroscopy, molecular genomic, and cellular patterns.[14,48–54]

Systemic Sclerosis–Specific Antibodies

Considerable attention has been given to subsetting SSc by autoantibody profile. It has long been recognized that SSc is associated with specific antibodies.[55] Autoantibodies are detected in more than 95% of patients with SSc.[55] Ten SSc-specific autoantibodies have been described, although not all are widely clinically available. In recent years, we have improved our understanding of SSc-specific antibodies and their clinical associations[55–61] (**Table 2**). These antibodies generally remain stable over time and are mutually exclusive in most of the patients.[62] SSc-specific antibodies are increasingly accessible in routine practice. SSc-specific antibodies are also helpful in the assessment of patients with Raynaud phenomenon without any SSc skin thickening in predicting future development of SSc in patients with Raynaud phenomenon without any scleroderma skin changes.[63] SSc-specific autoantibody production often precedes onset of SSc symptoms, whereas the absence of antibodies suggests a higher probability of primary Raynaud phenomenon, especially in the setting of normal capillaroscopy. A small proportion (6.4%) of patients with SSc do not have antinuclear antibodies detectable by commercial assays. This SSc subset more frequently includes male and has less frequent and less severe vasculopathy and more frequent lower gastrointestinal involvement.[64]

Gene Expression Profiling

Three distinct gene expression patterns have been identified among diffuse SSc and 2 groups among patients with limited SSc. The gene expression patterns from diffuse SSc and limited SSc are distinct from the skin gene expression of healthy controls.[65] The unique gene expression signatures indicate proliferating cells, immune infiltrates, and a fibrosis.[65] The intrinsic groups are statistically significant ($P<.001$) and associated with the modified Rodnan skin score, interstitial lung disease, gastrointestinal involvement, digital ulcers, Raynaud phenomenon, and disease duration.[65] Molecular signatures obtained from SSc skin biopsies have been associated with a beneficial response to treatment with mycophenolate.[66] The ability to subset patients with SSc based on gene expression profiling may have the potential to inform which individual level patients are most likely to respond to therapy.

Nailfold Capillaries

SSc is characterized by distinct pattern of nailfold capillary abnormalities. The presence of SSc pattern of capillary abnormalities may assist in predicting the development

Table 2
Systemic sclerosis–related autoantibodies and systemic sclerosis manifestations

Autoantibodies	Associations	Reference
ACA	SSc type: a higher frequency of ACA in type 1 SSc sclerodactyly only (60.8%), followed by type 2 sclerosis proximal to MCP, but excluding trunk (29.7%) and type 3 diffuse skin sclerosis including trunk (9.5%)	Barnett et al,[75] 1988
Anti-Th/To	lcSSc and mild slowly progressive ILD Compared with ACA"+" subset, anti –Th/Th "+" subset was associated with higher frequency of pericarditis, lower FVC, male gender, younger patients with SSc, and less frequent telangiectasia	Ceribelli et al,[76] 2010
ACA, ATA, anti-Th/To, anti-RNAP I, II, III, anti-U1 RNP, unidentified ANA, ANA negative	ACA: older at disease onset, isolated reduction in DLCO, reduced creatinine clearance, telangiectasia, less frequent ILD ATA: more extensive skin involvement, lung fibrosis Anti-U1 RNP: younger at disease onset, rare esophageal involvement, less frequent telangiectasia	Gliddon et al,[77] 2011
ACA, ATA, anti-Th/To, anti-RNAP III, anti-fibrillarin, unidentified ANA	ACA and anti-Th/To: lcSSc	Falkner et al,[78] 2000
Ten serological subtypes studied	dcSSc: ATA: ILD, reduced survival Anti-RNAP III: SRC, reduced survival lcSSc: ACA: no ILD Anti-Th/To: PAH Anti-Ku: myositis (NS) Overlap: Anti-U1-RNP: frequent PAH, reduced survival, younger at disease onset Anti-PM/Scl: ILD (NS)	Graf et al,[79] 2012

(continued on next page)

Table 2
(continued)

Autoantibodies	Associations	Reference
ACA; ATA; anti-U1-RNP, anti-RNAP; anti-Th/To (small number of pts); anti-U3 RNP (small number of pts)	ATA: dcSSc, high mRSS, diffuse skin hyperpigmentation, pulmonary fibrosis, decreased survival rate Anti-RNAP: dcSSc, high mRSS, finger contractures ACA: lcSSc, low mRSS, less frequent ILD Anti-U3-RNP: dcSSc, rarely decreased DLCO Anti-U1-RNP: low mRSS Anti-Th/To: low mRSS, rarely decreased DLCO and upper GI involvement Negative ANA: low mRSS dcSSc positive for anti-RNAP (compared to dcSSc positive for ATA): rapid skin progression, skin hyperpigmentation, less frequent pitting scars and ILD, lower serum IgG levels	Hamaguchi et al,[80] 2008
Anti-CENP-A or anti-CENP-B	ACA (anti-CENP-A or anti-CENP-B): lcSSc; less frequent ILD, cardiac involvement, skin ulcers	Hanke et al,[81] 2010
ACA, ATA	ACA: female predominance, lcSSc, calcinosis, telangiectasia ATA: intermediate and diffuse SSc, GI and heart involvement, myositis, skin ulcers, hyperpigmentation, shorter RP duration before skin changes	Ferri et al,[58] 1991
ACA, ATA, anti-RNAP I/II/III	ACA: lcSSc, rare renal disease and ILD ATA: ILD, renal involvement (compared with ACA) Anti-RNAP I/II/III: dcSSc	Harvey et al,[82] 1999
ACA, ATA, anti-RNAP I, II, III, anti-U1-RNP, anti-histone	ACA: less frequent ILD, female predominance, vascular changes (finger systolic pressure), reduced GFR ATA: dcSSc, higher % of men, ILD Anti-RNAP I, II, III: ILD Anti-U1-RNP: younger at disease onset, vasospasm Anti-histone: more frequent cardiac, pulmonary and renal involvement, reduced survival	Hesselstrand et al,[59] 2003
ACA*(anti-CENP-B and anti-CENP-Q)	Less frequent ILD	Song et al,[83] 2013

ACA	ACA: older at disease onset, women predominance, lcSSc and lower mRSS, pulmonary hypertension, lower overall disease severity, less likely to have finger ulcers, digital tuft resorption, or finger contractures, ILD, SRC, inflammatory arthritis, and myositis. ACA status was predictive of the extent of skin involvement over time. Patients with lcSSc who were CENP-A-negative at baseline were more likely to progress to diffuse disease compared with CENP-A–positive patients	Hudson et al,[84] 2012
Anti-RNAP III	dcSSc, higher maximum mRSS, and increased frequency of tendon friction rubs, SRC.	Kuwana et al,[85] 2005
ACA	Better prognosis, less frequent major renal, cardiac, pulmonary, and lower GI tract involvement compared with speckled or nucleolar ANA patterns	McCarty et al,[86] 1983
ACA (CENP-B)	CREST	Vazquez-Abad et al,[87] 1994
Anti-CCP3 in combination with ACA	CREST	Wu et al,[88] 2007
ACA	ACA: sclerodactyly with/without minimal skin involvement in other areas—armpits, eyelids, neck. ACA-negative (most were ATA-positive): arms, legs ± trunk involvement, lower cumulative survival rate, and higher severity of internal organ involvement	Giordano et al,[89] 1986
Anti-RNAP III	Risk of SRC	Santiago et al,[90] 2007
ANA negative	Less frequent vasculopathic manifestations	Salazar et al,[64] 2015
Anti-RNAP III	Severe skin and renal involvement	Satoh et al,[91] 2009
Anti-calpastatin antibodies	Higher ESR and inflammatory muscle involvement	Sato et al,[92] 2009
ATA fragment F1	No clinical associations	Simon et al,[93] 2009
ACA, ATA, and anti-RNAP III positive	ACA: female predominance, less common dcSSc and ILD, longer time from onset to SSc diagnosis; ATA: higher prevalence of ILD, less frequent lcSSc, and sine scleroderma subtypes; Anti-RNAPIII: dcSSc, malignancies more frequent, especially synchronous neoplasia. No difference in terms of survival rate at 5 y and 30 y and causes of death.	Iniesta Arandia et al,[94] 2017

(continued on next page)

Table 2
(continued)

Autoantibodies	Associations	Reference
5 clusters based on clinical and serological features	Autoantibodies improved detection of lung involvement, PAH and renal crisis, as well as patients with actual severe disease course, when shifting from clinical subgrouping to combined autoantibody and clinical subgrouping. High-risk (mortality around 10%): Subgroup 1: dcSSc and renal crisis, less often women, ATA+ Subgroup 2: dcSSc, PAH, GAVE, less often Caucasians, ATA+, ACA-. Intermediate (mortality risk 7.2%): Subgroup 5: less frequent ILD and vasculopathy (pitting scars, digital ulcers), anti-RNAPIII+, Pm/Scl- Low-risk: Subgroup 3: GI, ACA+, ATA- Subgroup 4: miscellaneous, Pm/Scl+, RNAP-	Boonstra et al,[95] 2018
ACA+dcSSc, ACA+lcSSc and ACA-dcSSc	dcSSc ACA+ is a distinct clinical subtype with more insidious onset of skin and major organ involvement, a lower incidence of ILD and SRC and better survival than expected for dcSSc	Caetano et al,[96] 2018
ACA, ATA, anti-RNAPIII, Th/To, PM/Scl	ACA: older, longer disease duration and time from RP onset ATA: ILD Anti-RNAPII: SRC	Caramaschi et al,[97] 2015
Anti-HP1 positive	CREST	Coppo et al,[98] 2013
ACA, anti-RNAP III dcSSc, and anti-RNAP lcSSc	Anti-RNAPIII+, ATA-, ACA-, anti-RNAPII: increased risk of cancer ACA+: lowest cancer risk dcSSc anti-RNAPII: breast cancer lcSSc anti-RNAPIII: lung cancer	Igusa et al,[99] 2018
ATA, ACA (CENP A, CENP B), anti-PM/Scl-100, anti-M/Scl-75, arti-Ku, anti-Ro52, anti-RNAP III (RP11 and RP155), anti-fibrillarin (U3RNP), anti-NOR-90, ant -Th/To, anti-PDGFR	ATA: female, dcSSc, high peak mRSS, RP, hand deformity ACA: negative association with hand deformity Anti-Ku: overlap syndrome SSc/PM	Foocharoen et al,[100] 2017

Autoantibody	Clinical association	Reference
Anti-RNAPIII	Anti-RNAPIII: SRC Subgrouping: the presence of anti-RNAPII in combination with anti-RNAPI/III (anti-RNAPI/II/III) and a higher ELISA index for anti-RNAPIII may be associated with the development of SRC in patients with SSc with anti-RNAPIII	Hamaguchi et al,[101] 2015
Anti-PM/Scl-100 as a part of the signature, also based on levels of CD40 ligand, chemokine (C-X-C motif) ligand 4 (CXCL4)	Clinical improvement	Haddon et al,[102] 2017
ATA, ACA	ATA: hand deformity ACA: negative association with hand deformity ATA+dcSSc: earlier ILD ATA−lcSSc: RP	Foocharoen et al,[100] 2016
Anti-Ku*	Anti-Ku: ILD, increased creatine kinase levels. No difference in survival	Hoa et al,[60] 2016
Anti-RNAP III	dcSSc, higher mRSS, renal involvement	Terras et al,[103] 2016
ACA cross-reacting with FOXE3p53-62	Less likely to develop active disease	Perosa et al,[104] 2013
Anti-Ro52/TRIM21 antibodies	Less likely Caucasians, ILD, poor survival	Wodkowski et al,[105] 2015
Anti-RNAP I/III	Temporal relationship with the onset of cancer	Shah et al,[106] 2010
Anti-SSA/Ro52	No clinical associations	Sánchez-Montalvá et al,[107] 2014
Anti-RPA194 (subgrouping among anti-RPC155 antibodies)	Cancer, less severe GI disease	Shah et al,[108] 2019
Anti-U1RNP	lcSSc (91%), digital ulcers/scars (50%), ILD (63%), joint (65%), and muscle (43%) involvement	Shayakhmetova & Ananyeva,[109] 2019
ACA, anti-RNAP III strong, anti-RNAP III weak, ATA, anti-RNAP III, anti-NOR-90, anti-fibrillarin, anti-Th/To, anti-PM/Scl-75, anti-PM/Scl-100, anti-Ku, ATA, anti-Ro 52, anti-PDGFR	lSSc: ACA dcSSc: RNAPIII, ATA Anti-Th/To: less likely joint contractures and reflux esophagitis Anti-fibrillarin: digital amputation and a trend toward GAVE Anti-TRIM-21/Ro 52: telangiectasia, dry eyes, PAH, and calcinosis Anti-PM/Scl-75/100: digital ulcers and a trend toward lcSSc Subgrouping RNAP III into 2 clusters: a strong cluster with increased risk of GAVE, lower risk of esophageal dysmotility The rest: male sex, smoking, malignancy, less likely telangiectasia, RP, and contractures	Patterson et al,[110] 2015

(continued on next page)

Table 2
(continued)

Autoantibodies	Associations	Reference
Subspecificities of anti-CANPA:anti-pc4.2 antibodies, anti-pc14.1 antibodies	Anti-pc4.2 antibodies: sPAP and inversely associated with DLCO Anti-pc14.1 antibodies: inversely sPAP and positively with DLCO	Perosa et al,[111] 2016
ACA, ATA, anti-RNAP	ACA: higher MiR-409-3p expression levels ATA, anti-RNAPIII: higher MiR-184 ATA, anti-RNP: lower MiR-92a	Wuttge et al,[112] 2015
anti-PM75 and anti-PM100	Anti-PM75 and anti-PM100: myositis Anti-PM75: ILD, calcinosis Anti-PM100: calcinosis, better survival	Wodkowski et al,[113] 2015
ATA, ACA, a-RNAP III (RP11, RP155), anti-fibrillarin, anti-Ku, anti-NOR90, anti-PM-Scl100, anti-PM-Scl75	ATA: dcSSc, ILD, PH and ILD-PH, digital ulcers Anti-CENPB: lcSSc, negatively ILD Anti-RP11: male sex Anti-NOR90: male sex, ILD Anti-Ro52: arthritis	Liaskos et al,[114] 2017

Abbreviations: a-RNAP, antibodies to RNA polymerase; ACA, anticentromere autoantibodies; ANA, antinuclear autoantibodies; ATA, antibodies to topoisomerase I; dcSSc, diffuse cutaneous systemic sclerosis; DLCO, diffusing capacity for carbon monoxide; ESR, erythrocyte sedimentation rate; FVC, forced vital capacity; GAVE, gastric antral vascular ectasia; GFR, glomerular filtration rate; GI, gastrointestinal; ILD, interstitial lung disease; lcSSc, limited cutaneous systemic sclerosis; MCP, metacarpophalangeal joints; mRSS, modified Rodnan skin score; PAH, pulmonary arterial hypertension; PH, pulmonary hypertension; RP, Raynaud phenomenon; sPAP, systolic pulmonary artery pressure; SRC, scleroderma renal crisis.

Adapted from Nevskaya T, Pope JE, Turk MA, et al. Systematic Analysis of the Literature in Search of Defining Systemic Sclerosis Subsets. J Rheumatol. 2021;48(11):1698-1717.

of SSc in patients with Raynaud phenomenon or those with an undifferentiated connective tissue disease. Nailfold videocapillaroscopic techniques have been used to describe 3 patterns of microangiopathy in SSc that correlate with disease duration: early, active, and late.[53,54] The early pattern is defined by fewer than 4 altered capillaries per millimeter, enlarged or giant capillaries, few capillary hemorrhages, relatively well-preserved capillary distribution, and no evident loss of capillaries. The active pattern has more than 6 altered capillaries per millimeter, giant capillaries, frequent capillary hemorrhages, 20% to 30% loss of capillaries, mild (between 4 and 6 altered capillaries per millimeter) disorganization of the capillary architecture, and absent or mild ramified capillaries. The late pattern shows irregular enlargement of the capillaries, few or absent giant capillaries and hemorrhages, 50% to 70% loss of capillaries with large avascular areas, disorganization of the normal capillary array, and ramified or bushy capillaries.[53,54] The late pattern is associated with older age and longer duration of Raynaud phenomenon and SSc when compared with the early and active patterns.[53] In the pediatric population the normal findings can incorporate "pathologic" capillaries; only giant capillaries and avascular regions are clearly pathologic. The number of capillaries correlates with age.[67,68]

The combination of autoantibodies and nailfold capillaroscopic abnormalities may be helpful in the early detection of SSc.[14] Patients with Raynaud phenomenon, normal nailfold capillaroscopy, and negative SSc-specific autoantibodies have a probability of 1.6% to develop SSc. In contrast, patients with Raynaud phenomenon, SSc pattern on nailfold capillaroscopy, and positive SSc-specific autoantibodies have a 73% probability of developing SSc over 10 years. A normal nailfold capillaroscopy pattern is rarely seen in SSc (4%–12%), nearly exclusively in the limited cutaneous subset.[69,70] Classifying patients into nailfold videocapillaroscopic subsets may be important early in the disease course because capillary loss is a reliable indicator of rapidly progressive early disease.[71,72] Shenavandeh and colleagues[71] showed that late pattern in patients with early SSc was associated with severity of finger contractures and significantly reduced pulmonary function, compared with "active" and "early" patterns.

THE NEXT ITERATION OF SYSTEMIC SCLEROSIS SUBSETS

New SSc subset criteria are under development.[73] There are a variety of opinions regarding the ideal number of subsets.[74] More than 90% of international experts believe there are more than 2 subsets for classifying SSc.[74] There is an expectation that the ability to subset patients with SSc should be able to perform several functions, which include the following:

- Guide baseline investigations
- Guide monitoring over time
- Inform treatment options
- Inform intensity of treatment
- Inform response to treatment
- Predict course of the disease
- Predict internal organ involvement
- Predict survival
- Assist with risk stratification
- Reduce heterogeneity
- Education tool for health care providers, trainees, and patients
- Facilitate communication

It is unlikely that one subsetting system will be able to perform all of these functions well. Trade-offs will be required: scientific advancement versus accessibility/feasibility; comprehensiveness versus simplicity. The community may need to consider new approaches to subsetting. One approach may be hierarchical clustering of a few key features (eg, rate of skin progression and SSc-specific antibodies). Purely data-driven methods of identifying SSc subsets (machine learning predictive modeling and clustering algorithms) are being explored. It may be that SSc represents a family of closely related diseases. With improvements in our ability to accurately identify subsets, we will improve our understanding of the members of this family and how they are related.

CLINICS CARE POINTS

- Subsetting SSc based on extent of skin involvement into limited and diffuse is the most widely used and have demonstrable predictive validity
- Testing for SSc-associated antibodies can identify subsets of patients at increaed risk of specific internal organ involvement and inform prognosis

DISCLOSURES

The authors have nothing to disclose.

REFERENCES

1. Johnson SR, Goek ON, Singh-Grewal D, et al. Classification criteria in rheumatic diseases: a review of methodologic properties. Arthritis Rheum 2007;57:1119–33.
2. Foeldvari I, Klotsche J, Kasapcopur O, et al. Differences sustained between diffuse and limited forms of juvenile systemic sclerosis in expanded international cohort. Arthritis Care Res (Hoboken) 2022;74(10):1575–84.
3. Alba MA, Velasco C, Simeon CP, et al. Early- versus late-onset systemic sclerosis: differences in clinical presentation and outcome in 1037 patients. Medicine (Baltimore) 2014;93:73–81.
4. Hussein H, Lee P, Chau C, et al. The effect of male sex on survival in systemic sclerosis. J Rheumatol 2014;41:2193–200.
5. Pasarikovski CR, Granton JT, Roos AM, et al. Sex disparities in systemic sclerosis-associated pulmonary arterial hypertension: a cohort study. Arthritis Res Ther 2016;18:30.
6. Low AH, Johnson SR, Lee P. Ethnic influence on disease manifestations and autoantibodies in Chinese-descent patients with systemic sclerosis. J Rheumatol 2009;36:787–93.
7. Al-Sheikh H, Ahmad Z, Johnson SR. Ethnic variations in systemic sclerosis disease manifestations, internal organ involvement, and mortality. J Rheumatol 2019;46(9):1103–8.
8. Johnson SR, Glaman DD, Schentag CT, et al. Quality of life and functional status in systemic sclerosis compared to other rheumatic diseases. J Rheumatol 2006;33:1117–22.
9. Hesselstrand R, Scheja A, Akesson A. Mortality and causes of death in a Swedish series of systemic sclerosis patients. Ann Rheum Dis 1998;57:682–6.

10. Jacobsen S, Halberg P, Ullman S. Mortality and causes of death of 344 Danish patients with systemic sclerosis (scleroderma). Br J Rheumatol 1998;37:750–5.
11. Aggarwal R, Ringold S, Khanna D, et al. Distinctions between diagnostic and classification criteria? Arthritis Care Res 2015;67:891–7.
12. Dougados M, Gossec L. Classification criteria for rheumatic diseases: why and how? Arthritis Rheum 2007;57:1112–5.
13. Johnson SR, Laxer RM. Classification in systemic sclerosis. J Rheumatol 2006; 33:840–1.
14. Nevskaya T, Pope J, Turk M, et al. Systematic analysis of the literature in search of defining systemic sclerosis subsets. J Rheumatol 2021;48:1698–717.
15. Johnson SR, Feldman BM, Hawker GA. Classification criteria for systemic sclerosis subsets. J Rheumatol 2007;34:1855–63.
16. van den Hoogen F, Khanna D, Fransen J, et al. 2013 classification criteria for systemic sclerosis: an American College of Rheumatology/European League against Rheumatism collaborative initiative. Arthritis Rheum 2013;65:2737–47.
17. van den Hoogen F, Khanna D, Fransen J, et al. 2013 classification criteria for systemic sclerosis: an American college of rheumatology/European league against rheumatism collaborative initiative. Ann Rheum Dis 2013;72:1747–55.
18. Pope JE, Johnson SR. New classification criteria for systemic sclerosis (Scleroderma). Rheum Dis Clin North Am 2015;41:383–98.
19. Johnson SR. New ACR EULAR guidelines for systemic sclerosis classification. Curr Rheumatol Rep 2015;17:32.
20. Johnson SR, Fransen J, Khanna D, et al. Validation of potential classification criteria for systemic sclerosis. Arthritis Care Res 2012;64:358–67.
21. Johnson SR, Naden RP, Fransen J, et al. Multicriteria decision analysis methods with 1000Minds for developing systemic sclerosis classification criteria. J Clin Epidemiol 2014;67:706–14.
22. Fransen J, Johnson SR, van den Hoogen F, et al. Items for developing revised classification criteria in systemic sclerosis: Results of a consensus exercise. Arthritis Care Res 2012;64:351–7.
23. Coulter C, Baron M, Pope JE. A Delphi exercise and cluster analysis to aid in the development of potential classification criteria for systemic sclerosis using SSc experts and databases. Clin Exp Rheumatol 2013;31:24–30.
24. Preliminary criteria for the classification of systemic sclerosis (scleroderma). Subcommittee for scleroderma criteria of the American Rheumatism Association Diagnostic and Therapeutic Criteria Committee. Arthritis Rheum 1980;23: 581–90.
25. Preliminary criteria for the classification of systemic sclerosis (scleroderma). Bull Rheum Dis 1981;31:1–6.
26. Barnett AJ, Miller M, Littlejohn GO. The diagnosis and classification of scleroderma (systemic sclerosis). Postgrad Med J 1988;64:121–5.
27. Masi AT, Medsger TA Jr, Rodnan GP, et al. Methods and preliminary results of the scleroderma criteria cooperative study of the American Rheumatology Association. Clin Rheum Dis 1979;5:27–48.
28. Jordan S, Maurer B, Toniolo M, et al. Performance of the new ACR/EULAR classification criteria for systemic sclerosis in clinical practice. Rheumatology (Oxford) 2015;54:1454–8.
29. Alhajeri H, Hudson M, Fritzler M, et al. The 2013 ACR/EULAR Classification Criteria for Systemic Sclerosis Out-perform the 1980 Criteria. Data from the Canadian Scleroderma Research Group. Arthritis Care Res (Hoboken) 2015;67(4): 582–7.

30. Hoffmann-Vold AM, Gunnarsson R, Garen T, et al. Performance of the 2013 American College of Rheumatology/European League Against Rheumatism Classification Criteria for Systemic Sclerosis (SSc) in large, well-defined cohorts of SSc and mixed connective tissue disease. J Rheumatol 2015;42:60–3.
31. Melchor S, Joven BE, Andreu JL, et al. Validation of the 2013 American College of Rheumatology/European League Against Rheumatism classification criteria for systemic sclerosis in patients from a capillaroscopy clinic. Semin Arthritis Rheum 2016;46:350–5.
32. Zulian F, Woo P, Athreya BH, et al. The Pediatric Rheumatology European Society/American College of Rheumatology/European League against Rheumatism provisional classification criteria for juvenile systemic sclerosis. Arthritis Rheum 2007;57:203–12.
33. LeRoy EC, Black C, Fleischmajer R, et al. Scleroderma (systemic sclerosis): classification, subsets and pathogenesis. J Rheumatol 1988;15:202–5.
34. Allanore Y. Limited cutaneous systemic sclerosis: the unfairly neglected subset. J Scleroderma Relat Disord 2016;1:241–6.
35. Avouac J, Fransen J, Walker UA, et al. Preliminary criteria for the very early diagnosis of systemic sclerosis: results of a Delphi Consensus Study from EULAR Scleroderma Trials and Research Group. Ann Rheum Dis 2011;70:476–81.
36. Matucci-Cerinic M, Bellando-Randone S, Lepri G, et al. Very early versus early disease: the evolving definition of the 'many faces' of systemic sclerosis. Ann Rheum Dis 2013;72:319–21.
37. Minier T, Guiducci S, Bellando-Randone S, et al. Preliminary analysis of the very early diagnosis of systemic sclerosis (VEDOSS) EUSTAR multicentre study: evidence for puffy fingers as a pivotal sign for suspicion of systemic sclerosis. Ann Rheum Dis 2014;73:2087–93.
38. Ferri C, Giuggioli D, Guiducci S, et al. Systemic sclerosis Progression INvestiGation (SPRING) Italian registry: demographic and clinico-serological features of the scleroderma spectrum. Clin Exp Rheumatol 2020;38(Suppl 125):40–7.
39. Omair MA, Mohamed N, Johnson SR, et al. ANCA-associated vasculitis in systemic sclerosis report of 3 cases. Rheumatol Int 2013;33:139–43.
40. Alharbi S, Ahmad Z, Bookman AA, et al. Epidemiology and survival of systemic sclerosis-systemic lupus erythematosus overlap syndrome. J Rheumatol 2018;45:1406–10.
41. Bowyer SL, Blane CE, Sullivan DB, et al. Childhood dermatomyositis: factors predicting functional outcome and development of dystrophic calcification. J Pediatr 1983;103:882–8.
42. Chung MP, Richardson C, Kirakossian D, et al. Calcinosis biomarkers in adult and juvenile dermatomyositis. Autoimmun Rev 2020;19:102533.
43. Tabarki B, Ponsot G, Prieur AM, et al. Childhood dermatomyositis: clinical course of 36 patients treated with low doses of corticosteroids. Eur J Paediatr Neurol 1998;2:205–11.
44. Elahmar H, Feldman BM, Johnson SR. Management of calcinosis cutis in rheumatic diseases. J Rheumatol 2022;49(9):980–9.
45. Klotsche J, Foeldvari I, Kasapcopur O, et al. Performance of juvenile scleroderma classification criteria for juvenile systemic sclerosis. results from the jssc inception cohort. Arthritis Rheumatol 2017;69(Suppl10):1777–8.
46. Foeldvari I, Klotsche J, Torok KS, et al. Are diffuse and limited juvenile systemic sclerosis different in clinical presentation? clinical characteristics of a juvenile systemic sclerosis cohort. J Scleroderma Relat Disord 2018;4(1):49–61.

47. Johnson S, Hinchcliff M, Asano Y. Controversies: molecular vs. clinical systemic sclerosis classification. J Scleroderma Relat Disord 2016;1:277–85.
48. Anders HJ, Sigl T, Schattenkirchner M. Differentiation between primary and secondary Raynaud's phenomenon: a prospective study comparing nailfold capillaroscopy using an ophthalmoscope or stereomicroscope. Ann Rheum Dis 2001;60:407–9.
49. Arnett FC, Reveille JD, Goldstein R, et al. Autoantibodies to fibrillarin in systemic sclerosis (scleroderma). an immunogenetic, serologic, and clinical analysis. Arthritis Rheum 1996;39:1151–60.
50. Assassi S, Radstake TR, Mayes MD, et al. Genetics of scleroderma: implications for personalized medicine? BMC Med 2013;11:9.
51. Barturen G, Beretta L, Cervera R, et al. Moving towards a molecular taxonomy of autoimmune rheumatic diseases. Nat Rev Rheumatol 2018;14:180.
52. Burgos-Vargas R, Martinez-Cordero E, Reyes-Lopez PA, et al. Antibody pattern and other criteria for diagnosis and classification of PSS. J Rheumatol 1988;15: 153–4.
53. Cutolo M, Pizzorni C, Tuccio M, et al. Nailfold videocapillaroscopic patterns and serum autoantibodies in systemic sclerosis. Rheumatology (Oxford) 2004;43: 719–26.
54. Cutolo M, Sulli A, Pizzorni C, et al. Nailfold videocapillaroscopy assessment of microvascular damage in systemic sclerosis. J Rheumatol 2000;27:155–60.
55. Steen VD. Autoantibodies in systemic sclerosis. Semin Arthritis Rheum 2005;35: 35–42.
56. Cavazzana I, Fredi M, Taraborelli M, et al. A subset of systemic sclerosis but not of systemic lupus erythematosus is defined by isolated anti-Ku autoantibodies. Clin Exp Rheumatol 2013;31:118–21.
57. Domsic RT. Scleroderma: the role of serum autoantibodies in defining specific clinical phenotypes and organ system involvement. Curr Opin Rheumatol 2014;26:646–52.
58. Ferri C, Bernini L, Cecchetti R, et al. Cutaneous and serologic subsets of systemic sclerosis. J Rheumatol 1991;18:1826–32.
59. Hesselstrand R, Scheja A, Shen GQ, et al. The association of antinuclear antibodies with organ involvement and survival in systemic sclerosis. Rheumatology (Oxford) 2003;42:534–40.
60. Hoa S, Hudson M, Troyanov Y, et al. Single-specificity anti-Ku antibodies in an international cohort of 2140 systemic sclerosis subjects: clinical associations. Medicine (Baltimore) 2016;95:e4713.
61. Kaji K, Fertig N, Medsger TA Jr, et al. Autoantibodies to RuvBL1 and RuvBL2: a novel systemic sclerosis-related antibody associated with diffuse cutaneous and skeletal muscle involvement. Arthritis Care Res 2014;66:575–84.
62. Reveille JD, Solomon DH. American College of Rheumatology Ad Hoc Committee of Immunologic Testing G. Evidence-based guidelines for the use of immunologic tests: anticentromere, Scl-70, and nucleolar antibodies. Arthritis Rheum 2003;49:399–412.
63. Kuwana M. Circulating anti-nuclear antibodies in systemic sclerosis: utility in diagnosis and disease subsetting. J Nippon Med Sch 2017;84:56–63.
64. Salazar GA, Assassi S, Wigley F, et al. Antinuclear antibody-negative systemic sclerosis. Semin Arthritis Rheum 2015;44:680–6.
65. Milano A, Pendergrass SA, Sargent JL, et al. Molecular subsets in the gene expression signatures of scleroderma skin. PLoS One 2008;3:e2696.

66. Hinchcliff M, Huang CC, Wood TA, et al. Molecular signatures in skin associated with clinical improvement during mycophenolate treatment in systemic sclerosis. J Invest Dermatol 2013;133:1979–89.
67. Terreri MT, Andrade LE, Puccinelli ML, et al. Nail fold capillaroscopy: normal findings in children and adolescents. Semin Arthritis Rheum 1999;29:36–42.
68. Piotto DP, Sekiyama J, Kayser C, et al. Nailfold videocapillaroscopy in healthy children and adolescents: description of normal patterns. Clin Exp Rheumatol 2016;34(Suppl 100):193–9.
69. Markusse IM, Meijs J, de Boer B, et al. Predicting cardiopulmonary involvement in patients with systemic sclerosis: complementary value of nailfold videocapillaroscopy patterns and disease-specific autoantibodies. Rheumatology (Oxford) 2017;56:1081–8.
70. Ostojic P, Damjanov N. Different clinical features in patients with limited and diffuse cutaneous systemic sclerosis. Clin Rheumatol 2006;25:453–7.
71. Shenavandeh SHM, Nazarinia MA. Nailfold digital capillaroscopic findings in patients with diffuse and limited cutaneous systemic sclerosis. Reumatologia 2017;55:15–23.
72. Scussel-Lonzetti L, Joyal F, Raynauld JP, et al. Predicting mortality in systemic sclerosis: analysis of a cohort of 309 French Canadian patients with emphasis on features at diagnosis as predictive factors for survival. Medicine (Baltimore) 2002;81:154–67.
73. Johnson SR. Progress in the clinical classification of systemic sclerosis. Curr Opin Rheumatol 2017;29:568–73.
74. Johnson SR, Soowamber ML, Fransen J, et al. There is a need for new systemic sclerosis subset criteria. a content analytic approach. Scand J Rheumatol 2018; 47:62–70.
75. Barnett AJ, Miller MH, Littlejohn GO. A survival study of patients with scleroderma diagnosed over 30 years (1953-1983): the value of a simple cutaneous classification in the early stages of the disease. J Rheumatol 1988;15:276–83.
76. Ceribelli A, Cavazzana I, Franceschini F, et al. Anti-Th/To are common antinucleolar autoantibodies in Italian patients with scleroderma. J Rheumatol 2010; 37:2071–5.
77. Gliddon AE, Dore CJ, Dunphy J, et al. Antinuclear antibodies and clinical associations in a british cohort with limited cutaneous systemic sclerosis. J Rheumatol 2011;38:702–5.
78. Falkner D, Wilson J, Fertig N, et al. Studies of HLA-DR and DQ alleles in systemic sclerosis patients with autoantibodies to RNA polymerases and U3-RNP (fibrillarin). J Rheumatol 2000;27:1196–202.
79. Graf SW, Hakendorf P, Lester S, et al. South Australian Scleroderma Register: autoantibodies as predictive biomarkers of phenotype and outcome. Int J Rheum Dis 2012;15:102–9.
80. Hamaguchi Y, Hasegawa M, Fujimoto M, et al. The clinical relevance of serum antinuclear antibodies in Japanese patients with systemic sclerosis. Br J Dermatol 2008;158:487–95.
81. Hanke K, Becker MO, Brueckner CS, et al. Anticentromere-A and anticentromere-B antibodies show high concordance and similar clinical associations in patients with systemic sclerosis. J Rheumatol 2010;37:2548–52.
82. Harvey GR, Butts S, Rands AL, et al. Clinical and serological associations with anti-RNA polymerase antibodies in systemic sclerosis. Clin Exp Immunol 1999; 117:395–402.

83. Song G, Hu C, Zhu H, et al. New centromere autoantigens identified in systemic sclerosis using centromere protein microarrays. J Rheumatol 2013;40:461–8.
84. Hudson M, Mahler M, Pope J, et al. Clinical correlates of CENP-A and CENP-B antibodies in a large cohort of patients with systemic sclerosis. J Rheumatol 2012;39:787–94.
85. Kuwana M, Okano Y, Pandey JP, et al. Enzyme-linked immunosorbent assay for detection of anti-RNA polymerase III antibody: analytical accuracy and clinical associations in systemic sclerosis. Arthritis Rheum 2005;52:2425–32.
86. McCarty GA, Rice JR, Bembe ML, et al. Anticentromere antibody. clinical correlations and association with favorable prognosis in patients with scleroderma variants. Arthritis Rheum 1983;26:1–7.
87. Vazquez-Abad D, Wallace S, Senecal JL, et al. Anticentromere autoantibodies. Evaluation of an ELISA using recombinant fusion protein CENP-B as antigen. Arthritis Rheum 1994;37:248–52.
88. Wu R, Shovman O, Zhang Y, et al. Increased prevalence of anti-third generation cyclic citrullinated peptide antibodies in patients with rheumatoid arthritis and CREST syndrome. Clin Rev Allergy Immunol 2007;32:47–56.
89. Giordano M, Valentini G, Migliaresi S, et al. Different antibody patterns and different prognoses in patients with scleroderma with various extent of skin sclerosis. J Rheumatol 1986;13:911–6.
90. Santiago M, Baron M, Hudson M, et al. Antibodies to RNA polymerase III in systemic sclerosis detected by ELISA. J Rheumatol 2007;34:1528–34.
91. Satoh T, Ishikawa O, Ihn H, et al. Clinical usefulness of anti-RNA polymerase III antibody measurement by enzyme-linked immunosorbent assay. Rheumatology (Oxford) 2009;48:1570–4.
92. Sato LT, Kayser C, Andrade LE. Nailfold capillaroscopy abnormalities correlate with cutaneous and visceral involvement in systemic sclerosis patients. Acta Reumatol Port 2009;34:219–27.
93. Simon D, Czompoly T, Berki T, et al. Naturally occurring and disease-associated auto-antibodies against topoisomerase I: a fine epitope mapping study in systemic sclerosis and systemic lupus erythematosus. Int Immunol 2009;21:415–22.
94. Iniesta Arandia N, Simeon-Aznar CP, Guillen Del Castillo A, et al. Influence of antibody profile in clinical features and prognosis in a cohort of Spanish patients with systemic sclerosis. Clin Exp Rheumatol 2017;35(Suppl 106):98–105.
95. Boonstra M, Mertens BJA, Bakker JA, et al. To what extent do autoantibodies help to identify high-risk patients in systemic sclerosis? Clin Exp Rheumatol 2018;36(Suppl 113):109–17.
96. Caetano J, Nihtyanova SI, Harvey J, et al. Distinctive clinical phenotype of anti-centromere antibody-positive diffuse systemic sclerosis. Rheumatol Adv Pract 2018;2:rky002.
97. Caramaschi P, Tonolli E, Biasi D, et al. Antinuclear autoantibody profile in systemic sclerosis patients who are negative for anticentromere and anti-topoisomerase I specificities. Joint Bone Spine 2015;82:209–10.
98. Coppo P, Henry-Dessailly I, Rochette J, et al. Clinical significance of autoantibodies to the pericentromeric heterochromatin protein 1a protein. Eur J Intern Med 2013;24:868–71.
99. Igusa T, Hummers LK, Visvanathan K, et al. Autoantibodies and scleroderma phenotype define subgroups at high-risk and low-risk for cancer. Ann Rheum Dis 2018;77:1179–86.

100. Foocharoen C, Watcharenwong P, Netwijitpan S, et al. Relevance of clinical and autoantibody profiles in systemic sclerosis among Thais. Int J Rheum Dis 2017; 20:1572–81.
101. Hamaguchi Y, Kodera M, Matsushita T, et al. Clinical and immunologic predictors of scleroderma renal crisis in Japanese systemic sclerosis patients with anti-RNA polymerase III autoantibodies. Arthritis Rheumatol 2015;67:1045–52.
102. Haddon DJ, Wand HE, Jarrell JA, et al. Proteomic analysis of sera from individuals with diffuse cutaneous systemic sclerosis reveals a multianalyte signature associated with clinical improvement during imatinib mesylate treatment. J Rheumatol 2017;44:631–8.
103. Terras S, Hartenstein H, Hoxtermann S, et al. RNA polymerase III autoantibodies may indicate renal and more severe skin involvement in systemic sclerosis. Int J Dermatol 2016;55:882–5.
104. Perosa F, Favoino E, Cuomo G, et al. Clinical correlates of a subset of anti-CENP-A antibodies cross-reacting with FOXE3p53-62 in systemic sclerosis. Arthritis Res Ther 2013;15:R72.
105. Wodkowski M, Hudson M, Proudman S, et al. Clinical correlates of monospecific anti-PM75 and anti-PM100 antibodies in a tri-nation cohort of 1574 systemic sclerosis subjects. Autoimmunity 2015;48:542–51.
106. Shah AA, Rosen A, Hummers L, et al. Close temporal relationship between onset of cancer and scleroderma in patients with RNA polymerase I/III antibodies. Arthritis Rheum 2010;62:2787–95.
107. Sanchez-Montalva A, Fernandez-Luque A, Simeon CP, et al. Anti-SSA/Ro52 autoantibodies in scleroderma: results of an observational, cross-sectional study. Clin Exp Rheumatol 2014;32:S-177–182.
108. Shah AA, Laiho M, Rosen A, et al. Protective effect against cancer of antibodies to the large subunits of both RNA polymerases I and III in scleroderma. Arthritis Rheumatol 2019;71:1571–9.
109. Shayakhmetova RU, Ananyeva LP. Mixed connective tissue disease. Mod Rheumatol 2019;13:11–8.
110. Patterson KA, Roberts-Thomson PJ, Lester S, et al. Interpretation of an extended autoantibody profile in a well-characterized australian systemic sclerosis (scleroderma) cohort using principal components analysis. Arthritis Rheumatol 2015;67:3234–44.
111. Perosa F, Favoino E, Favia IE, et al. Subspecificities of anticentromeric protein A antibodies identify systemic sclerosis patients at higher risk of pulmonary vascular disease. Medicine (Baltimore) 2016;95:e3931.
112. Wuttge DM, Carlsen AL, Teku G, et al. Specific autoantibody profiles and disease subgroups correlate with circulating micro-RNA in systemic sclerosis. Rheumatology (Oxford) 2015;54:2100–7.
113. Wodkowski M, Hudson M, Proudman S, et al. Monospecific anti-Ro52/TRIM21 antibodies in a tri-nation cohort of 1574 systemic sclerosis subjects: evidence of an association with interstitial lung disease and worse survival. Clin Exp Rheumatol 2015;33:S131–5.
114. Liaskos C, Marou E, Simopoulou T, et al. Disease-related autoantibody profile in patients with systemic sclerosis. Autoimmunity 2017;50:414–21.

Multi-Organ System Screening, Care, and Patient Support in Systemic Sclerosis

Cecília Varjú, MD, PhD[a], John D. Pauling, BMedSci, BMBS, PhD, FRCP[b,c],
Lesley Ann Saketkoo, MD, MPH[d,e,f,g],*

KEYWORDS

- Interstitial lung disease • Pulmonary hypertension • Ischemic
- Health-related quality of life • Patient-centred • Gastrointestinal disease
- Renal crisis • Shared decision-making

KEY POINTS

- Systemic sclerosis is a multi-organ system disease portending high risk of severe disability and death; and thus requires a global approach to prevention and management of complications.
- Standardized screening, anticipatory guidance and counselling are needed for early detection and appropriate treatement of SSc organ involvement.
- Screening for psycho-social well-being, includng sexual health, may reveal the most pressing biophysical influences for a person living with SSc.
- This article provides a reference to support a global approach to caring for people living with SSc.

INTRODUCTION

Systemic sclerosis (SSc) is a relatively rare heterogenous systemic autoimmune disease with complex multi-organ manifestations. Greater than 50% of deaths are directly attributable to SSc. The patient journey is commonly fraught with severe, diverse, and diffuse physical impairment as well as multiple causes impacting psychological burden, and greatly diminishing health-related quality of life (HRQoL).

The intricacies of care and guidance required in SSc remain unfamiliar territory for many clinicians; leaving patients feeling further isolated and unsupported. Delayed

[a] Department of Rheumatology and Immunology, Medical School, University of Pécs, Pécs, Hungary; [b] Department of Rheumatology, North Bristol NHS Trust, Bristol, UK; [c] Musculoskeletal Research Unit, Translational Health Sciences, Bristol Medical School, University of Bristol, Bristol, UK; [d] New Orleans Scleroderma and Sarcoidosis Patient Care and Research Center, New Orleans, LA 70112, USA; [e] University Medical Center – Comprehensive Pulmonary Hypertension Center and Interstitial Lung Disease Clinic Programs, New Orleans, LA, USA; [f] Section of Pulmonary Medicine, Louisiana State University School of Medicine, New Orleans, LA, USA; [g] Tulane University School of Medicine, New Orleans, LA, USA
* Corresponding author.
E-mail address: Lsaketk@tulane.edu

Rheum Dis Clin N Am 49 (2023) 211–248
https://doi.org/10.1016/j.rdc.2023.01.002
0889-857X/23/© 2023 Elsevier Inc. All rights reserved.

diagnosis, misdiagnosis, inadequate screening for common complications as well as insufficient recognition of and attention to common disabling features frequently occur contributing to potentially preventable disability and death.

This review outlines actionable standards in SSc care including screening, anticipatory guidance, and counseling in the context of patient-centered care. A reverse perspective to that traditionally found in disease state publications is presented here with a patient-forward sequence of SSc-relevant concerns. This sequence emphasizes psycho-social health as the underlying and overall central goal of care, whereas robust vigilance and efforts to improve biophysical health and survival are imperatives that support this goal.[1,2] This perspective naturally maintains shared decision-making (SDM; **Box 1**) in counseling and providing anticipatory guidance in treatment, preventive SSc care, and "red flag" situations (**Table 1**). The following are overall reference companions we hope will be useful: (a) **Fig. 1** is an aide memoire for a biophysical organizational approach for SSc's complex multi-organ system involvement. (b) Though SSc portends a high risk of severe disability and death for all patients—including those with an indolently progressive phenotypes—**Table 2** outlines biophysical factors that confer even higher risk associations. (c) **Table 3** provides an overview of recurrent anticipatory guidance and counseling essential in SSc care.

Psychosocial Experience of Living with Systemic Sclerosis

Screening for aspects psychosocial well-being in systemic sclerosis

Screening for and querying psycho-social well-being upfront can provide an informative entrée into the most pressing biophysical experiences for a patient with SSc. After which, it remains important that clinicians query biophysical aspects that the patient had not yet addressed (see **Fig. 1**). SSc pervasively influences patients' physical,

---

Box 1
Checklist to support shared decision-making

Shared Decision-Making Checklist

- Restate the patient's items of concern as expressed by the patient and if possible which are of the highest priority to them

- Ascertain patient's thoughts on the potential underlying cause/s of new concerns or symptom changes

- State the items of concern from the clinical perspective including short and long-term concerns (eg, potential progressive damage and associated abrupt complications)

- Respond to patient's perceptions of potential cause to gain further clinical insight, provide support, and clarify any divergence between patient and clinician perceptions.

- Remain transparent in what is known, unknown, yet to be known, and that requires researching by the clinician

- Name available treatment options, including any nonpharmacological options with particular attention to those suggested by the patient

- Discuss safety, side effects, and efficacy (including anticipated onset) of available therapies and those suggested by the patient.

- Assess the patient's expectations, priorities, and desires related to treatment

- Set treatment expectations including prognosis, anticipated degree of symptom/impairments resolution (*ie, cure vs regression vs slowing progression*), and disease activity versus damage

Courtesy of LA Saketkoo, MD, MPH, New Orleans, LA.

Table 1
Red flags in systemic sclerosis that patients should be aware of and report

Organ System	Red Flag	Potential Complication
General	Unexplained weight loss Decreased physical activity Loss of muscle mass	Cancer Infection Active progressive disease Significant GI involvement Deterioration of general health status (Frailty) Depression

Skin	Diffuse skin tenderness, ± pruritus
	Appearance of active
	  inflammation around calcinotic
	  lesions
		Rapidly progressive diffuse
		  cutaneous disease
		Infected calcinosis cutis
		Risk of osteolysis or joint
		  infection

Digital vascular	Increased pain, tenderness,
	  pressure, or appearance of
	  tissue inflammation
		Digital ulcer occurrence
		Critical digital ischemia
		  or gangrene
		Infection ± osteomyelitis

Cardiopulmonary	Reduced performance status
	Decreased physical activity
	Inspiratory dry cough
	Decreased trend in FVC and/or
	  DLCO even if within normal
	  range
		Arrhythmia, critical bradycardia
		Development and/or
		  progression of ILD or PH
		Ventricular dysfunction

Gastrointestinal	Onset of (severe) anemia
	Severe swallowing difficulty/
	  inability
	Unexplained weight loss
	Severe abdominal pain
	Change in bowel habit
	Elevated serum lactate
	Low BMI and poor nutritional
	  state
		Gastric vascular ectasia (GAVE)
		Esophageal stricture
		Pneumatosis Coli (risk of
		  perforation) GI malignancy
		GI ischemia
		Intestinal pseudo-obstruction
		
		Malnourishment

Sexual health in
  females
	Skin thickening, vaginal dryness,
	  stenosis, ulceration, multiple SSc
	  vascular features, and pain
		Sexual dysfunction

Sexual health in
  males
	Multiple SSc vascular features and
	  erectile dysfunction
		Sexual dysfunction

Psychological
  disorders
	Anxiety, depression, loneliness,
	  sleeping disorders, and work
	  disability
		Poor treatment adherence,
		  deteriorating HRQoL,
		  diminished perceived disease
		  impact regardless of
		  biophysical health status

Musculoskeletal	Presence of synovitis and/or joint
	  tenderness, tendon friction rubs
	  (TFRs), proximal muscle
	  weakness, or atrophy
		Joint contractures, arthritis,
		  permanent deterioration of
		  hand function, myopathy,
		  and weakness, myositis

Renal	Sudden onset of hypertension in
	  the early stage of dcSSc
		Scleroderma renal crisis:
		  hypertension,
		  azotemia-uremia

Secondary
  immunodeficiency
	Low white blood cell count and
	  neutropenia
		Side effects of DMARDs
		  (eg, MTX, MMF, CYC, and
		  tocilizumab)

Proposed Screening & Monitoring Algorithm for Clinically Significant SSc-ILD

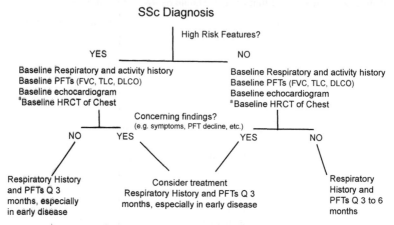

Fig. 1. Proposed screening for ILD in SSc. [a]Currently no absolute consensus on baseline HRCT upon new SSc diagnosis; however there is increasing support. HRCT is not routinely repeated for monitoring, but rather for unexplained or unexpected cardiopulmonary manifestations. (*Courtesy of* LA Saketkoo, MD, MPH, New Orleans, LA.)

psychological, and social well-being. Advances in diagnosis and treatment of SSc, are linked to increased median survival. However, the overall patient-perceived disease impact is influenced to a high degree by the psychological aspects of living with SSc and SSc-related disabilities. These include mood disorders, body image, fatigue, pain, family relations, and disease impact on professional and social life.[3,4] Targeted interventions that improve factors, especially pain and fatigue, can mitigate disease impact[5] (**Table 4**).

Anxiety and/or depression has a prevalence between 17% and 65% in people with SSc, compared with 4% to 10% among the general population.[3-9] Anxiety is associated with the severity of lung involvement, pain, and diminished body image.[6,7]

Appearance changes on visible body areas (eg, face, hands) in SSc are common and distressing. Greater dissatisfaction with appearance, body image, and social discomfort occur more frequently in people of younger age and when unmarried.[3,9-11] People with diffuse cutaneous systemic sclerosis (dcSSc) reported greater body image dissatisfaction than those with limited cutaneous systemic sclerosis, and expressed greater dissatisfaction in appearance with increased finger/hand skin involvement in dcSSc.[7,11]

Symptoms of depression are associated with disease severity, gastrointestinal function, pain, health status, education level, and ability to cope with psychological impact.[10,12-14] Simple self-administered questionnaires, as an integral part of overall SSc care, support the early recognition and treatment of various psychological distresses (**Table 5**).[10,12-14]

Fatigue and sleeping problems were among the five highest-rated symptoms in terms of severe impact on daily activities reported by 72% and 59% respectively.[15] *Sleeping disorders* have a higher prevalence in SSc patients, with decreased sleep quality further deteriorating fatigue and mental health symptoms that are common characteristics of chronic inflammatory diseases.[15,16]

Poor sleep quality impacts factors important in SSc such as inflammation levels, memory, cognition, anxiety, depression, well-being, wound healing, pain perception, muscle health, and also correlates with a degree of loneliness which in turn influences

Table 2
Risk factors for death, disability, and rapidly progressive disease and for severe organ involvement

Risk Factor	Clinical Measures	Indication of Rapidly Progressive SSc or Severe Disease
Demographics	Inquiry	African ancestry Asian ancestry Hispanic ancestry Male sex
Diffuse skin involvement	modified Rodnan Skin Score (mRSS)	Increasing diffuse scleroderma skin, mRSS > 29
Tendon friction rub	Palpable presence on examination	Palpable presence on examination
Anti-topoisomerase-1	See measures for ILD, dcSSc, renal crisis, and cardiac fibrosis	
Anti-RNA polymerase III	See measures for SSc renal crisis, dcSSc, GAVE, rapidly development of joint contractures; Malignancies synchronous to SSc onset	
Interstitial lung disease	PFT: spirometry PFT: DLCO HRCT: Extent of ground-glass opacity and honeycombing fibrosis	FVC<70% DLCO<70% >20% extent of disease on HRCT
Pulmonary hypertension (PH)	Echocardiography Right heart catheterization WHO/NYHA Classification	sPAP >40 mm Hg Right atrial or ventricular enlargement Septal flattening mPAP>20 mm Hg PVR > 3 wood units Class III/IV
Cardiac involvement	ECG Echocardiography	ECG arrhythmia Diastolic dysfunction > grade 2 left ventricular ejection fraction <45%
Digital ulcers and gangrene	Nailfold capillaroscopy	Severe capillary loss, fibrotic infiltration
Scleroderma renal Crisis	Hypertension Serum biomarkers	Abnormal or an unusually elevated value for the patient Normotensive if on prednisone Elevated serum creatinine ? Anti-topoisomerase ? Anti-polymerase III
GAVE	Gastric bleeding Anemia	Frank blood on inspection Hb < 9.6 g/dL
Severe malabsorption	Weight loss Muscle atrophy Stool frequency Electrolytes Albumin/prealbumin	

(continued on next page)

Table 2
(continued)

Risk Factor	Clinical Measures	Indication of Rapidly Progressive SSc or Severe Disease

Polyarthritis	HAQ-DI
	DAS-28
	Cochin Hand Function Scale
		Active joint disease:
		  HAQ-DI≥1.0, Cochin Hand
		  Function Scale ≥10 and/or
		  28-tender joint count ≥6

General health status	Weight loss/BMI Serum biomarkers Loss of muscle mass	Weight loss > 10% Low albumin, low Hb
Comorbidities	Presence of: COPD, malignancy, diabetes mellitus	

Organ Manifestation	Risk Factors
Heart	Pericarditis Arrhythmia Right bundle branch block (RBBB) Left ventricular dysfunction Myopathy Tendon friction rubs
Kidney (renal crisis)	Diffuse cutaneous SSc Rapid skin progression in the first year of the onset Presence of anti-RNA polymerase III autoantibodies Medium or high dose glucocorticoid therapy, that is, >10 mg prednisone daily Significant cardiac manifestation Joint contractures Tendon friction rubs
Interstitial lung disease (ILD)	Male gender High mRSS Diffuse cutaneous SSc Anti-topoisomerase 1 antibody Increased ESR FVC<70%, DLCO<70% Decrease of FVC ≥5% within 6 mo regardless of normal values Increased serum creatinine phosphokinase (CK)
Progressive ILD	Active polyarthritis Increased ESR Disease onset over 55 y High mRSS Reflux (GERD) NYHA III-IV heart disease Decreased SpO$_2$ during 6MWT
Pulmonary hypertension	Disease onset over 55 y Long disease duration African ancestry for early onset of PH Skin telangiectasias Isolated DLCO decrease in trend—*even with normal values* FVC/DLCO ratio > 1.6 Severe Raynaud's Severe digital ulcers Decreased capillary density by nail fold capillaroscopy

(continued on next page)

Table 2 *(continued)*	
Organ Manifestation	**Risk Factors**
	Increased serum uric acid
	Presence of Th/To, U3 RNP, or RNA Polymerase III autoantibodies
Digital ulcers	Diffuse scleroderma
	High mRSS
	Male gender
	Polyarthritis
	Early non-Raynaud's first symptom
	Increased capillary loss by capillary-microscopy
Arthritis, contractures, tendon friction rubs	Early manifestation in diffuse cutaneous SSc
	Presence of overlap SSc
	Presence of RNA Polymerase III and Topoisomerase I autoantibodies
	Lack of early referral to Occupational and Physical Therapy

Abbreviations: 6MWT, 6-min walk test; DLCO, diffusion capacity of the lung for carbon monoxide; ESR, erythrocyte sedimentation rate; FVC, forced vital capacity; GAVE, gastric antral vascular ectasia; GERD, gastroesophageal reflux disorder; HAQ-DI, health assessment questionnaire-disability index; ILD, interstitial lung disease; mRSS, modified Rodnan Skin Score; NYHA, New York Heart Association; PAS, estimated pulmonary artery systolic pressure by Doppler echo; SpO2, blood oxygen saturation; WHO, World Health Organization.

Courtesy of C Varju, MD, PhD, Pécs, Hungary and LA Saketkoo, MD, MPH, New Orleans, LA.

health status and inflammation levels.[17] Screening for and addressing issues related to sleep quality creates opportunities to greatly effect overall perceived disease impact.[10,18–25]

Engagement in remunerative work is greatly impacted by SSc with 18% to 61% of patients discontinuing work.[26] *Work disability* correlates with more severe lung function parameters, less social support, higher fatigue severity scores, and lower education level.[27,28] Awareness of these risk factors, initiation of early appropriate treatment, and nonpharmacological therapy, may mitigate SSc-disease impact on work ability.[29]

Sexual health in people living with systemic sclerosis

Sexual health concerns are common and greatly impact HRQoL *for both women and men* with SSc, with the prevalence of sexual dysfunction (SDF) varying from 46.7% to 86.6% in women and 76.9% to 81.4% in men.[30–38] Yet sexual health is rarely addressed in clinical practice,[30–32] with only 9.6% of patients with SSc ever having discussed sexual problems with their physicians.[31] SDF in SSc is a multifactorial concern influenced by disease-related, treatment-associated, and psychological factors. SDF in SSc may involve any phase of the sexual activity response cycle: desire/libido, arousal/excitement before or during intercourse/activity (such as erectile dysfunction, dyspareunia or vaginismus), orgasm (disorders inhibiting male or female orgasm, premature ejaculation in men) and resolution (physical or psychological dissatisfaction).[30–34,36] Early introduction of pelvic floor muscle exercises may help both men and women to maintain urinary and fecal continence, increase local blood supply, and responsiveness during sexual activity.[39,40]

Sexual health in female patients

The assessment and complex problem-solving regarding female sexual function benefit from collaboration between rheumatology and gynecology. Vaginal dryness, mucosal stenosis, and pain are of the most problematic concerns for women with SSc.[30,31,34] The Female Sexual Function Index Scoring (FSFI) is the most commonly

Table 3
Key elements of recurrent multi-organ system counseling and anticipatory guidance in systemic sclerosis

Category	Subcategory	Item	Advisements for Patients
Vascular	Raynaud	Prevention is key	• Related complications include DUs, calcinosis, osteolysis and core temperature loss • Initiate protective measure in anticipation of and upon noticing a cold atmosphere, before allowing oneself to "feel" cold • Immediate action can result in decreased recovery time, pain and the sequela associated with loss of core warmth (fatigue, headache, incapacity, etc.) • Avoid extreme temperature changes, for example, from cold to warmth • Anticipate cold environments, for example, air conditioning in summer, grocery store freezer aisle, hospitals, etc.
		Core Temperature	• Exercise/movement increases circulation and body heat • Clothes layering and use of insulated vests • Hand warmers, can be placed in pockets, undergarments
		Peripheral	• Gloves/socks always at hand • Should allow for a thin space to trap a warming layer of air • Hand warmers, can be placed in pockets, gloves, socks • Heated gloves/insoles/shoes
	Digital ulcers/calcinosis	Protection	Cushioned bandages for high friction areas Waterproof gloves for washing or handling wet items Bandage and gloves for handling dry household items potentially snagging healing ulcers and to protect from bacteria and chemical irritants Exercise gloves for use of gym equipment as needed • Protection as above
		Pain management	• Topical lidocaine • Wound cleansing routine
		Signs of infection	• Increased pain/tenderness • Redness • Purulence
		Prevention	As much as possible avoid: *Cold exposure* and *Trauma* Use topical antibiotics with signs of infection

	Additional calcinosis	Advisement	• Avoid digging to prevent infection • If pain intolerable can try repeated soaking in warm Epsom salt water • Topical antibiotics • Seek help if seems infected or ulceration occurs
	Erectile dysfunction		• Increased physical activity helps protect circulatory and neuronal function • *RP* and *Core Temperature* preventive measures may have a protective effect
Nutrition	Calorie intake	Nutritious	• Avocado • Nuts, nut butters, sprinkling nut and protein powders • Adding cheeses (soft or hard as tolerated), butter, creams • Potatoes, rice • Olive and other oils • Plant-based high calorie formulas eg, *Kate Farms* • Thoroughly chewing/macerating food to liquid/paste
	Food tolerance	Nutritious	• Pureed foods (soups, dips, stews) • Smaller amounts of a food type • Variation of food type, for example, sliced, pureed, grated, cooked, etc. • Foods softened (marinated) with small amounts of citrus or vinegar • Mobility after eating to increase motility
Heent	Oro-facial		Facial Exercises and Massage for skin tightness, mobility and circulation
	Oral		High risk for dental complications: • Essential follow-up with a dental clinician sensitive to SSc care or perhaps pediatric dentist • Proactive dental care • Topical Fluoride Rinse to protect against dental caries • Keeping mouth moist • Adapted and powered devices for teeth and oral care
	SICCA		Wetting and pro-salivation products Singing, humming, chanting and exercise to increase salivation and oral, facial and diaphragmatic muscle mass

(continued on next page)

Table 3
(continued)

Category	Subcategory	Item	Advisements for Patients
Cardiopulmonary	PH and cardiac		Graded exercise essential to health Control of GERD and PND to avoid lung injury from micro-aspiration Vaccination for prevention of infection (see **Table 7**) Daily weights as needed Alert MD of new-onset lower extremity edema
Gastrointestinal	GERD	Esophageal injury and lung risks	Reflux in SSc is a serious issue of which related injury can lead to multiple complications that impact mortality. • Often exists without pain • Pain does not equate severity • Esophagitis • Esophageal cancer • Dysphagia and potential loss of swallow function • Strictures & Webbing • Need for esophageal stretching • Acid aggravates lung disease • CPAP use can inhibit reflux
		Medications	• PPI daily or twice daily, especially with esophagitis or esophageal ulcer • it is perceived that in SSc the benefits of PPIs greatly outweigh associated risks • Adding PRN or OTC agents (eg, sucralfate, H2 blockade) • Advise on the timing of administration to avoid drug-drug interactions
		Sleep essentials	• Head of Bed Elevation (wedge pillow, leveraging mattress, bricks/books under bed legs) • Avoid right-side lying
		Reflux hygiene	• Smaller, more frequent meals

Gastroparesis		• Avoid meals 2 to 3 h before lying down • Avoid sphincter relaxants at end of day, for example, alcohol, chocolate, caffeine, mint, etc. • Sleep and hygiene as for GERD • Exercise/walking may help • Gravity strategies for passive digestion • Upright position • Attention to food consistency, for example, thinner foods • Gastroparesis dietary suggestions for food tolerance
Bloating		• Exercise for motility • Small frequent meals • Simethicone or *IBGard* are safe over-the-counter options for possible relief
Nausea	SSc or medication related	• Mobility/exercise to decrease nausea • Ginger-based sweets, tea, and drinks • Sucking candies • Cold pops • Instruction on PRN anti-emetics
Diarrhea	SSc or medication related	Logistics until controlled: change of clothes, time planning Medication use, for example, anti-motility agents: risks/benefits/ when to use/limited use
Key element to SSc care	Counseling at each visit for support, guidance, and consideration for therapeutic referral Early OT/PT referral can have a critical impact on function and disability prevention	
Exercise		Improves: • Circulation and vascular responsiveness • Body warmth • Sleep • Energy • Self-esteem • Breathlessness • Hand function • Joint mobility stiffness and lubrication • Skin function and health • GI function and microbiome diversity • Nausea • Salivation

(continued on next page)

Table 3
(continued)

Category	Subcategory	Item	Advisements for Patients
			• Respiratory performance
			• Cognitive clarity
			Decreases:
			• inflammation
			• Pain (anywhere)
			• Joint stiffness
			• Possibly contractures
			• Possibly skin tightness
			• Depression
			• Stress
			• Fatigue
			• Cancer risk
Women of Child-Bearing Age	Medication toxicity		• Use of contraception essential with specific IS and PAH medications
			• Discontinuation of specific IS or PAH medications before conception
	Conception		• Should be a planned event
			• Medication washout pre-conception
			• Discuss assessing the extent of ILD, PH, cardiac or renal involvement in light of safe pregnancy
	Care of children		• Adaptations for childcare
			• Strategies to manage fatigue
Psychological			Advocacy/education groups
			Local support groups
			Online self-management program eg, *Dr. Janet Poole*
			Referral for professional psychological support

Courtesy of LA Saketkoo, MD, MPH, New Orleans, LA.

Table 4
Modifiable causes and treatment of fatigue and pain in systemic sclerosis

Symptom	System/Origin	Potential Causes	Team Involvement/Interventions
Fatigue	Anemia	GI loss, chronic inflammatory disease	
	Cardiac	PH, diastolic HF, CAD, and physical deconditioning	PT and PR teach adapted aerobic and muscular exercises and breath pattern training OT teaches energy conservation strategies such as pacing, prioritizing, and accommodating devices
	Respiratory	PH, ILD, and OSA	OT, PT, PR, as for cardiac above
	Muscular	Low muscle endurance, muscle strength, or reduced aerobic capacity	MT, MMM, PR-PTr, PT for Aerobic exercises, muscle strengthening and endurance exercises, and education
	Systemic inflammation	Effects on hypothalamic axis, causing systemic malaise, effects on muscle	Immunosuppression, exercise
	Psychological	Anxiety, depression, fear, impact of reduced self-esteem, and self-image	MT, MMM, PR-PTr, PT, OT, Breath pattern training, Psychologist, Social Worker
	Neurologic	Pain: ischemic, edematous skin, articular, restless leg syndrome	Assess treatable causes, MT MMM, and PR
	Malnutrition	Weight loss, and malabsorption	
	Sleep-related	OSA, nocturnal pain, pruritus, GI symptoms, depression, anxiety, steroid, or opioid use	SH, RSS, MMM, and MT
	Medication-related	Methotrexate, MMF, nintedanib, etc.	
Pain/dysesthesia	Vascular	Raynaud	EC preventive strategies, MT, vasodilators, sympathectomy, PT for aerobic exercise to improve blood flow
		Digital ulcers	EC wound care, protective dressing, anesthetics, OT for daily activities, MT, PT as for RP
		Calcinosis	As above, UTPRM: soaking for relief
		Infected digital ulcers/calcinosis	EC red flags, Aerobic exercise to improve circulation
		Skin tightening	PT, ST, and OT for stretching and manipulation
	Dermal	Subcutaneous edema and pressure	MT, ST, OT as above
		Pruritus	MT, SH, ST, opioid receptor blocker, and phototherapy

(continued on next page)

Table 4
(continued)

Symptom	System/Origin	Potential Causes	Team Involvement/Interventions
	Musculoskeletal	Myopathy/myalgias	MMM, OT, PT, PR-PTr, for strength, endurance, and anti-inflammatory effects of exercise
		Fibrous tendinopathy	MMM, OT, PT, THE as above
		Inflammatory arthropathy/tendinopathy	MMM, OT, PT, ST, and local injections, muscle strengthening, stretching, and targeted hand exercises
		Secondary fibromyalgia	MMM, PR-PTr, SH, and education
	Gastrointestinal	Heartburn	EC, RH, NH, and anti-acid and PPI
		Abdominal cramping	Assessment with Giessen GI Questionnaire or UCLA GIT[106,107]
		Abdominal bloating	
	Genitourinary	Dyspareunia	Pelvic floor therapies and sometimes systemic treatment
		Vaginal dryness	Lubricants, topical estrogen
		Erectile dysfunction	Vasodilators, PT for aerobic exercise, and specialist referral

Abbreviations: AG, anticipatory guidance; ATT, assessment with targeted treatment; DHS, dental hygiene strategies; EC, education/counseling; ILD, interstitial lung disease; MMM, mindful movement modalities (e; g; gentle yoga; tai chi etc.); MT, mindfulness training strategies; NH, nutrition hygiene (EC on attention to selection, volume; texture, preparation; combination strategies of foods); OSA, obstructive sleep apnea; OT, occupational therapy; PAH, pulmonary arterial hypertension; POS, practical organizational strategies; PPI, proton pump inhibitors; PR, pulmonary rehabilitation; PR-EC, pulmonary rehabilitation educational component; PR-PTr, PR physical training component; PT, physiotherapy; RH, reflux hygiene (including head of bed elevation); RHS, refer to hand specialist; RME, refer to motility expert; RSS, refer to sleep specialist; SH, sleep hygiene; SR, specialist referral; ST, systemic treatment; THE, the targeted home exercises; UTPRM, untested patient-reported management.[2]

Courtesy of LA Saketkoo, MD, MPH, New Orleans, LA.

Table 5
Selected questionnaires for psychosocial status in patients with systemic sclerosis

Instrument	Item Breakdown Qualities	Demonstrated Use in SSc
Psychological Impact		
Beck Depression Inventory[14,15,17]	A simple 13-items self-report questionnaire	Reliably Discriminates Between Depressed and Nondepressed Medical patients
The Hospital Anxiety and Depression Scale (HADS)[10,11]	A simple 14-item self-administered questionnaire, with 7 anxiety items and 7 depression items, on a 4-point (0 to 3) scale	Feasibility, validity, and responsiveness in SSc
Patient-Reported Outcomes Measurement Information System PROMIS-29[19,99,129]	https://www.promishealth.org Assesses 8 HRQoL domains: physical function, anxiety, depression, ability to participate in social roles, sleep disturbances, pain interference, pain intensity, fatigue	Internal consistency, reliability, and construct validity in SSc-ILD; uncertain discrimination and change over time
Center for Epidemiologic Studies-Depression scale (CES-D)[4,5,20]	CES-D is a 20-item questionnaire that measures depressive symptomatology using Likert scales of 0 to 3, and the total score ranges from 0 to 60. Scoring above 16 denotes possible depression	CES-D is a reliable and valid instrument for measuring depressive symptoms in SSc. Specific cut-off scores need to be established.
Ten-Item Personality Inventory (TIPI)[6,21]	TIPI is assessing five major personality dimensions on a 7-point scale	Not specifically tested in SSc
UCLA—Loneliness Scale[22]	20-item questionnaire, a commonly used measure of loneliness. There are shorter versions, for example, ULS-8 (8-item version)	Not specifically tested in SSc
Body Image		
The Brief-Satisfaction with Appearance Scale (Brief SWAP)[11,16]	Easy 6-item self-administered questionnaire Items are scored on a seven-point scale ranging from 0 to 7. Higher scores indicate greater dissatisfaction or social discomfort.	Internal consistency, reliability, and construct validity in SSc; Sensitivity to change has not been studied.
Derriford Appearance Scale short-form[7]	DAS-24 is a 24-item questionnaire that measures distress and dysfunction related to physical appearance	Internal consistency, reliability, and construct validity in SSc

(continued on next page)

Page 226 — Varjú et al

Table 5 (continued)

Instrument	Item Breakdown Qualities	Demonstrated Use in SSc
Sexual Dysfunction		
The International Index of Erectile Function (IIEF)—for male patients[45]	The IIEF includes five questions on erectile function, orgasmic function, sexual desire, intercourse satisfaction, and overall sexual satisfaction with each item being scored from 1 to 5. A scoring <22 denotes possible erectile dysfunction (ED)	IIEF is a fully validated measure of ED in the general population. IIEF has been used in some clinical studies with SSc patients; uncertain discrimination and change over time
Female Sexual Function Index Scoring (FSFI)[32,41]	19 items that easily assess desire, arousal, satisfaction, lubrication, orgasm, and pain on vaginal penetration	Fully validated instrument of sexual function in the general population. In some clinical studies with SSc patients, FSFI has been used.
Qualisex[35,130]	10-item questionnaire with less intimate questions on the influence of the respective disease on sexual function. The score ranges from 0 to 10 with higher scores indicating more sexual impairment.	No validation process has been performed in patients with SSc. In one clinical study, Qualisex has been used in patients with SSc.[130]
Pelvic Floor Impact Questionnaire Short Form 7 (PFIQ-7)[34,43]	7-item self-administered questionnaire to evaluate sexual function in women	No validation process has been performed in patients with SSc. In one clinical study with SSc patients, PFIQ-7 has been used.
Pelvic Organ Prolapse/Urinary Incontinence Sexual Questionnaire Short Form (PISQ-12)[34,42]	12-item self-administered questionnaire to evaluate sexual function and urinary incontinence in women	Validated measure in the general population. In some clinical studies with SSc patients, PISQ-12 has been used
Fatigue, Sleeping Disorders		
Functional Assessment of Chronic Illness Therapy Fatigue Scale (FACIT-F)[16,17]	FACIT-F is a 13-item measure designed to assess tiredness, weakness, and difficulty managing daily activities due to fatigue in the past 7 d. Items are scored on a 5-point Likert-type scale Total scores range from 0 to 52, with higher scores indicating less fatigue.	Internal consistency, reliability, and construct validity in SSc; Sensitivity to change has not been studied.

Multidimensional Assessment of Fatigue (MAF)[168]	MAF, with 16 items, is used to evaluate fatigue. The score ranges from 1 to 50 and higher scores signify greater fatigue.	The MAF in Swedish has been validated in SSc (internal consistency, reliability, and construct validity).
Pittsburgh Sleep Quality Index (PSQI)[15,169]	PSQI has 19 items and measures 7 components of sleep quality: subjective sleep quality, sleep latency, duration, habitual sleep efficiency, sleep disturbances, use of sleeping medication, and daytime dysfunction (each domain score ranges between 0 and 3).	No validation process has been performed in patients with SSc. In some clinical studies with SSc patients, PSQI has been used.
Family relations, social functioning, Disease impact on professional and social life		
PROMIS-29[19,129]	See above	See above
Scleroderma Health Assessment Questionnaire (SHAQ)	A 30-item questionnaire that assesses the global impact of SSc addressing overall perceived disease severity, pain, fatigue, organ-based physical impairment, and SSc-specific symptom interference in daily life and self-care as well as need for assistance.	Widely validated in SSc. Routinely used in SSc centers and in SSc clinical trials. The most global and specific PROM in SSc.
Short Form 36	HRQoL generic measure with 36 items evaluating the physical function, energy, pain, mental health, social participation, and perceived health status,	Widely used to assess HRQoL in SSc
Short Form of Social Support (SSq)[5,23]	A 6-item questionnaire, which consists of two parts: the number of persons that provide support to each participant (min. 0, max. 9) and the level of satisfaction from that support, measured on a 6-point scale (1 to 6).	Clinical studies with SSc patients have used SSq.
The Ways of Coping Checklist—Revised (WCCL-R)[24,25]	WCCL-R is a 57-item self-report measure, it yields 8 coping subscales: problem-focused, wishful thinking, seeking social support, avoidance, self-blame, blaming others, counting one's blessings, and religiosity.	WCCL-R has been used in one clinical study of patients with SSc.

used self-administrated questionnaire in clinical practice and studies.[41] The association of impaired sexual function and pelvic floor function in women with SSc has been recently shown.[42] The Pelvic Floor Impact Questionnaire (PFIQ-7) and Pelvic Organ Prolapse/Urinary Incontinence Sexual Questionnaire (PISQ-12)[43] easily assess the severity and impact of pelvic floor muscle impairment. Clitoral circulation as assessed by resistive index (RI) and the systolic/diastolic (S/D) ratio of clitoral blood defined by color Doppler ultrasound have uncertain clinical significance.[37,38]

Sexual health in male patients
SDF in men with SSc, especially ED, is highly prevalent ($\sim$80%) and an early occurring symptom within 4 years of SSc onset.[30,32,39,44,45] Impairment of endothelial-dependent smooth muscle relaxation (functional vascular ED, initial stages), the occlusion of the corpus cavernosa arteries by fibrotic lesions (structural vascular ED, late stages) or a combination of these processes contribute to SSc-related ED.[45,46] Complex interactions between subclinical autoimmune inflammation, myo-intimal proliferation of the small penile arteries and corporal fibrosis underlie SSc-related ED pathophysiology.[32,39] Common risk factors for ED include hypertension, diabetes mellitus, obesity, and smoking, whereby endothelial dysfunction and low level of inflammation has been identified.[32,39,45] However, progressive SSc vascular disease is associated with rapidly developing ED, underscoring the importance of routine screening in the "very early" phase of SSc.[32,39,45] The International Index of Erectile Function (IIEF), a widely used, easily self-administered assessment tool[46] that investigates erectile function, orgasmic function, sexual desire, intercourse satisfaction, and overall sexual satisfaction.[47] A lower IIEF score is associated with higher scores on the Beck Depression Inventory.[44,48] Early urologic referral and initiation of ED treatment may prevent progression to arterial occlusion. Penile color Doppler ultrasound and hormone panel comprise the routine workup.[32,39,46,47]

Vascular Experience in Systemic Sclerosis

Raynaud's phenomenon
Raynaud's phenomenon (RP), being a hallmark SSc feature, its absence prompts consideration of 'scleroderma mimics'.[49] The sub-absolute reporting of RP prevalence of $\sim$96% in SSc likely reflects either strict adherence to a report of bi-phasic color changes which are not present in all patients with SSc-RP, or non-standardized history-taking, especially for non-whites.[50,51]

Preserving core temperature facilitates maximal digital vasodilatation of thermoregulatory arteriovenous anastomoses.[52,53] SSc-RP symptom burden doubles over winter,[54,55] and exposure to drastic temperature changes such as air-conditioning or during grocery-shopping. Counseling on the importance of vigilance for cold situations, carrying hand warmers, gloves, and extra layers of clothing and, if needed, smoking cessation can help avoid and/or ameliorate SSc-RP symptoms.[50,53,56,57]

Digital ulceration and calcinosis cutis
Digital ulcers (DUs) occur in over half of SSc patients and contributes largely to SSc disease-related morbidity.[58] Previous DU, dcSSc sub-type, elevated inflammatory response, early-onset RP and anti-topoisomerase antibody presence increase DU occurrence risk.[59,60] Categorizations of DU etiopathogenesis have been attempted without consensus that includes purely/true ischemic (typically digital tip), mechanical or friction (typically over extensor aspects held in fixed flexion) and mixed etiology (eg, those overlying calcinotic deposits).[61] Patterns of DU occurrence, with or without calcinosis present, show $\sim$50% of patients with recurrence, 1/3 solitary DU, $\sim$10% infrequent episodic DU, and $\sim$10% "chronic" refractory DU.[62]

SSc-DUs are scleroderma emergencies. Digital ischemic lesions and calcinosis warrant documentation at routine clinic visits, with vasodilator and other approaches optimized to reduce DU and pain burden.[53] DU emergence and healing are often influenced by modifiable exposures such as cold exposure, local trauma, or soft tissue (or deep) infection.[58,63–66] Calcinosis cutis forms at the foci of ischemic injury, often at sites overlying the extensor aspects of joints that are regularly subject to local pressure or the blanching effects of taught skin.[67,68]

Anticipatory guidance and early intervention with hand therapy, counseling on RP management and skin care, and protection against trauma and microtraumas by joint cushioning or work glove use (especially in people with known flexion contractures or evidence of tissue vulnerability by visible blanching of sclerotic skin). Smoking, being an independent risk factor for DU occurrence, makes smoking cessation an imperative.[52,53,66,69,70]

Prodromal symptoms of ischemic pain, "pressure" and local inflammatory symptoms help patients predict DU emergence.[64] Counseling patients on red flag symptoms and complications such as infection or calcinosis[71] along with contact details for prompt reporting and assessment of new lesions is critical. Patient education in infection prevention, wound care, and dressing strategies are crucial to healing, that is, wet ulcers managed with alginates and antimicrobial dressing to promote drying, and dry ulcers kept moistened with local application of hydrogel or hydrocolloid dressings.[53,71]

Cutaneous Experience in Systemic Sclerosis

Skin thickening

Skin thickening or subcutaneous edema reflecting the inflammatory transformation to fibrosis is a classic consideration in SSc that is *not always present*. The *pattern* of skin thickening provides the basis for SSc disease subsets.[72] All subsets including *sine scleroderma* are serious life-threatening illnesses. However, documenting changes in the extent and severity of skin involvement (eg, telangiectasias, skin score), especially in early disease, can guide prognostication and aggressivity of investigation and systemic treatment.

Skin thickening in early phases often gives rise to subcutaneous inflammation and edema resulting in diffuse pain/tenderness (often mistaken for fibromyalgia) and pruritus. In addition to counseling on general skincare (eg, moisturizing, sun-protection), anti-pruritus strategies, early referral to occupational and physical therapy for face/mouth and joint exercises to prevent/mitigate contracture formation and microstomia[66,73] may be pivotal to HRQoL.

Soft tissue vulnerability, pigment, and vascular changes

SSc results in vulnerability to soft tissue injury, ulceration, and infection; warranting guidance on skin protection, for example, wearing gloves when gardening, handling chemicals, or activities prone to microtrauma. Pigmentary changes and telangiectasia are associated with body image dissatisfaction and emotional distress. If dissatisfaction is detected, counseling on laser treatments, camouflage cosmetics, and other mitigating strategies might be introduced.[66,74,75]

Musculoskeletal Experience in Systemic Sclerosis

Most patients with SSc develop disabling musculoskeletal (MSK) symptoms with joint, tendon and muscle involvement. Early referral of and maintaining intermittent care from occupational and physical therapy can preserve function and mitigate progression.

Articular involvement

Extent of synovitis, chronic tendinitis and tendon friction rubs (TFRs) are independent predictors for overall disease progression, development of new DUs, and decreased left ventricular ejection fraction in early-phase SSc.[76] Arthritis-related disability and diminished HRQoL is most strongly experienced in the hands resulting in pain, stiffness, contractures, and extensive disability. Progressive articular involvement is a marker of active disease—*even if slowly progressive*—and without early intervention can become irreversible regardless of antibody presence/specification.[77]

The Health Assessment Questionnaire Disability Index (HAQ-DI), the Cochin Hand Function Scale[78] are validated simple instruments for measuring hand function and disability in SSc.[79,80] Similarly in RA, inflammatory articular involvement is easily monitored using the Disease Activity Scores of 28 joints (DAS28),[81] except that in SSc the number of tender and swollen joints is expectedly less. Interestingly, on ultrasound, joint effusions do not appear to differ between SSc and RA patients, but SSc patients show lower prevalence of synovial proliferation.[82] Progressive and, in many cases, irreversible joint erosions and other MSK involvement often occur sub-clinically, making color Doppler ultrasonography, MRI, and MR angiography (MRA) useful techniques to evaluate joint, muscle and synovial vascularity, thus the active MSK inflammation.[83]

Muscle involvement

Myopathy in SSc is frequently under-recognized with prevalence varying from 5% to 96%[84] SSc-myopathy can reflect atrophy, inflammatory, vasculopathic, fibrotic, or necrotic pathology. Both muscle strength and endurance in proximal muscles are commonly reduced[85] especially in patients with significant lung disease and predicts SSc-related cardiac involvement.[85–92]

Several auto-antibodies are predictive of SSc-myopathy: anti-PM-Scl, anti-topoisomerase-1, anti-Ku, anti-U1-RNP, anti-U3-RNP, anti-Jo, and anti-RuvBL1/2.[93] Basic diagnostic testing includes serum creatine kinase (CK), aldolase, inflammatory markers, and transaminases. However, a normal CK value does not exclude the presence of inflammatory myopathy.[84,93] Supportive investigations include electromyography (EMG), imaging modalities (US, MRI), and muscle biopsy.

Although the Manual Muscle Test (MMT-8) assesses moment muscle strength (on a 0 to 10 scale) of eight muscle groups commonly affected in idiopathic inflammatory myopathies (IIMs),[93] the Functional Index-2 (FI-2) and FI-3 evaluates muscle weakness and endurance in IIMs. Muscle endurance is the more sensitive performance outcome in IIM. FI-2 uses time-controlled repetitive movements such as shoulder flexion, shoulder abduction, head lift, and hip flexion, whereas FI-3 is equally validated and focuses on three muscle groups requiring 3 minutes to administer.[93]

Maintaining muscle mass, strength, and physical activity are key predictors of frailty and mortality across health conditions including SSc.[94–96] During muscle contraction hundreds of pro- or anti-inflammatory and metabolic cytokines (myokines) are synthetized, for example, interleukin-6, Irisin, and Meteorin-like adipomyokine.[97] Optimally dosed aerobic and strengthening exercises have positive effects on the whole organism through myokine production and maintenance of physical capacity in many chronic diseases.

Gastrointestinal Experience in Systemic Sclerosis

Oral and gastrointestinal involvement occurs in virtually all SSc patients from the oral cavity through the upper and lower GI tract and anus and remains a leading cause of SSc death with the most common causes being malabsorption, malnutrition, hyperalimentation, hemorrhage from ectasias along the GI tract, or obstruction[98,99] **(Fig. 2)**. GI involvement correlates with patient-perceived disease severity, distress, and lower HRQoL that is worse even than that associated with severe PH, ILD, renal and cardiac involvement.[100,101] Reduced esophageal motility with lower esophageal sphincter relaxation (LES), gastroesophageal reflux disorder (GERD), lower intestinal dysmotility leading to bloating, diarrhea, and/or constipation, small intestinal bacterial overgrowth (SIBO) and malabsorption, and fecal incontinence are frequently reported SSc-GI manifestations.[102] GI symptoms often progress over the disease course.[103] Patients express frustration that despite the extent and severity of their GI manifestations, they often lack support from rheumatologists generally avoiding GI-related discussion.[1] Diagnostic and therapeutic interventions can be guided by a dietician, speech therapist, and gastroenterologist.[104]

Of note, GERD has far-reaching detrimental impacts on the esophagus and the lung. Premalignant and malignant injury, structural abnormalities such as webbing, scarring, strictures, and esophageal dysmotility were more common before proton pump inhibitor (PPI) use; with severe esophageal dysfunction, being a major cause of malnutrition and mortality. Endoscopic findings of esophageal injury can occur in the absence of heartburn or regurgitation. Further, GERD plays an inciting role in the extent of ILD, as may post-nasal drip.[105] **Table 3** provides essential SSc-GI and oral health counseling points, the Giessen GI Questionnaire is a direct and simple GI assessment for the detection and severity of symptoms clinical use[106]; however, the UCLA GIT is more elaborate and helpful to monitor the frequency of symptoms.[107]

Cardiopulmonary Experience in Systemic Sclerosis

Respiratory-type symptoms

Breathlessness, exercise intolerance, and cough in SSc is often multifactorial and can be related to diverse, severe complications other than the onset or worsening ILD or PH; and require careful consideration as to cause (**Table 6**). ILD, PH, anemia, heart

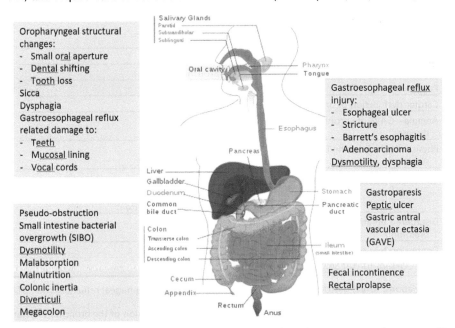

Fig. 2. Depiction of the diffuse nature of gastrointestinal involvement in SSc. (*Courtesy of* T Frech, MD, MS, Nashville, TN.)

involvement, physical deconditioning, GERD, and anxiety are common causes of SSc respiratory symptoms and are not mutually exclusive. Cylindrical bronchiectasis, bronchiole wall weakening resulting in mucous stasis and sub-acute infection, as well as pneumonia, occurs not uncommonly in SSc.

Symptom development is often quite subtle. When symptoms become apparent to the patient, lung involvement is usually significantly progressed. Patients may not recognize or explicitly complain of breathlessness; instead, they unwittingly modify pace, intensity, and types of activities to avoid the biophysical stress creating the symptoms. Careful historical probing may reveal experiences of decreased exercise tolerance, intensity, speed and/or duration of daily activities, and an unconscious slowing of movement (**Table 7**). Queries on "change over time" of these parameters are necessary to facilitate patient (and their loved ones) recall.

Queries more specific to ILD include breathlessness and coughing with deep inspiration or activities requiring deeper inspiration such as laughing, sneezing, walking-talking, or a catching sensation with inspiration which suggest a restrictive process like ILD.[108–111] Patients often restrict inspiration to avoid symptoms, which often results in incomplete inspiration during the physical examination and therefore ILD physical examination findings (ie, basilar crackles) and tell-tale inspiratory cough[108–111] are missed on clinical assessment.

Cough in SSc is associated with increased ILD severity and worse HRQoL.[112,113] Exertion and/or inspiration can trigger frightening, embarrassing, exhausting, and inconvenient episodes of dyspneic coughing with prolonged recovery phases.[108–111]

Table 6 Common causes of dyspnea and cough in systemic sclerosis	
ILD	**ILD—Dry Inspiratory**
Pulmonary hypertension—any or any combination of the following: Groups I, II, III, and IV	
Heart failure	Heart failure
Bronchiectasis[a]	Bronchiectasis[a]
Pneumonia	Pneumonia
Cardiac dysfunction or arrhythmia	
Anemia—*GAVE* or chronic inflammatory disease	
Physical deconditioning/Lack of Physical Activity	
	GERD—can be "wet" cough/gastroparesis
	PND—possible drip sensation, often in the morning, sore throat
Disordered breathing patterns/dysfunctional breathing	
Depression/fear of physical activity	
CAD, COPD/history of Smoking	

Abbreviations: GAVE, gastric antral vascular ectasia; GERD, gastroesophageal reflux disorder; ILD, interstitial lung disease; PND, post-nasal drip.

[a] *Bronchiectasis* can be either *traction* (extrinsic pulling and distortion of the bronchioles often seen in pulmonary fibrosis on HRCT) or *cylindrical* (laxity of the bronchiole wall either due to infection or perhaps CTD itself, creating a stasis environment for bacteria cough is often productive).

Courtesy of LA Saketkoo, MD, MPH, New Orleans, LA.

Table 7
Screening questions to help patients reflect on potential onset and changes in dyspnea and cough

DYSPNEA Screening	COUGH Screening for ILD
Do you notice being more short-winded now than 1 mo ago? 3 mo ago? 6 mo ago? last year? while doing activities (consider activities likely for the patient)?	Have you been coughing? Do you feel it's been the same or worse in the past 3 mo? 6 mo?
Do you notice you are becoming shorter of breath when vacuuming, making the bed, or mowing the lawn?	Are you coughing anything up? Is your cough dry?
Do you notice it takes you longer to, for example, vacuum, mop, make the bed, and mowing the lawn?	Do you cough when taking a deep breath in?
Do you notice that you need to take more breaks when going upstairs, walking, vacuuming, mopping, making the bed, and mowing the lawn?	Do you cough with laughing or sneezing?
Are you able to keep up with family members/peers when walking? Do you feel they slow their pace for you? Do you find it difficult to walk and talk at the same time?	Do you cough while talking?
Do you feel that bending over takes your breath away?	Does coughing make you feel short-winded?
Do you notice a "catching" sensation when taking a deep breath in?	

See **Table 5** for potential causes of respiratory symptoms in systemic sclerosis.
Courtesy of LA Saketkoo, MD, MPH, New Orleans, LA.

Lung involvement in systemic sclerosis

Cardio-respiratory manifestations are associated with deterioration of the physical condition and early mortality in SSc.[114–116] ILD and PH are the leading causes of SSc-related death. Early identification and initiation of early appropriate treatment prolongs survival.[117–119] Careful history, pulmonary function testing (PFTs) including diffusion capacity of the lung for carbon monoxide (DLCO), high-resolution CT scan (HRCT), echocardiogram and exercise tolerance testing (6-min walk test (6MWT)) for distance and oxygen saturation (preferentially by forehead oximeter[115,120]) are key assessments (**Figs. 3** and **4**).

HRCT is the gold standard to screen for and diagnose SSc-ILD and with a typical pattern that is, usual or nonspecific interstitial pneumonitis (UIP or NSIP) makes lung biopsy unnecessary. PFTs, though crucial for trending baseline and follow-up studies, are inadequate in detecting ILD particularly in the early stages.[121] Repeat HRCT is reserved to investigate unexplained symptoms or PFT worsening to ascertain other possible causes versus progressive ILD. Bronchoscopy helps investigate co-existent concerns of infection or malignancy.

ILD behavior is highly variable and requires a vigilant individualized approach. Maintaining a chart trajectory from the first available studies affords insights into behavior patterns that is, rapidly progressive versus stable versus slowly progressing ILD.[122] Trajectory charting prevents ignoring progressing disease as any ≥5% decrease in FVC or DLCO over 6 months despite normal range values warrants investigation and likely treatment.

Organ-Based Screening & Education Begun by Patient-Centered Queries

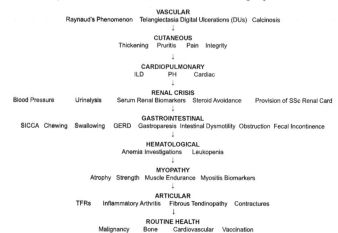

Initial Enquiries Guided by Patient-Centered Priorities / Concerns including Psycho-Social-Emotional-Physical

VASCULAR
Raynaud's Phenomenon   Telangiectasia Digital Ulcerations (DUs)   Calcinosis
↓
CUTANEOUS
Thickening   Pruritis   Pain   Integrity
↓
CARDIOPULMONARY
ILD   PH   Cardiac
↓
RENAL CRISIS
Blood Pressure   Urinalysis   Serum Renal Biomarkers   Steroid Avoidance   Provision of SSc Renal Card
↓
GASTROINTESTINAL
SICCA   Chewing   Swallowing   GERD   Gastroparesis   Intestinal Dysmotility   Obstruction   Fecal Incontinence
↓
HEMATOLOGICAL
Anemia Investigations   Leukopenia
↓
MYOPATHY
Atrophy   Strength   Muscle Endurance   Myositis Biomarkers
↓
ARTICULAR
TFRs   Inflammatory Arthritis   Fibrous Tendinopathy   Contractures
↓
ROUTINE HEALTH
Malignancy   Bone   Cardiovascular   Vaccination

Fig. 3. Overall framework to approach biophysical assessment.

ILD and PH often coexist, and can be temporally coincident in early SSc, especially in patients of African descent. PH in SSc can be of either WHO Group 1, 2, 3, or 4; and more commonly PH group types coexist together. Right heart catheterization is required to diagnose PH. However, annual echocardiogram without following trends of patient symptoms (*dyspnea, fatigue, exercise tolerance*), serum NT-pro-BNP, 6MWT *distance,* and *oxygen saturation levels,* is unreliable missing up to 40% of RHC-confirmed SSc-PH cases.[123]

DLCO provides an early detection mechanism for PH and when compared with FVC or TLC can differentiate parenchymal from vascular lung disease. DLCO reflects gas

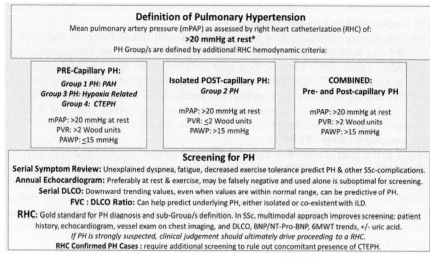

Fig. 4. Screening and characterization of pulmonary hypertension in SSc. (*Courtesy of* LA Saket-koo, MD, MPH, New Orleans, LA.) *'Exercise Induced PH' is defined by mPAP/Cardiac Output slope between rest and exercise; 'Unclassified PH' is defined as mPAP >20mmHg but low PVR (≤2 Wood units) and low PAWP (≤15mmHg); >3mmHg/L/min. Humbert, M., Kovacs, G., Hoeper, M. M., et al. ESC/ERS Scientific Document Group (2022). 2022 ESC/ERS Guidelines for the diagnosis and treatment of pulmonary hypertension. European heart journal, 43(38), 3618–3731.

transfer from airspace to the bloodstream which requires gas to diffuse across *two barriers*: the *lung parenchyma* and the *vascular wall*. Resistance to permeable gas of either or both barriers causes reduction in DLCO. In ILD the FVC and DLCO trend downward in parallel; however, in PH the DLCO declines more steeply than FVC. However, in early SSc-ILD, the FVC may be stable, whereas the DLCO decreases, but generally FVC:DLCO ratio helps distinguish between the presence/predominance of PH from ILD.[124,125]

Lung transplantation in SSc is safe, for patients with progressive lung disease despite maximal therapy. Early discussions on transplant evaluation permits time for familiarization with the transplant process, make informed unhurried decisions, and adjust to psychosocial and financial pressures related to transplant. It also provides lead time for habituation of healthy life practices including optimizing fitness supported by pulmonary rehabilitation.[116]

Cardiac involvement in systemic sclerosis
Microvascular insufficiency, or inflammatory-fibrotic infiltration of the myocardium, may underlie SSc-cardiac involvement causing arrhythmias, diastolic or systolic dysfunction, pericarditis, or myocarditis. Cardiac involvement is often associated with SSc-myopathy.[89–91] Noncontrast cardiovascular magnetic resonance (CMR) may play a role in early diagnosis and has shown a 45% prevalence of myocardial fibrosis unexplained by other causes. Cardiac involvement is often associated with diffuse skin involvement, elevated CRP, and upward-trending NT-Pro-BNP.[126,127]

Renal Experience in Systemic Sclerosis

Before the recognition of risk factors and *early* effective intervention with angiotensin-converting-enzyme inhibition (ACEi), scleroderma renal crisis (SRC) was the leading cause of SSc-related mortality.[99,128–130] Delayed ACEi continues to lead to poorer outcomes.[130] However, the prophylactic role of ACEi has been associated with increased incidence of SRC and with poorer outcomes.[131,132]

Clinical and serologic risk factors for SRC[130] can be nonmodifiable such as dcSSc subset, early rapidly progressing skin disease and the presence of anti-RNA-polymerase III antibodies[133]; or modifiable such as corticosteroid exposure (prednisolone >10 to 15 mg daily).[133–135]

Notwithstanding the lack of clear SRC screening standards, educating high-risk patients about SRC and the provision of the SRC prevention card (**Fig. 5**) can help patients and other health care professionals, especially emergency and primary care physicians, recognize SRC.[136] Despite the apparent rapidity of presentation, SRC likely has a protracted asymptomatic prodromal period, providing an opportunity to avert renal injury. Monitoring trends in routine simple point-of-care assessments such as blood pressure (BP) and urine-dipstick, and at-home blood pressure recording 2 to 3 times weekly can help identify SRC in the absence of symptoms. Red flags such as increased systolic BP 20 mm Hg above usual values, and features of malignant hypertension such as headaches or visual disturbance[137] are prompts to seek medical attention.

Additional Health Maintenance in Systemic Sclerosis

Vaccination
Dysregulated immune responses and widespread use of immunomodulatory drugs predispose to serious infection in SSc, thrusting rheumatologists into the pivotal role of advocating for vaccine adherence in SSc[138,139] (**Table 8**). However, lack of specialist recommendation (36.1%) topped the list, along with fear of side effects (23.1%) or of inefficacy (4%), in reported reasons for influenza vaccine noncompliance in SSc.[140] Similarly, poor vaccine compliance with pneumococcal vaccine[140]; occurs

```
┌─────────────────────────────────────────────────────────┐
│     SCLERODERMA RENAL CRISIS PREVENTION                   │
│       << Please fill out this card and keep it with you. >> │
│   ▶ You have been identified as a person at risk of RENAL CRISIS, │
│     a preventable problem.                                │
│   ▶ Warning signs: New onset headaches, blurred vision, shortness │
│     of breath, confusion, abrupt elevation of blood pressure. │
│   ▶ Monitor your blood pressure and know and record your usual │
│     readings _____ │
│   ▶ Call Dr. _____ if BP is greater │
│     than _____ or seek urgent care.             │
│                                                           │
│   Show any treating physician this card.                  │
└─────────────────────────────────────────────────────────┘
```

```
┌─────────────────────────────────────────────────────────┐
│            SCLERODERMA RENAL CRISIS:                      │
│          PREVENTION AND TREATMENT                         │
│   ▶ This is a patient at risk of scleroderma renal crisis. │
│   ▶ If hypertensive or blood pressure is acutely          │
│     increased, ACE INHIBITORS are the only drugs          │
│     predictably effective at aborting renal crisis.       │
│   ▶ If unable to administer orally, give I.V. enaprilat.  │
│   ▶ Check creatinine as renal failure may occur abruptly. │
│   ▶ Please call this patient's rheumatologist,            │
│     Dr. _____           │
│     Phone # _____           │
└─────────────────────────────────────────────────────────┘
```

Fig. 5. Renal crisis prevention card may help patients direct emergency health care providers to abort a crisis and avoid adverse outcomes.[136] (*From* Shapiro, L, Saketkoo, L, Farrell, J et al AB0712 Development of a "Renal Crisis Prevention Card" as an Education Tool to Improve Outcomes in High Risk Patients with Systemic Sclerosis (SSC). Annals of the Rheumatic Diseases 2015: 74: 1136.)

despite a higher rate ratio of pneumococcal-related hospitalization in SSc (4.2 vs 3.7 for diabetes).[141]

SSc immunomodulatory treatments create concern for vaccine efficacy, but regardless whenever possible adherence to vaccination schedules is essential to SSc care vaccination timing (eg, around rituximab therapy use) informed by most current approaches.[142–146] Hematopoietic stem cell transplant (HSCT) requires re-vaccination as immunologic memory to vaccines is often lost (>24 months for live vaccines).[147–149] Administration of "killed" (pneumococcal, influenza, hepatitis B, and zoster) vaccinations, including for SARS-CoV-2, are key in patients receiving immunosuppressants.[150,151] The malignancy risk associated with SSc, makes the recombinant (human papillomavirus, HPV) vaccination an important consideration.[152]

Cancer screening

A close temporal relationship exists between cancer and SSc. SSc confers relative risks (RR) ranging from 1.55 to 1.81[153,154] with 7.1% to 14.2% of patients having a history of cancer. Cancer accounts for ~16% of deaths in SSc[155]; with breast,

Table 8
Health maintenance screening in systemic sclerosis

Immunizations	Inactive formulations of vaccines: Influenza (annually) COVID-19 according to guidelines for vulnerable/ immunocompromised Hepatitis B series Pneumococcal series Diphtheria/tetanus/pertussis Varicella Zoster vaccine/Shingles (Shingrix) HPV series for females

Age-appropriate
  malignancy screening
	Gynecologic
	Breast
	Prostate
	Colon
	Annual skin cancer screening
	Smoking history with cognizance of lung and oral malignancy
	  potential
	Lung cancer screening

Cardiovascular	Appropriate assessment and treatment to target hypertension,
	  diabetes, and high cholesterol
	Routine screening for pulmonary hypertension and heart failure
	Consider screening for OSA
	Weight trends especially in those with pulmonary hypertension or
	  heart failure
	Regular assessments of volume status

Bone health	Risk factors for DEXA screening earlier than 65 years old: Osteopenia on radiographs History of fracture History of malabsorption Corticosteroid use Low serum testosterone Prolonged use of proton pump inhibitors
Ophthalmologic health	Evaluation and management of SICCA-type symptoms Hydroxychloroquine toxicity screening, as applicable Visual acuity
Dental health	Twice-yearly routine dental visits are advised Evaluation and management of SICCA-type symptoms Evaluate for impact on nutritional intake

Courtesy of LA Saketkoo, MD, MPH, New Orleans, LA.

hematological, skin, and lung cancers being most prevalent,[156,157] particularly with anti-RNA-polymerase III and anti-topoisomerase antibody positivity.[153,156,158–160] Though formal guidelines are not yet established, age-appropriate malignancy screening should be rigorously adhered to, and symptoms suggestive of possible malignancy should be met with a low threshold for investigative imaging.

Cardiovascular disease
Vasculopathy, having an indisputable central role in SSc pathology, provides a strong rationale for screening and modification of traditional cardiovascular risk factors (such as prioritizing smoking cessation) to avert additive damage to already vulnerable vasculature.[53] Beyond this, enhanced cardiovascular risk in SSc[161] is suggested by increased carotid intima-medial thickness with reduced flow-mediated dilatation,[162] increased coronary calcifications,[163] and the risks of MI and stroke being approximately 2-fold in SSc compared with controls.[164]

Bone health in systemic sclerosis

Patients with SSc seems to be at greater risk of low bone mineral density and fracture, with risk highest amongst patients with known risk factors for reduced bone density for example, corticosteroid use, and fracture history.[165,166] No formal guidance exists for osteoporosis screening in SSc. Thus prevention rests on the recognition and modification of risk factors such as nutritional impairment, immobility, sedentary indoor lifestyle, corticosteroid exposure, and smoking cessation counseling.[166] Long-term proton pump inhibitor use in SSc also increases concerns around fracture risk.[167]

SUMMARY

Presented here is a paradigm of philosophic approach to prioritize HRQoL with biophysical elements being a crucial pillar in attaining this priority. Though the clinician's level of care and vigilance of the biophysical aspect may not alter, this patient-centered approach may sensitize us to the importance of SDM, empowering patients with anticipatory guidance and counseling, and the value of more readily and proactively integrate the experience of living with SSc into clinical decision-making.

CLINICS CARE POINTS

- Routine assessment of HRQoL in SSc may provide clinical guidance to pressing and treatable patient concerns.
- Screening for depression, anxiety, sleep, fatigue and sexual dysfunction in people with SSc may reveal treatable conditions that markedly improve HRQoL in SSc.
- Pain and Fatigue are each multi-factorial experiences in SSc and require careful assessment to identify and treat their cause/s.
- Raynauds, digital vascular complications and hand impairment are key sources of disability in people with SSc. Proactive history, assessment, counselling and early referral to occupational therapy are key to controlling symptoms and preserving function.
- Gastrointestinal impairment and dysfunction is a leading cause of poor HRQoL in people living with SSc. Routine assessment of symptoms, proactive management and counselling may markedly improve HRQoL in SSc.
- Screening for ILD and PH requires a vigilant multi-modal approach that combines history, pulmonary function, exercise testing and imaging for all SSc sub-types.
- DLCO trend is an important predictor of ILD and/or PH in people with SSc.
- RHC is the gold standard for diagnosis and classification of PH. Though multiple diagnostic variables should be considered, the decision to perform a RHC relies heavily upon a clinician's judgement.
- Multiple types of PH can co-exist in a person with SSc.
- A wallet card, anticipatory counselling and home blood pressure monitoring may help prevent death and disability for people with SSc who are at higher risk for Scleroderma Renal Crisis (SRC).

DISCLOSURES

J.D. Pauling has received personal support from Janssen, Astra Zeneca, Permeatus Inc, Boehringher-Ingelheim and Sojournix Pharma. L.A. Saketkoo has received consultancy and research support from Abbvie, Boehringer Ingelheim, Corbus, Eicos, Kadmon, Horizon, Janssen, Johnson and Johnson Pharmaceutical companies.

ACKNOWLEDGMENTS

The authors thank Mr Humza Ahmad Chaudhry, MD, MBA candidate at Tulane University School of Medicine for his interest in multi-organ system diseases and invaluable assistance in the production of this paper.

REFERENCES

1. Saketkoo LA, Frech T, Varjú C, et al. A comprehensive framework for navigating patient care in systemic sclerosis: A global response to the need for improving the practice of diagnostic and preventive strategies in SSc. Best Pract Res Clin Rheumatol 2021 Sep;35(3):101707.
2. Saketkoo LA. Wildflowers abundant in the garden of systemic sclerosis research, while hopeful exotics will one day bloom. Rheumatology 2018;57(3): 410–3.
3. Malcarne VL, Fox RS, Mills SD, et al. Psychosocial aspects of systemic sclerosis. Curr Opin Rheumatol 2013;25:707–13.
4. Golemati CV, Moutsopoulos HM, Vlachoyiannopoulos PG. Psychological characteristics of systemic sclerosis patients and their correlation with major organ involvement and disease activity. Clin Exp Rheumatol 2013;31(2 Suppl 76): 37–45.
5. Santiago T, Santos E, Duarte AC, et al. Happiness, quality of life and their determinants among people with systemic sclerosis: a structural equation modelling approach. Rheumatology 2021;60:4717–27.
6. Gholizadeh S, Meier A, Malcarne VL. Measuring and managing appearance anxiety in patients with systemic sclerosis. Expert Rev Clin Immunol 2019;15: 341–6.
7. Merz EL, Kwakkenbos L, Carrier ME, et al. Factor structure and convergent validity of the Derriford Appearance Scale-24 using standard scoring versus treating 'not applicable' responses as missing data: a Scleroderma Patient-centered Intervention Network (SPIN). BMJ Open 2018;8:e018641.
8. Thombs BD, Taillefer SS, Hudson M, et al. Depression in patients with systemic sclerosis: a systematic review of the evidence. Arthritis Rheum 2007;57: 1089–97.
9. Bassel M, Hudson M, Taillefer SS, et al. Frequency and impact of symptoms experienced by patients with systemic sclerosis: results from a Canadian National Survey. Rheumatology 2011;50:762–7.
10. Garaiman A, Mihai C, Dobrota R, et al. The Hospital Anxiety and Depression Scale in patients with systemic sclerosis: a psychometric and factor analysis in a monocentric cohort. Clin Exp Rheumatol 2021;39(Suppl 131):34–42.
11. Fox RS, Mills SD, Gholizadeh S, et al. Validity and correlates of the Brief Satisfaction With Appearance Scale for patients with limited and diffuse systemic sclerosis: Analysis from the University of California, Los Angeles Scleroderma Quality of Life Study. J Scleroderma Relat Disord 2020;5:143–51.
12. Angelopoulos NV, Drosos AA, Moutsopoulos HM. Psychiatric symptoms associated with scleroderma. Psychother Psychosom 2001;70:145–50.
13. Türk İ, Cüzdan N, Çiftçi V, et al. Malnutrition, associated clinical factors, and depression in systemic sclerosis: a cross-sectional study. Clin Rheumatol 2020;39:57–67.

14. Ostojic P, Jankovic K, Djurovic N, et al. Common Causes of Pain in Systemic Sclerosis: Frequency, Severity, and Relationship to Disease Status, Depression, and Quality of Life. Pain Manag Nurs 2019;20:331–6.

15. Figueiredo FP, Aires GD, Nisihara R, et al. Sleep Disturbance in Scleroderma. J Clin Rheumatol 2021;27:S242–5.

16. Strickland G, Pauling J, Cavill C, et al. Predictors of health-related quality of life and fatigue in systemic sclerosis: evaluation of the EuroQol-5D and FACIT-F assessment tools. Clin Rheumatol 2012;31:1215–22.

17. Vingeliene S, Hiyoshi A, Lentjes M, et al. Longitudinal analysis of loneliness and inflammation at older ages: English longitudinal study of ageing. Psychoneuroendocrinology 2019 Dec;110:104421.

18. Ostojic P, Damjanov N. The impact of depression, microvasculopathy, and fibrosis on development of erectile dysfunction in men with systemic sclerosis. Clin Rheumatol 2007;26(10):1671–4.

19. Hinchcliff ME, Beaumont JL, Carns MA, et al. Longitudinal evaluation of PROMIS-29 and FACIT-dyspnea short forms in systemic sclerosis. J Rheumatol 2015;42(1):64–72.

20. Thombs BD, Hudson M, Schieir O, et al, Canadian Scleroderma Research Group. Reliability and validity of the center for epidemiologic studies depression scale in patients with systemic sclerosis. Arthritis Rheum 2008;59(3):438–43.

21. Santos EF, Duarte CM, Ferreira RO, et al. Multifactorial explanatory model of depression in patients with rheumatoid arthritis: a structural equation approach. Clin Exp Rheumatol 2019;37(4):641–8.

22. Emmungil H, İlgen U, Turan S, et al. Assessment of loneliness in patients with inflammatory arthritis. Int J Rheum Dis 2021;24(2):223–30.

23. Kwakkenbos L, Carboni-Jiménez A, Carrier ME, et al. Reasons for not participating in scleroderma patient support groups: a comparison of results from the North American and European scleroderma support group surveys. Disabil Rehabil 2021;43(9):1279–86.

24. Condon SE, Roesch SC, Clements PJ, et al. Coping profiles and health outcomes among individuals with systemic sclerosis: A latent profile analysis approach. J Scleroderma Relat Disord 2020;5(3):231–6.

25. DiRenzo DD, Smith TR, Frech TM, et al. Effect of Coping Strategies on Patient and Physician Perceptions of Disease Severity and Disability in Systemic Sclerosis. J Rheumatol 2021;48(10):1569–73.

26. Decuman S, Smith V, Verhaeghe ST, et al. Work participation in patients with systemic sclerosis: a systematic review. Clin Exp Rheumatol 2014;32(6 Suppl 86): 206–13.

27. Lee JJY, Gignac MAM, Johnson SR. Employment outcomes in systemic sclerosis. Best Pract Res Clin Rheumatol 2021;35:101667.

28. Schouffoer AA, Schoones JW, Terwee CB, et al. Work status and its determinants among patients with systemic sclerosis: a systematic review. Rheumatology 2012;51:1304–14.

29. Ł Mokros, Świtaj P, Bieńkowski P, et al. Depression and loneliness may predict work inefficiency among professionally active adults. Int Arch Occup Environ Health 2022;3:1–9.

30. Gao R, Qing P, Sun X, et al. Prevalence of Sexual Dysfunction in People With Systemic Sclerosis and the Associated Risk Factors: A Systematic Review. Sex Med 2021;9:100392.

31. Levis B, Hudson M, Knafo R, et al. Rates and correlates of sexual activity and impairment among women with systemic sclerosis. Arthritis Care Res 2012; 64:340–50.
32. Jaeger VK, Walker UA. Erectile Dysfunction in Systemic Sclerosis. Curr Rheumatol Rep 2016;18:49.
33. Bhadauria S, Moser DK, Clements PJ, et al. Genital tract abnormalities and female sexual function impairment in systemic sclerosis. Am J Obstet Gynecol 1995;172:580–7.
34. Bongi MS, Del Rosso A, Mikhaylova S, et al. Sexual function in Italian women with systemic sclerosis is affected by disease-related and psychological concerns. J Rheumatol 2013;40:1697–705.
35. Schmalzing M, Nau LF, Gernert M, et al. Sexual function in German women with systemic sclerosis compared with women with systemic lupus erythematosus and evaluation of a screening test. Clin Exp Rheumatol 2020;38(Suppl 125): 59–64.
36. Schouffoer AA, van der Marel J, Ter Kuile MM, et al. Impaired sexual function in women with systemic sclerosis: a cross-sectional study. Arthritis Rheum 2009; 61:1601–8.
37. Rosato E, Gigante A, Barbano B, et al. Clitoral blood flow in systemic sclerosis women: correlation with disease clinical variables and female sexual dysfunction. Rheumatology 2013;52:2238–42.
38. Gigante A, Navarini L, Margiotta D, et al. Female sexual dysfunction in systemic sclerosis: The role of endothelial growth factor and endostatin. J Scleroderma Relat Disord 2019;4:71–6.
39. Bruni C, Raja J, Denton CP, et al. The clinical relevance of sexual dysfunction in systemic sclerosis. Autoimmun Rev 2015;14:1111–5.
40. Dorey G. Restoring pelvic floor function in men: review of RCTs. Br J Nurs 2005; 14:1014–21.
41. Rosen R, Brown C, Heiman J, et al. The Female Sexual Function Index (FSFI): a multidimensional self-report instrument for the assessment of female sexual function. J Sex Marital Ther 2000;26:191–208.
42. Heřmánková B, Špiritović M, Šmucrová H, et al. Female Sexual Dysfunction and Pelvic Floor Muscle Function Associated with Systemic Sclerosis: A Cross-Sectional Study. Int J Environ Res Public Health 2022;19:612.
43. Barber MD, Walters MD, Bump RC. Short forms of two condition-specific quality-of-life questionnaires for women with pelvic floor disorders (PFDI-20 and PFIQ-7). Am J Obstet Gynecol 2005;193:103–13.
44. Sanchez K, Denys P, Giuliano F, et al. Systemic sclerosis: Sexual dysfunction and lower urinary tract symptoms in 73 patients. Presse Med 2016;45(4Pt1): e79–89.
45. Foocharoen C, Tyndall A, Hachulla E, et al. Erectile dysfunction is frequent in systemic sclerosis and associated with severe disease: a study of the EULAR Scleroderma Trial and Research group. Arthritis Res Ther 2012;14:R37.
46. Krittian SM, Saur SJ, Schloegl A, et al. Erectile function and connective tissue diseases. Prevalence of erectile dysfunction in German men with systemic sclerosis compared with other connective tissue diseases and healthy subjects. Clin Exp Rheumatol 2021;39(Suppl 131):52–6.
47. Rosen RC, Cappelleri JC, Smith MD, et al. Development and evaluation of an abridged, 5-item version of the International Index of Erectile Function (IIEF-5) as a diagnostic tool for erectile dysfunction. Int J Impot Res 1999;11:319–26.

48. Proietti M, Aversa A, Letizia C, et al. Erectile dysfunction in systemic sclerosis: effects of longterm inhibition of phosphodiesterase type-5 on erectile function and plasma endothelin-1 levels. J Rheumatol 2007;34:1712–7.

49. Schneeberger D, Tyndall A, Kay J, et al. Systemic sclerosis without antinuclear antibodies or Raynaud's phenomenon: a multicentre study in the prospective EULAR Scleroderma Trials and Research (EUSTAR) database. *Rheumatology (Oxford)*. Mar 2013;52(3):560–7.

50. Pauling JD, Reilly E, Smith T, et al. Evolving Symptom Characteristics of Raynaud's Phenomenon in Systemic Sclerosis and Their Association With Physician and Patient-Reported Assessments of Disease Severity. Arthritis Care Res (Hoboken) 2019;71(8):1119–26.

51. Murphy SL, Lescoat A, Alore M, et al. How do patients define Raynaud's phenomenon? Differences between primary and secondary disease. Clin Rheumatol 2021;40(4):1611–6.

52. Hudson M, Lo E, Lu Y, et al. Cigarette smoking in patients with systemic sclerosis. Arthritis Rheum 2011;63(1):230–8.

53. Hughes M, Ong VH, Anderson ME, et al. Consensus best practice pathway of the UK Scleroderma Study Group: digital vasculopathy in systemic sclerosis. Rheumatology (Oxford) 2015;54(11):2015–24.

54. Pauling JD, Reilly E, Smith T, et al. Factors Influencing Raynaud Condition Score Diary Outcomes in Systemic Sclerosis. J Rheumatol 2019;46(10):1326–34.

55. Watson HR, Robb R, Belcher G, et al. Seasonal variation of Raynaud's phenomenon secondary to systemic sclerosis. J Rheumatol 1999;26(8):1734–7.

56. Pauling JD, Saketkoo LA, Matucci-Cerinic M, et al. The patient experience of Raynaud's phenomenon in systemic sclerosis. Rheumatology Jan 1 2019; 58(1):18–26.

57. Pauling JD, Domsic RT, Saketkoo LA, et al. Multinational Qualitative Research Study Exploring the Patient Experience of Raynaud's Phenomenon in Systemic Sclerosis. Arthritis Care Res (Hoboken) 2018;70(9):1373–84.

58. Hughes M, Pauling JD. Exploring the patient experience of digital ulcers in systemic sclerosis. Semin Arthritis Rheum 2019;48(5):888–94.

59. Morrisroe K, Stevens W, Sahhar J, et al. Digital ulcers in systemic sclerosis: their epidemiology, clinical characteristics, and associated clinical and economic burden. Arthritis Res Ther Dec 23 2019;21(1):299.

60. Sunderkotter C, Herrgott I, Bruckner C, et al. Comparison of patients with and without digital ulcers in systemic sclerosis: detection of possible risk factors. Br J Dermatol 2009;160(4):835–43.

61. Hachulla E, Clerson P, Launay D, et al. Natural history of ischemic digital ulcers in systemic sclerosis: single-center retrospective longitudinal study. J Rheumatol 2007;34(12):2423–30.

62. Matucci-Cerinic M, Krieg T, Guillevin L, et al. Elucidating the burden of recurrent and chronic digital ulcers in systemic sclerosis: long-term results from the DUO Registry. Ann Rheum Dis 2016;75(10):1770–6.

63. Hughes M, Pauling JD, Jones J, et al. Multicenter Qualitative Study Exploring the Patient Experience of Digital Ulcers in Systemic Sclerosis. Arthritis Care Res (Hoboken) 2020;72(5):723–33.

64. Hughes M, Pauling JD, Jones J, et al. Patient experiences of digital ulcer development and evolution in systemic sclerosis. Rheumatology Aug 1 2020;59(8): 2156–8. https://doi.org/10.1093/rheumatology/keaa037.

65. Giuggioli D, Manfredi A, Colaci M, et al. Scleroderma digital ulcers complicated by infection with fecal pathogens. Arthritis Care Res (Hoboken) 2012;64(2): 295–7.
66. Denton CP, Hughes M, Gak N, et al. BSR and BHPR guideline for the treatment of systemic sclerosis. Rheumatology Oct 2016;55(10):1906–10.
67. Baron M, Pope J, Robinson D, et al. Calcinosis is associated with digital ischaemia in systemic sclerosis-a longitudinal study. Rheumatology Dec 2016; 55(12):2148–55.
68. Christensen A, Khalique S, Cenac S, et al. Systemic Sclerosis Related Calcinosis: Patients Provide What Specialists Want to Learn. J La State Med Soc May-Jun 2015;167(3):158–9.
69. Jaeger VK, Valentini G, Hachulla E, et al. Brief Report: Smoking in Systemic Sclerosis: A Longitudinal European Scleroderma Trials and Research Group Study. Arthritis Rheumatol 2018;70(11):1829–34.
70. Harrison BJ, Silman AJ, Hider SL, et al. Cigarette smoking as a significant risk factor for digital vascular disease in patients with systemic sclerosis. Arthritis Rheum 2002;46(12):3312–6.
71. Saketkoo LA, Frech TM, Gordon JK, et al. Patient Experience of Systemic Sclerosis related Calcinosis: An International Study Informing Clinical Trials, Practice and the Development of the Mawdsley Calcinosis Questionnaire. Rheum Dis Clin 2022.
72. LeRoy EC, Black C, Fleischmajer R, et al. Scleroderma (systemic sclerosis): classification, subsets and pathogenesis. J Rheumatol 1988;15(2):202–5.
73. Poole JL, Macintyre NJ, Deboer HN. Evidence-based management of hand and mouth disability in a woman living with diffuse systemic sclerosis (scleroderma). *Physiother Can*. Fall 2013;65(4):317–20.
74. Jewett LR, Hudson M, Malcarne VL, et al. Canadian Scleroderma Research G. Sociodemographic and disease correlates of body image distress among patients with systemic sclerosis. PLoS One 2012;7(3):e33281.
75. Pauling JD. The challenge of establishing treatment efficacy for cutaneous vascular manifestations of systemic sclerosis. Expert Rev Clin Immunol 2018; 14(5):431–42.
76. Avouac J, Walker UA, Hachulla E, et al. Joint and tendon involvement predict disease progression in systemic sclerosis: a EUSTAR prospective study. Ann Rheum Dis 2016;75:103–9.
77. Sandler RD, Matucci-Cerinic M, Hughes M. Musculoskeletal hand involvement in systemic sclerosis. Semin Arthritis Rheum 2020;50:329–34.
78. Ernste FC, Chong C, Crowson CS, et al. Functional index-3: a valid and reliable functional outcome assessment measure in patients with dermatomyositis and polymyositis. J Rheumatol 2021;48(1):94–100.
79. Pauling JD, Caetano J, Campochiaro C, et al. Patient-reported outcome instruments in clinical trials of systemic sclerosis. Journal of Scleroderma and Related Disorders 2020;5:90–102.
80. Clements P, Allanore Y, Furst DE, et al. Points to consider for designing trials in systemic sclerosis patients with arthritic involvement. Rheumatology 2017; 56(suppl_5):v23–6.
81. Lóránd V, Nagy G, Bálint Z, et al. Sensitivity to change of joint count composite indices in 72 patients with systemic sclerosis. Clin Exp Rheumatol 2021; 39(Suppl 131):77–84.
82. Cuomo G, Zappia M, Abignano G, et al. Ultrasonographic features of the hand and wrist in systemic sclerosis. Rheumatology 2009;48:1414–7.

83. Boutry N, Hachulla E, Zanetti-Musielak C, et al. Imaging features of musculo-skeletal involvement in systemic sclerosis. Eur Radiol 2007;17:1172–80.

84. Varjú C, Péntek M, Lóránd V, et al. Musculoskeletal Involvement in Systemic Sclerosis: An Unexplored Aspect of the Disease. Journal of Scleroderma and Related disorders 2017;2:19–32.

85. Pettersson H, Bostrom C, Bringby F, et al. Muscle endurance, strength, and active range of motion in patients with different subphenotypes in systemic sclerosis: a cross-sectional cohort study. Scand J Rheumatol 2019;48(2):141e8.

86. Nie L-Y, Wang X-D, Zhang T, et al. Cardiac complications in systemic sclerosis: early diagnosis and treatment. Chin Med J (Engl). 2019;132(23):2865e71.

87. Rodríguez-Reyna TS, Morelos-Guzman M, Hernandez-Reyes P, et al. Assessment of myocardial fibrosis and microvascular damage in systemic sclerosis by magnetic resonance imaging and coronary angiotomography. Rheumatol Oxf Engl 2015;54(4):647e54.

88. Rodríguez-Reyna TS, Rosales-Uvera SG, Kimura-Hayama E, et al. Myocardial fibrosis detected by magnetic resonance imaging, elevated U-CRP and higher mRSS are predictors of cardiovascular complications in systemic sclerosis (SSc) patients. Semin Arthritis Rheum 2019;49(2):273e8.

89. Follansbee WP, Zerbe TR, Medsger TA. Cardiac and skeletal muscle disease in systemic sclerosis (scleroderma): a high risk association. Am Heart J 1993; 125(1):194e203.

90. Ranque B, Authier F-J, Le-Guern V, et al. A descriptive and prognostic study of systemic sclerosis-associated myopathies. Ann Rheum Dis 2009;68(9):1474e7.

91. Ranque B, Berezne A, Le-Guern V, et al. Myopathies related to systemic sclerosis: a case-control study of associated clinical and immunological features. Scand J Rheumatol 2010;39(6):498e505.

92. West SG, Killian PJ, Lawless OJ. Association of myositis and myocarditis in progressive systemic sclerosis. Arthritis Rheum 1981;24(5):662e8.

93. Baumberger R, Jordan S, Distler O, et al. Diagnostic measures for patients with systemic sclerosis-associated myopathy. Clin Exp Rheumatol 2021;39(Suppl 131):85–93.

94. Sepehri K, Low H, Hoang J, et al. Promoting early management of frailty in the new normal: An updated software tool in addressing the need of virtual assessment of frailty at points of care. Aging Med (Milton) 2022;5(1):4–9.

95. Guler SA, Kwan JM, Winstone TA, et al. Severity and features of frailty in systemic sclerosis-associated interstitial lung disease. Respir Med 2017;129:1–7.

96. Farooqi MAM, O'Hoski S, Goodwin S, et al. Prevalence and prognostic impact of physical frailty in interstitial lung disease: A prospective cohort study. Respirology 2021;26(7):683–9.

97. Zunner BEM, Wachsmuth NB, Eckstein ML, et al. Myokines and Resistance Training: A Narrative Review. Int J Mol Sci 2022;23:3501.

98. Elhai M, Meune C, Boubaya M, et al. Mapping and predicting mortality from systemic sclerosis. Ann Rheum Dis 2017;76(11):1897–905.

99. Steen VD, Medsger TA. Changes in causes of death in systemic sclerosis, 1972-2002. Ann Rheum Dis 2007;66(7):940–4.

100. Jaeger VK, Distler O, Maurer B, et al. Functional disability and its predictors in systemic sclerosis: a study from the DeSScipher project within the EUSTAR group. Rheumatol Oxf Engl 2018;57(3):441e50.

101. Saketkoo LA. Wildflowers abundant in the garden of systemic sclerosis research, while hopeful exotics will one day bloom. Rheumatol Oxf Engl 2018; 57(3):410e3.

102. Emmanuel A. Current management of the gastrointestinal complications of systemic sclerosis. Nat Rev Gastroenterol Hepatol 2016;13(8):461–72.
103. McMahan ZH, Paik JJ, Wigley FM, et al. Determining the risk factors and clinical features associated with severe gastrointestinal dysmotility in systemic sclerosis. Arthritis Care Res 2018;70(9):1385–92.
104. Gyger G, Baron M. Systemic sclerosis: gastrointestinal disease and its management. Rheum Dis Clin North Am 2015;41(3):459e73.
105. Hansi N, Thoua N, Carulli M, et al. Consensus best practice pathway of the UK scleroderma study group: gastrointestinal manifestations of systemic sclerosis. Clin Exp Rheumatol 2014;32(6 Suppl 86):214e21.
106. Schmeiser T, Saar P, Jin D, et al. Profile of gastrointestinal involvement in patients with systemic sclerosis. Rheumatol Int 2012;32(8):2471–8.
107. Khanna D, Hays RD, Maranian P, et al. Reliability and validity of the University of California, Los Angeles Scleroderma Clinical Trial Consortium Gastrointestinal Tract Instrument. Arthritis Rheum 2009;61(9):1257–63.
108. Lammi M, Baughman R, Birring S, et al. Outcome measures for clinical trials in interstitial lung diseases. Curr Respir Med Rev 2015;11(2):163e74.
109. Saketkoo LA, Mittoo S, Huscher D, et al. Connective tissue disease related interstitial lung diseases and idiopathic pulmonary fibrosis: provisional core sets of domains and instruments for use in clinical trials. Thorax 2014 May;69(5): 428–36.
110. Saketkoo LA, Mittoo S, Frankel S, et al. Reconciling healthcare professional and patient perspectives in the development of disease activity and response criteria in connective tissue disease-related interstitial lung diseases. J Rheumatol 2014;41(4):792–8.
111. Mittoo S, Frankel S, LeSage D, et al. Patient perspectives in OMERACT provide an anchor for future metric development and improved approaches to healthcare delivery in connective tissue disease related interstitial lung disease (CTD-ILD). Curr Respir Med Rev 2015;11(2):175e83.
112. Theodore AC, Tseng C-H, Li N, et al. Correlation of cough with disease activity and treatment with cyclophosphamide in scleroderma interstitial lung disease: findings from the Scleroderma Lung Study. Chest 2012;142(3):614e21.
113. Tashkin DP, Volkmann ER, Tseng C-H, et al. Improved cough and cough-specific quality of life in patients treated for scleroderma-related interstitial lung disease: results of scleroderma lung study II. Chest 2017;151(4):813e20.
114. Saketkoo LA, Magnus JH, Doyle MK. The primary care physician in the early diagnosis of systemic sclerosis: the cornerstone of recognition and hope. Am J Med Sci 2014;347:54–63.
115. Wilsher M, Good N, Hopkins R, et al. The six-minute walk test using forehead oximetry is reliable in the assessment of scleroderma lung disease. Respirology 2012;17:647–52.
116. Saketkoo LA, Obi ON, Patterson KC, et al. Ageing with Interstitial Lung Disease: Preserving Health and Well Being. Curr Opin Pulm Med 2022. https://doi.org/10.1097/MCP.0000000000000880.
117. Rodriguez-Pla A, Simms RW. Geographic disparity in systemic sclerosis mortality in the United States: 1999e2017. J Scleroderma Relat Disord 2021;6(2): 139e45.
118. Tashkin DP, Roth MD, Clements PJ, et al. Mycophenolate mofetil versus oral cyclophosphamide in scleroderma-related interstitial lung disease (SLS II): a randomised controlled, double-blind, parallel group trial. Lancet Respir Med 2016;4(9):708e19.

119. Tashkin DP, Elashoff R, Clements PJ, et al. Cyclophosphamide versus placebo in scleroderma lung disease. N Engl J Med 2006;354(25):2655e66.
120. Guber A, Epstein Shochet G, Kohn S, et al. Wrist-Sensor Pulse Oximeter Enables Prolonged Patient Monitoring in Chronic Lung Diseases. J Med Syst 2019;43:230.
121. Bernstein EJ, Jaafar S, Assassi S, et al. Performance characteristics of pulmonary function tests for the detection of interstitial lung disease in adults with early diffuse cutaneous systemic sclerosis. Arthritis Rheumatol Hoboken NJ 2020; 72(11):1892e6.
122. Volkmann ER. Natural history of systemic sclerosis-related interstitial lung disease: how to identify a progressive fibrosing phenotype. J Scleroderma Relat Disord 2020;5(2 Suppl):31e40.
123. Coghlan JG, Denton CP, Grünig E, et al. Evidence-based detection of pulmonary arterial hypertension in systemic sclerosis: the DETECT study. Ann Rheum Dis 2014;73(7):1340–9.
124. Steen VD, Graham G, Conte C, et al. Isolated diffusing capacity reduction in systemic sclerosis. Arthritis Rheum 1992;35(7):765e70.
125. Chung L, Domsic RT, Lingala B, et al. Survival and predictors of mortality in systemic sclerosis-associated pulmonary arterial hypertension: outcomes from the pulmonary hypertension assessment and recognition of outcomes in scleroderma registry. Arthritis Care Res 2014;66(3):489e95.
126. Rodríguez-Reyna TS, Morelos-Guzman M, Hern'andez-Reyes P, et al. Assessment of myocardial fibrosis and microvascular damage in systemic sclerosis by magnetic resonance imaging and coronary angiotomography. Rheumatol Oxf Engl 2015;54(4):647e54.
127. Rodríguez-Reyna TS, Rosales-Uvera SG, Kimura-Hayama E, et al. Myocardial fibrosis detected by magnetic resonance imaging, elevated U-CRP and higher mRSS are predictors of cardiovascular complications in systemic sclerosis (SSc) patients. Semin Arthritis Rheum 2019;49(2):273e8.
128. Lazzaroni MG, Airò P. Anti-RNA polymerase III antibodies in patients with suspected and definite systemic sclerosis: Why and how to screen. J Scleroderma Relat Disord 2018;3(3):214–20.
129. Jaafar S, Lescoat A, Huang S, et al. Clinical characteristics, visceral involvement, and mortality in at-risk or early diffuse systemic sclerosis: a longitudinal analysis of an observational prospective multicenter US cohort. Arthritis Res Ther 2021;23(1):170.
130. Penn H, Howie AJ, Kingdon EJ, et al. Scleroderma renal crisis: patient characteristics and long-term outcomes. QJM Aug 2007;100(8):485–94.
131. Butikofer L, Varisco PA, Distler O, et al. ACE inhibitors in SSc patients display a risk factor for scleroderma renal crisis-a EUSTAR analysis. Arthritis Res Ther 2020;22(1):59.
132. Hudson M, Baron M, Tatibouet S, et al. International Scleroderma Renal Crisis Study I. Exposure to ACE inhibitors prior to the onset of scleroderma renal crisis-results from the International Scleroderma Renal Crisis Survey. Semin Arthritis Rheum 2014;43(5):666–72.
133. Penn H, Denton CP. Diagnosis, management and prevention of scleroderma renal disease. Curr Opin Rheumatol 2008;20(6):692–6.
134. Steen VD, Medsger TA Jr. Case-control study of corticosteroids and other drugs that either precipitate or protect from the development of scleroderma renal crisis. Arthritis Rheum 1998;41(9):1613–9.

135. Nikpour M, Hissaria P, Byron J, et al. Prevalence, correlates and clinical useful-ness of antibodies to RNA polymerase III in systemic sclerosis: a cross-sectional analysis of data from an Australian cohort. Arthritis Res Ther 2011;13(6):R211.

136. Shapiro L, Saketkoo LA, Farrell J, et al. AB0712 Development of a "Renal Crisis Prevention Card" as an Education Tool to Improve Outcomes in High Risk Pa-tients with Systemic Sclerosis (SSC). Ann Rheum Dis 2015;74(Suppl 2):1136.

137. Lynch BM, Stern EP, Ong V, et al. UK Scleroderma Study Group (UKSSG) guide-lines on the diagnosis and management of scleroderma renal crisis. Clin Exp Rheumatol 2016;34(Suppl 100):106–9.

138. Bizjak M, Blazina S, Zajc Avramovic M, et al. Vaccination coverage in children with rheumatic diseases. Clin Exp Rheumatol 2020;38(1):164–70.

139. Assala M, Groh M, Blanche P, et al. Pneumococcal and influenza vaccination rates in patients treated with corticosteroids and/or immunosuppressive thera-pies for systemic autoimmune diseases: A cross-sectional study. Joint Bone Spine 2017;84(3):365–6.

140. Mouthon L, Mestre C, Berezne A, et al. Low influenza vaccination rate among patients with systemic sclerosis. Rheumatology 2010;49(3):600–6.

141. Wotton CJ, Goldacre MJ. Risk of invasive pneumococcal disease in people admitted to hospital with selected immune-mediated diseases: record linkage cohort analyses. J Epidemiol Community Health Dec 2012;66(12):1177–81.

142. Torrelo A, Suarez J, Colmenero I, et al. Deep morphea after vaccination in two young children. Pediatr Dermatol 2006;23(5):484–7.

143. Khaled A, Kharfi M, Zaouek A, et al. Postvaccination morphea profunda in a child. Pediatr Dermatol 2012;29(4):525–7.

144. Adler S, Krivine A, Weix J, et al. Protective effect of A/H1N1 vaccination in immune-mediated disease–a prospectively controlled vaccination study. Rheu-matology 2012;51(4):695–700.

145. Smith KG, Isbel NM, Catton MG, et al. Suppression of the humoral immune response by mycophenolate mofetil. Nephrol Dial Transplant 1998;13(1):160–4.

146. Md Yusof MY, Vital EM, McElvenny DM, et al. Predicting Severe Infection and Effects of Hypogammaglobulinemia During Therapy With Rituximab in Rheu-matic and Musculoskeletal Diseases. Arthritis Rheumatol 2019;71(11):1812–23.

147. Brinkman DM, Jol-van der Zijde CM, ten Dam MM, et al. Resetting the adaptive immune system after autologous stem cell transplantation: lessons from responses to vaccines. J Clin Immunol 2007;27(6):647–58.

148. Rubin LG, Levin MJ, Ljungman P, et al. 2013 IDSA clinical practice guideline for vaccination of the immunocompromised host. Clin Infect Dis 2014;58(3): e44–100.

149. CfDCa Prevention. General Best Practice Guidelines for Immunization: Best Practices Guidance of the Advisory Committee on Immunization Practices (ACIP). Available at: https://www.cdc.gov/vaccines/hcp/acip-recs/general-recs/immunocompetence.html. Updated November 18, 2020. Accessed December 23, 2020.

150. Singh JA, Furst DE, Bharat A, et al. 2012 update of the 2008 American College of Rheumatology recommendations for the use of disease-modifying antirheu-matic drugs and biologic agents in the treatment of rheumatoid arthritis. Arthritis Care Res 2012;64(5):625–39.

151. Singh JA, Saag KG, Bridges SL Jr, et al. 2015 American College of Rheuma-tology Guideline for the Treatment of Rheumatoid Arthritis. Arthritis Rheumatol 2016;68(1):1–26.

152. Martin M, Mougin C, Pretet JL, et al. Screening of human papillomavirus infection in women with systemic sclerosis. Clin Exp Rheumatol 2014;32(6 Suppl 86): 145–8.
153. Roumm AD, Medsger TA Jr. Cancer and systemic sclerosis. An epidemiologic study. Arthritis Rheum 1985;28(12):1336–40.
154. Derk CT, Rasheed M, Artlett CM, et al. A cohort study of cancer incidence in systemic sclerosis. J Rheumatol 2006;33(6):1113–6 [pii].
155. Elhai M, Meune C, Avouac J, et al. Trends in mortality in patients with systemic sclerosis over 40 years: a systematic review and meta-analysis of cohort studies. Rheumatology Jun 2012;51(6):1017–26.
156. Moinzadeh P, Fonseca C, Hellmich M, et al. Association of anti-RNA polymerase III autoantibodies and cancer in scleroderma. Arthritis Res Ther 2014;16(1):R53.
157. Morrisroe K, Hansen D, Huq M, et al. Incidence, Risk Factors, and Outcomes of Cancer in Systemic Sclerosis. Arthritis Care Res (Hoboken) 2020;72(11): 1625–35.
158. Shah AA, Xu G, Rosen A, et al. Brief Report: Anti-RNPC-3 Antibodies As a Marker of Cancer-Associated Scleroderma. Arthritis Rheumatol 2017;69(6): 1306–12.
159. Shah AA, Hummers LK, Casciola-Rosen L, et al. Examination of autoantibody status and clinical features associated with cancer risk and cancer-associated scleroderma. Arthritis Rheumatol 2015;67(4):1053–61.
160. Shah AA, Rosen A. Cancer and systemic sclerosis: novel insights into pathogenesis and clinical implications. Curr Opin Rheumatol 2011;23(6):530–5.
161. Ngian GS, Sahhar J, Proudman SM, et al. Prevalence of coronary heart disease and cardiovascular risk factors in a national cross-sectional cohort study of systemic sclerosis. Ann Rheum Dis 2012;71(12):1980–3.
162. Au K, Singh MK, Bodukam V, et al. Atherosclerosis in systemic sclerosis: a systematic review and meta-analysis. Arthritis Rheum 2011;63(7):2078–90.
163. Khurma V, Meyer C, Park GS, et al. A pilot study of subclinical coronary atherosclerosis in systemic sclerosis: coronary artery calcification in cases and controls. Arthritis Rheum Apr 15 2008;59(4):591–7.
164. Man A, Zhu Y, Zhang Y, et al. The risk of cardiovascular disease in systemic sclerosis: a population-based cohort study. Ann Rheum Dis 2013;72(7): 1188–93.
165. Omair MA, Pagnoux C, McDonald-Blumer H, et al. Low bone density in systemic sclerosis. A systematic review. J Rheumatol 2013;40(11):1881–90.
166. Bimal G, Sahhar J, Savanur M, et al. Screening rates and prevalence of osteoporosis in a real-world, Australian systemic sclerosis cohort. Int J Rheum Dis 2022;25(2):175–81.
167. Targownik LE, Lix LM, Metge CJ, et al. Use of proton pump inhibitors and risk of osteoporosis-related fractures. CMAJ (Can Med Assoc J) Aug 12 2008;179(4): 319–26.
168. Mattsson M, Sandqvist G, Hesselstrand R, et al. Validity and reliability of the Swedish version of the Self-Efficacy for Managing Chronic Disease scale for individuals with systemic sclerosis. Scand J Rheumatol 2022;51(2):110–9.
169. Sariyildiz MA, Batmaz I, Budulgan M, et al. Sleep quality in patients with systemic sclerosis: relationship between the clinical variables, depressive symptoms, functional status, and the quality of life. Rheumatol Int 2013;33(8): 1973–9.

Scleroderma Skin
How Is Treatment Best Guided by Data and Implemented in Clinical Practice?

Madelon C. Vonk, MD, PhD[a,*], Shervin Assassi, MD, MS[b],
Anna-Maria Hoffmann-Vold, MD, PhD[c]

KEYWORDS

- Systemic sclerosis • Skin involvement • Modified Rodnan skin score • Biomarkers
- Skin severity • Response to treatment

KEY POINTS

- Determination of systemic sclerosis (SSc) subsets and early trajectory of skin involvement provide insights into the general disease course, including other organ manifestation of SSc.
- The most used method of assessing skin involvement is the modified Rodnan skin score, which is a validated instrument but is hampered by high interobserver variability and requires extensive training.
- Studies with novel imaging modalities are needed to evaluate the content validity of examining a reduced number of body areas as a surrogate for the overall skin disease severity.
- Future predictive biomarker studies examine the predictive role of skin transcript profile after adjustment for clinical predictors such as baseline modified Rodnan Skin score, disease duration, and antibody profile.

NATURAL DISEASE COURSE OF SKIN INVOLVEMENT AND ITS IMPACT ON OUTCOME IN SYSTEMIC SCLEROSIS

Skin involvement is the hallmark and most clinically evident aspect of systemic sclerosis (SSc).[1] Even the disease name is derived from skin involvement; "scleroderma" originates from the Greek "sklerosis," meaning hardness, and "derma," meaning skin.[1] Physicians use the skin findings in SSc as key determinants of disease classification and diagnosis and for the classification of patients into SSc subtypes.[2] The 2 main subtypes of SSc are defined according to the extent of skin involvement: diffuse cutaneous (dcSSc) and limited cutaneous (lcSSc) SSc.[1] Skin hardening and thickening has a high impact on patient's perception of the disease and on quality of life.[3] Especially early

[a] Department of Rheumatology, Radboud University Nijmegen Medical Centre, Huispost 667, PO Box 9101, Nijmegen 6500HB, the Netherlands; [b] Division of Rheumatology, The University of Texas Health Science Center at Houston, 6431 Fannin, Houston, TX, USA; [c] Department of Rheumatology, Oslo University Hospital - Rikshospitalet, Pb 4950, Nydalen, Oslo 0424, Norway
* Corresponding author.
E-mail address: Madelon.Vonk@Radboudumc.nl

Rheum Dis Clin N Am 49 (2023) 249–262
https://doi.org/10.1016/j.rdc.2023.01.003
0889-857X/23/© 2023 Elsevier Inc. All rights reserved.

in the disease course, it causes pain, itching, and functional disability.[3,4] In clinical practice, dcSSc is the subtype considered as more severe, because it is characterized by rapid progression of the skin and a high prevalence of early internal organ involvement (including lung, heart, and renal involvement), which can be life-threatening.[5,6] The determination of SSc subsets as well as early trajectory of skin fibrosis provide insights into the general disease course, including other organ manifestation of SSc as well as for treatment approaches.[5] Therefore, all patients should be assessed for skin manifestation at time of diagnosis and regularly at each follow-up visit.[7]

Clinical Assessment of Skin Involvement

The skin is assessed by the modified Rodnan Skin score (mRSS). To assess the mRSS, skin thickness is evaluated by palpitation of 17 body parts and scored as 0 (normal skin), 1 (mild skin thickness), 2 (moderate skin thickness), and 3 (severe skin thickness)[8] (**Fig. 1**).[9] The method of global average of an area is advocated, as this method is more sensitive to change.[9] The interobserver and intraobserver mean within patient standard deviations was found to be 17.7 ($\pm$4.6) and 20.7 ($\pm$2.5), respectively.[8] The scleroderma lung studies I and II have provided patient-anchored evidence on the minimal clinically important difference of the mRSS, which was found to be 3 to 4 units for all patients and 5 units for patients with dcSSc.[10] For clinicians this minimal clinically important difference helps guide treatment. Furthermore, there exist exact definitions for stable, improving, and worsening skin, where skin worsening is defined as change in mRSS greater than or equal to 5 units or greater than or equal to 25% over a 12-month period.[11] Most skin worsening appears early in the disease

Modified Rodnan Skin Score (MRSS) Document

Subject ID: _____

Date of Examination: _____

	Right				Left			
Fingers	0☐	1☐	2☐	3☐	0☐	1☐	2☐	3☐
Hands	0☐	1☐	2☐	3☐	0☐	1☐	2☐	3☐
Forearms	0☐	1☐	2☐	3☐	0☐	1☐	2☐	3☐
Upper Arms	0☐	1☐	2☐	3☐	0☐	1☐	2☐	3☐
Face		0☐	1☐	2☐	3☐			
Anterior Chest		0☐	1☐	2☐	3☐			
Abdomen		0☐	1☐	2☐	3☐			
Thighs	0☐	1☐	2☐	3☐	0☐	1☐	2☐	3☐
Legs	0☐	1☐	2☐	3☐	0☐	1☐	2☐	3☐
Feet	0☐	1☐	2☐	3☐	0☐	1☐	2☐	3☐
Column Totals								
Total:								

Key: 0 – No Thickening   1 – Mild Thickening   2 – Moderate Thickening   3 – Severe Thickening

Notes:

Examiner:

Printed Name: _____

Signature: _____ Date: _____

Fig. 1. Modified Rodnan skin score. (*From* Khanna D, Furst DE, Clements PJ, Allanore Y, Baron M, Czirjak L, et al. Standardization of the modified Rodnan skin score for use in clinical trials of systemic sclerosis. J Scleroderma Relat Disord. 2017;2(1):11-8.)

course. After the initial worsening of the skin disease (as assessed by the mRSS) the skin involvement will generally plateau, followed by improvement with gradual softening and atrophying of the skin usually within 3 to 5 years after disease onset.[12] However, it has recently been shown in a European Scleroderma Trials and Research (EUSTAR) study assessing 1043 patients with SSc that also late skin worsening appears frequently in patients with SSc with approximately 20% after more than 5 years onset of the disease.[13] The reason for late skin fibrosis in that study was due to new worsening of skin disease or due to failure of skin to improve. Approximately two-thirds with new worsening or failure of skin to improve were antitopoisomerase I antibody (ATA)-positive patients.[13] Identifying progressive skin disease early in patients with SSc is important not only to manage patients symptoms adequately but also because skin worsening is associated with more severe disease and increased mortality.[14] The disease course of skin manifestation, especially skin worsening, also guides the development or worsening of other SSc-specific organ manifestations such as scleroderma renal crisis and interstitial lung disease (ILD).[15,16] On the other hand, improving skin has shown to be associated with less frequent ILD worsening, less new cardiac involvement, peripheral vascular and musculoskeletal involvement as well as a better outcome and improved survival.[17,18]

THE COMPOSITE RESPONSE INDEX IN DIFFUSE CUTANEOUS SYSTEMIC SCLEROSIS

Reliable outcome measures that are feasible and sensitive to change are prerequisite to assess disease progression and response to treatment in clinical trials and practice. Although mRSS is a validated outcome measure according to OMERACT criteria, it has a high interobserver variability and requires extensive training.[9] These limitations might have contributed to the fact that there are currently no approved medications for treatment of skin involvement in SSc. Furthermore, the complexity and heterogeneity of SSc necessitates a composite response measure that captures the different organ systems that are involved as well as patient-reported outcomes. The CRISS was developed for outcome assessment of early dcSSc in clinical trials and consists of the mRSS, forced vital capacity, the patient and physician global assessments, and Health Assessment Questionnaire disability index. Patients with significant worsening of renal or cardiopulmonary involvement are classified as not improved regardless of the score.[19] Although the CRISS has shown a good sensitivity and specificity, it is not suitable to use in patients with late dcSSc or lcSSc to date. Recently, the revised CRISS was published, which is easier to interpret and has reduced ceiling and floor effects.[20] The revised CRISS is currently chosen as the primary endpoint in medication clinical trials.

NONINVASIVE, OBJECTIVE METHODS FOR ASSESSMENT OF SKIN SEVERITY

There are ongoing studies to develop objective and accurate assessment for SSc skin involvement severity. Herein, the authors discuss 3 methods: durometry, ultrasonography, and optical coherence tomography/elastography.

Durometer is a handheld and easy-to-use device for measurement of skin hardness. In a multicenter study, durometry in 6 body sites (forearms, thighs, and legs/calves) showed excellent interobserver reliability in patients with early dcSSc. Moreover, the durometry score showed moderate correlation with the corresponding 6-site mRSS ($r = 0.52$), and change in durometer scores was also highly correlated with change in the 6-site mRSS ($r = 0.7$).[21] In a more recent study, durometry was performed in all 17 body sites assessed by mRSS in patients with dcSSc, showing again that durometry had an excellent interrater reliability. However, the correlation between durometry and mRSS was poor in the body areas in which skin was close to the underlying bone (fingers, face, and shins), as durometry cannot differentiate hardness in skin or the underlying bone tissue.[22]

Ultrasonography can assess SSc skin involvement in 3 domains: thickness, echogenicity, and elasticity. Variable approaches have been taken in measuring skin thickness with ultrasonography but ideally dermal thickness should be assessed because fibrosis in SSc primarily occurs in the dermal layer and epidermal thickness measurement seems to be less reliable.[23] However, discerning epidermal-dermal junction requires utilization of high frequency ultrasound. On the other hand, echogenicity can be influenced not only by dermal thickness but also the water content of skin, which can vary based on the stage of skin disease, starting with the edematous phase progressing to fibrotic and atrophic phases.[24] Lastly, ultrasound-based shear-wave elastography can measure skin stiffness/hardness using acoustic radiation force impulse imaging.[25] A recent systematic review on accuracy of the 3 aforementioned ultrasonography domains for skin assessment in SSc evaluated 46 studies. The interobserver reliability for skin thickness ranged from 0.65 to 0.94 (median intraclass correlation coefficient), and this measurement showed a low to moderate correlation with the local site–specific mRSS. Skin stiffness as assessed by shear-wave elastography showed moderate to strong correlation with the local site–specific mRSS. Several studies have shown that ultrasonography-based skin measurements change over time but there are no studies reporting sensitivity to change of these longitudinal assessments based on statistical analyses such as effect size of standardized response mean.[26] Few studies have examined the criterion validity of skin ultrasonography measurements by comparing them with histologic findings. A recent study reported all 3 ultrasonographical domains showed weak to moderate correlations with histologic skin thickness (correlation coefficient ranging from 0.32 to 0.48) in 10 patients with SSc, which was in a similar range as the correlation coefficient observed for site-specific skin score (0.51). Interestingly, although both ultrasonographic skin thickness and elastography showed strong significant correlations with histologic dermal collagen content, echogenicity did show any significant correlations.[27] Few studies have reported on the time requirement for performing ultrasonographic assessment of 17 body areas; in 2 reports the time for assessment of skin thickness was 20 to 25 minutes.[23,28] There are no reports on reliability and feasibility of SSc skin assessment by ultrasonography in large, multicenter clinical trials.

Optical coherence imaging has substantially higher spatial resolution than ultrasonography and has been widely used in ophthalmology as a noninvasive, high-resolution imaging technique.[29] Three studies have examined the utility of optical coherence tomography in SSc, showing that SSc skin can be differentiated from healthy controls with this imaging technique.[30–32] Moreover, optical coherence elastography and tomography measurements outperformed site-specific skin scoring in their correlation with histologic dermal thickness (taken from forearm area) in a small pilot study.[32] However, the currently used optical coherence tomography technology has limited imaging depth of 0.3 mm, which usually corresponds to papillary dermal layer; an improved optical coherence technology will be needed to assess the deeper dermal layers (reticular dermis), which can be prominently affected in SSc.[33]

In general, additional multicenter, longitudinal studies are needed to establish the accuracy and feasibility of these novel technologies as skin outcome measurement tools in SSc. Future studies are also needed to evaluate the content validity of examining a reduced number of body areas instead of the 17 body areas used for mRSS as a surrogate for the overall skin disease severity. If valid, limiting the assessed body areas can make the utilization of these objective imaging techniques more feasible in clinical trials and practice.

Clinical Markers for Predicting and Tracking Skin Involvement Severity

Assessing skin involvement at diagnosis and every study visit is important to the patient to predict the disease course, the involvement of other organ manifestations, and for inclusion in clinical trials.[7,34] In the past, many randomized clinical trials applying the mRSS as endpoint have failed to show treatment efficacy on the skin,[35–38] and this has led to an extensive search for clinical markers, which can lead to enrichment for skin worsening.[39] There are now several clinical markers that can be helpful in predicting skin worsening. First, the autoantibody profile is helpful.[40] It has long been known that ATA is associated with more severe and more progressive skin disease in patients with dcSSc.[40] Also anti-RNA polymerase III antibodies (ARA) have been associated with severe and progressive skin disease in dcSSc, especially in early disease phases.[15] In clinical practice and also for inclusion into clinical trials, it is important to assess the extent of skin involvement and the SSc subtypes in association with antibodies, as ATA- and ARA-positive dcSSc patients will behave differently and show different disease courses. Patients with ARA-positive dcSSc have shown to reach the highest skin scores and peak earlier compared with patients with ATA-positive dcSSc.[41] Although most predictors for skin and skin subsets with organ involvement and progression have been assessed in patients with dcSSc, a recent EUSTAR study showed that also in patients with lcSSc, ATA was associated with progressive ILD.[42] It was not mentioned whether these patients also showed progressive skin disease, which is more unlikely, as this is rare in lcSSc. As for other organ manifestations in SSc, a combination of risk factors for progressive skin disease has shown to be most efficacious. An analysis again from the EUSTAR database showed that skin severity and skin progression was more frequent, if patients had low mRSS at baseline, short disease duration, and joint synovitis.[11] In contrast, patients with high baseline mRSS and absence of friction rubs were likely to improve in their skin.[43]

Disease duration has been shown to be a strong predictor of skin progression, but the definition of short has varied across the published studies. In the Pittsburgh cohort a disease duration of less than 18 months was the best disease duration to predict skin worsening and the investigators suggested this cut-off for clinical trials.[44] Other studies have focused on the combination of disease duration and the mRSS for predicting skin worsening. In a Japanese multicenter prospective cohort study a disease duration less than 12 months in the presence of an mRSS of less than or equal to 19 predicted progression.[45] In the Genetics versus Environment in Scleroderma Outcomes Study (GENISOS) cohort, the mRSS predictive of progression was less than or equal to 27 with a longer disease duration.[39] Interestingly, and again highlighting the role of the skin as a mirror for other organ involvement, the combination of a disease duration less than or equal to 60 months from first non-Raynaud's symptom, mRSS 10 to 35, and signs of active disease (with C-reactive protein ≥ 6 mg/L; erythrocyte sedimentation rate ≥ 28 mm/h; platelets $\geq 330 \times 109$/L) did not lead to a significant change in the mRSS as the primary endpoint in the FocuSSced trial but to a major enrichment for ILD progressors with forced vital capacity as the key secondary endpoint.[36] To overcome the hurdles of using clinical markers for severe and progressive skin disease, molecular biomarkers for predicting and tracking skin involvement severity have been assessed.

Molecular Biomarkers for Predicting and Tracking Skin Involvement Severity

Several global gene expression studies have shown that SSc skin has a distinct transcript profile, consisting of inflammatory and fibrotic signatures that can co-exist in the same skin sample.[46,47] Interestingly, a subgroup of SSc skin samples, mostly patients with lcSSc and dcSSc and longer disease duration, show a "normal-like" gene expression profile that resembles the skin transcript profile of healthy controls.[47–49] There is increasing evidence that SSc skin transcript profile in a given patient can change overtime and lose its fibroinflammatory profile, which is consistent with the observed natural history of SSc skin involvement, which normalizes over time. A recent study on longitudinal global gene expression of 105 patients with SSc showed that immune cell and fibroblast signatures decreased over time, and the overall SSc gene expression profile trended toward normalization in patients with early dcSSc[50] (Fig. 2). Although it might be possible that the trend toward normalization is partially driven by immunosuppressive treatment in this study, immune cell and fibroblast signatures were not significantly lower in patients taking immunosuppressive agents.[50] Moreover, a pathway analysis based on unsupervised machine learning approach indicated that SSc skin samples assigned to inflammatory cluster tended to switch to a more fibrotic cluster after 24 weeks in the placebo arm of a randomized controlled trial (RCT) of tocilizumab in which a background immunosuppressive treatment was not permitted.[51] There are also conflicting data on predictive significance of baseline SSc skin gene expression profile for the future course of mRSS. A 5-gene transcript signature consisting of genes associated with macrophage activation (CD14, IL13RA1) and transforming growth factor β activation (SERPINE1, CTGF, OSMR) was reported to predict the course of mRSS in patients with dcSSc in the placebo arm of a clinical trial, as well as an independent cohort with heterogenous treatment regimens.[52] However, neither these 5 transcripts nor cell-type signatures were predictive of future mRSS course in early patients with dcSSc enrolled in the Prospective Registry of Early Systemic Sclerosis (PRESS) cohort. However, immune cell type signatures in SSc skin in the PRESS cohort correlated with the preceding skin thickness progression rate, indicating the gene expression profile of this prominently affected end-organ reflected better the preceding rate of disease progression than the future

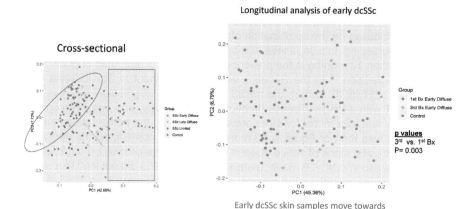

Early dcSSc skin samples move towards
normalization over time

Fig. 2. Principal component analysis of differentially expressed genes in SSc versus healthy control comparison. Left panel depicts cross-sectional comparison of early diffuse SSc, late diffuse SSc, limited SSc, and healthy control skin. Right panel shows the changes in the skin gene expression profile of early diffuse SSc samples over time with their trend to move toward healthy control skin samples. (*Modified from* Skaug B, Lyons MA, Swindell WR, Salazar GA, Wu M, Tran TM, et al. Large-scale analysis of longitudinal skin gene expression in systemic sclerosis reveals relationships of immune cell and fibroblast activity with skin thickness and a trend towards normalisation over time. Ann Rheum Dis. 2022;81(4):516-23.)

mRSS course.[49] There is some emerging evidence indicating that baseline skin transcript profile can predict response to immunosuppression. Using a machine learning approach, SSc skin samples were categorized into inflammatory, fibroproliferative, and normal-like intrinsic categories.[53] In a follow-up study based on a phase II RCT, patients with inflammatory, and normal-like base skin gene expression profile were more likely to respond to this immunosuppressive agent than those with fibroproliferative transcript signature.[54]

In addition to correlation of skin gene expression profile with disease duration, several studies have indicated that skin transcript profile highly correlates with concurrent local and overall skin score.[47,55] A recent study of patients with lcSSc and dcSSc indicated that baseline global gene expression profile in this mixed patient population had predictive significance for the serially obtained mRSS levels, in which high baseline immune cell and fibroblast signatures predicted higher mRSS over time. However, these signatures were not predictive of mRSS course after adjustment for baseline mRSS levels. Thus, it is important that future predictive biomarker studies examine the predictive role of skin transcript profile after adjustment for clinical predictors such as baseline mRSS, disease duration, and antibody profile (especially ARA positivity).

Molecular Biomarkers for Predicting Response to Treatment

Considering issues arising from limited reliability of mRSS in multicenter clinical trial, dynamic biomarkers that track accurately skin thickness severity represent an unmet clinical need, and as such, the role of skin transcript levels as dynamic surrogate biomarkers for assessment of response to treatment has been also investigated. Transforming growth factor beta (TGF-β) is a profibrotic factor that is implicated to play an important role in skin fibrosis.[56] Thrombospondin-1 (THBS1) and cartilage oligomeric protein (COMP) are TGF-β–regulated genes expressed by SSc dermal fibroblasts.[57] THBS1 and COMP in forearm skin biopsies correlated with mRSS cross-sectionally and longitudinally in an observational cohort and in an early phase II clinical trial.[58,59] In this trial, THBS1 and COMP skin expression levels declined after treatment and correlated with the decline in mRSS, supporting the notion that these 2-gene biomarkers are sensitive to change.[59] These biomarkers have also been used in other trials showing no movement, suggesting the observed dynamic changes in the transcript levels in this trial were specific to TGF-β blockade or the investigated medications in the other trials were ineffective.[60,61] This exemplifies the fact that longitudinal changes in the skin transcripts belonging to the targeted pathways are feasible and easily obtainable tools for verification of target engagement in clinical trials but there are currently no skin gene expression–based surrogate biomarkers that have been validated across several clinical trials.

Serum/plasma is the ideal source for biomarker development, as serial blood samples can be obtained during routine clinical practice. Recent studies have indicated that serum proteins reflect more accurately the molecular dysregulations at the end-organ level such as skin rather the biological processes in the surrounding peripheral blood cells in SSc.[62,63] Discovery of serum/plasma based surrogate biomarkers for skin severity is complicated by the fact that SSc is a multicompartment disease in which fibrosis in affected organs such as skin and lung can have a divergent course over time. Therefore, it is important that the discovered biomarkers specifically track skin severity. A study, using a proteomic platform that enabled simultaneous measurement of 1129 serum proteins in patients with dcSSc and controls, identified serum proteins that were differentially expressed between SSc and controls and correlated with concurrent mRSS. Two serum proteins, ST2 and Spondin-1, best described the longitudinal change in mRSS in linear mixed effect models. Using the generated coefficients from the discovery cohort, these 2 serum proteins showed moderate correlation with mRSS in 3 independent cohorts with Pearson's correlation ranging from 0.33 to 0.44.[64]

Treatment of Skin Involvement in Systemic Sclerosis

Although there is currently no cure for SSc, several immunomodulating therapies have shown efficacy in randomized RCTs regarding the skin involvement as assessed by mRSS. Methotrexate has shown in 2 RCT to improve skin scores in early dcSSc.[65,66] Cyclophosphamide has shown to improve skin in SSc in one RCT, and mycophenolate has shown to be noninferior to cyclophosphamide in an RCT as well.[67,68] Furthermore, 2 RCTs and a long-term follow-up study have shown the beneficial effect of hematopoietic stem cell transplantation in well-selected patients with early dcSSc.[69–71] In the last years, several RCTs were performed in SSc, mostly in early dcSSc, which are summarized in **Table 1**. Of those studies, the proof-of-concept study with romilkimab showed promising results warranting further investigation.[72]

DISCUSSION

As changes in skin involvement in patients with SSc, both improvement and progression are related to organ involvement and thus prognosis, an easily accessible, reliable measurement that is sensitive to change is necessary. However, mRSS has its pitfalls as primary endpoint in clinical trials and is not sufficient to use as sole efficacy parameter in clinical practice, as it does not capture all aspects of this complex and heterogenous disease. On one hand, research is focusing on composite endpoints including skin, lungs, patient-reported outcomes, and global impression of the patients, with promising results. Unfortunately, the first RCT with the CRISS as primary endpoint was found to be negative and which leaded among other reasons to the revised CRISS. On the other hand, dynamic biomarkers that track disease activity and skin severity represent an unmet clinical need and could facilitate drug approvals for this disease manifestation as well as guidance for clinicians. These biomarkers should be investigated after adjustment for clinical predictors such as antibody profile, disease duration, and baseline mRSS. As for treatment, no cure for SSc is available to date, but several treatment options are evidence based available for skin involvement.

Table 1
Published phase II/III randomized controlled trials for systemic sclerosis from 2019 onward

Compound	Phase	No of Subjects	Endpoint	Result
Nintedanib[73]	III	576	Secondary: mRSS wk 52	Placebo: −1.96 Nintedanib: −2.17 ($P = .58$)
Riociguat[38]	II	109	Primary: mRSS wk 52	Placebo: −0.77 Riociguat: −2.09 ($P = .08$)
Abatacept[54]	II	88	Primary: mRSS wk 52	Placebo: −4.49 Abatacept: −6.24 ($P = .28$)
Tocilizumab[36]	III	210	Primary: mRSS wk 48	Placebo: −4.41 Tocilizumab: −6.14 ($P = .10$)
Lenabasum[74]	II	363	Secondary mRSS wk 52	Placebo: −8.1 Lenabasum: −6.7
Romilkimab[72]	II	97	Primary: mRSS wk 24	Placebo −2.45 Romilkimab − 4.76 ($P = .03$)

The most striking reduction of mRSS and survival benefit is found with treatment with hematopoietic stem cell transplantation, which is unfortunately only available for a small minority of the patients. Therefore, research in the scleroderma community should focus on 2 goals: first to find a reliable disease activity measure and second to find a biomarker of prognosis for patients with both lcSSc and dcSSc, with early disease and longstanding disease, which is sensitive to change and easily assessable. In the current era, in which international collaboration is booming, patient engagement in research is common, and pharmaceutical companies are interested in pharmacologic trials in SSc that could foster researchers to reach those goals.

CLINICS CARE POINTS

- Identifying progression of skin involvement is important as it is associated with more severe disease and increased mortality.
- Currently, the revised CRISS is chosen as the primary endpoint in medication clinical trials.
- To date, multicenter, longitudinal studies are needed to establish the accuracy and feasibility of novel techniques to assess skin involvement in SSc such as durometry, ultrasonography and optical coherence imaging.
- Clinical markers for predicting skin progression are auto antibodie status, baseline mRSS, joint synovitis, disease duration and combinations of these factors. Future predictive biomarkers such as the skin transcript profile should be combined with theses clinical predictors.

DISCLOSURE

M.C. Vonk has received research funding and/or consulting fees from Boehringer Ingelheim, Bristol-Myers Squibb, Corbus, Ferrer, Galapagos, GSK, Janssen, Merk Sharp & Dohme, Novartis, and Roche. S. Assassi has received research funding and/or consulting fees from Boehringer Ingelheim, Janssen, Novartis, CSL Behring, Astra Zeneca, and Abbvie. A-M. Hoffmann-Vold has received research funding and/or consulting fees and/or other remuneration from Actelion, Arxx, Bayer, Boehringer Ingelheim, Janssen, Lilly, Medscape, Merck Sharp & Dohme, and Roche.

REFERENCES

1. Denton CP, Khanna D. Systemic sclerosis. Lancet 2017;390(10103):1685–99.
2. van den Hoogen F, Khanna D, Fransen J, et al. Classification criteria for systemic sclerosis: an American college of rheumatology/European league against rheumatism collaborative initiative. Ann Rheum Dis 2013;72(11):1747–55.
3. Frantz C, Avouac J, Distler O, et al. Impaired quality of life in systemic sclerosis and patient perception of the disease: A large international survey. Semin Arthritis Rheum 2016;46(1):115–23.
4. Herrick AL, Pan X, Peytrignet S, et al. Treatment outcome in early diffuse cutaneous systemic sclerosis: the European Scleroderma Observational Study (ESOS). Ann Rheum Dis 2017;76(7):1207–18.
5. Steen VMTJ. Severe organ involvement in systemic sclerosis with diffus scleroderma. Arthritis Rheum 2000;43(11):2437–44.
6. Elhai M, Meune C, Boubaya M, et al. Mapping and predicting mortality from systemic sclerosis. Ann Rheum Dis 2017;76(11):1897–905.

7. Hoffmann-Vold AM, Distler O, Murray B, et al. Setting the international standard for longitudinal follow-up of patients with systemic sclerosis: a Delphi-based expert consensus on core clinical features. RMD Open 2019;5(1):e000826.

8. Clements P, Lachenbruch P, Siebold J, et al. Inter and Intraobserver Variability of Total Skin Thickness Score (Modified Rodnan Tss) in Systemic-Sclerosis. J Rheumatol 1995;22(7):1281–5.

9. Khanna D, Furst DE, Clements PJ, et al. Standardization of the modified Rodnan skin score for use in clinical trials of systemic sclerosis. J Scleroderma Relat Disord 2017;2(1):11–8.

10. Khanna D, Clements PJ, Volkmann ER, et al. Minimal Clinically Important Differences for the Modified Rodnan Skin Score: Results from the Scleroderma Lung Studies (SLS-I and SLS-II). Arthritis Res Ther 2019;21(1):23.

11. Maurer B, Graf N, Michel BA, et al. Prediction of worsening of skin fibrosis in patients with diffuse cutaneous systemic sclerosis using the EUSTAR database. Ann Rheum Dis 2015;74(6):1124–31.

12. Amjadi S, Maranian P, Furst DE, et al. Course of the modified Rodnan skin thickness score in systemic sclerosis clinical trials: Analysis of three large multicenter, double-blind, randomized controlled trials. Arthritis Rheum 2009;60(8):2490–8.

13. Hughes M, Huang S, Alegre-Sancho JJ, et al. Late Skin Fibrosis in Systemic Sclerosis: A Study from the EUSTAR Cohort. Rheumatology (Oxford) 2023;62(SI): SI54–63.

14. Ledoult E, Launay D, Béhal H, et al. Early trajectories of skin thickening are associated with severity and mortality in systemic sclerosis. Arthritis Res Ther 2020; 22(1):30.

15. Domsic RT, Rodriguez-Reyna T, Lucas M, et al. Skin thickness progression rate: a predictor of mortality and early internal organ involvement in diffuse scleroderma. Ann Rheum Dis 2011;70(1):104–9.

16. Wu W, Jordan S, Graf N, et al. Progressive skin fibrosis is associated with a decline in lung function and worse survival in patients with diffuse cutaneous systemic sclerosis in the European Scleroderma Trials and Research (EUSTAR) cohort. Ann Rheum Dis 2019;78(5):648–56.

17. Steen VD, Medsger TA. Improvement in skin thickening in systemic sclerosis associated with improved survival. Arthritis Rheum 2001;44(12):2828–35.

18. Nevskaya T, Zheng B, Baxter CA, et al. Skin improvement is a surrogate for favourable changes in other organ systems in early diffuse cutaneous systemic sclerosis. Rheumatology 2020;59(7):1715–24.

19. Khanna D, Berrocal VJ, Giannini EH, et al. The American College of Rheumatology Provisional Composite Response Index for Clinical Trials in Early Diffuse Cutaneous Systemic Sclerosis. Arthritis Rheum 2016;68(2):299–311.

20. Khanna D, Huang S, Lin CJF, et al. New composite endpoint in early diffuse cutaneous systemic sclerosis: revisiting the provisional American College of Rheumatology Composite Response Index in Systemic Sclerosis. Ann Rheum Dis 2021; 80(5):641–50.

21. Merkel PA, Silliman NP, Denton CP, et al. Validity, reliability, and feasibility of durometer measurements of scleroderma skin disease in a multicenter treatment trial. Arthritis Rheum 2008;59(5):699–705.

22. de Oliveira MFC, Leopoldo VC, Pereira KRC, et al. Durometry as an alternative tool to the modified Rodnan's skin score in the assessment of diffuse systemic sclerosis patients: a cross-sectional study. Adv Rheumatol 2020;60(1):48.

23. Moore TL, Lunt M, McManus B, et al. Seventeen-point dermal ultrasound scoring system–a reliable measure of skin thickness in patients with systemic sclerosis. Rheumatology 2003;42(12):1559–63.
24. Hesselstrand R, Scheja A, Wildt M, et al. High-frequency ultrasound of skin involvement in systemic sclerosis reflects oedema, extension and severity in early disease. Rheumatology 2008;47(1):84–7.
25. Hou Y, Zhu QL, Liu H, et al. A preliminary study of acoustic radiation force impulse quantification for the assessment of skin in diffuse cutaneous systemic sclerosis. J Rheumatol 2015;42(3):449–55.
26. Santiago T, Santos E, Ruaro B, et al. Ultrasound and elastography in the assessment of skin involvement in systemic sclerosis: A systematic literature review focusing on validation and standardization - WSF Skin Ultrasound Group. Semin Arthritis Rheum 2022;52:151954.
27. Flower VA, Barratt SL, Hart DJ, et al. High frequency ultrasound assessment of systemic sclerosis skin involvement: intra-observer repeatability and relationship with clinician assessment and dermal collagen content. J Rheumatol 2020;48(6):867–76.
28. Sulli A, Ruaro B, Smith V, et al. Subclinical dermal involvement is detectable by high frequency ultrasound even in patients with limited cutaneous systemic sclerosis. Arthritis Res Ther 2017;19(1):61.
29. Ly A, Phu J, Katalinic P, et al. An evidence-based approach to the routine use of optical coherence tomography. Clin Exp Optom 2019;102(3):242–59.
30. Pires NSM, Dantas AT, Duarte A, et al. Optical coherence tomography as a method for quantitative skin evaluation in systemic sclerosis. Ann Rheum Dis 2018;77(3):465–6.
31. Abignano G, Aydin SZ, Castillo-Gallego C, et al. Virtual skin biopsy by optical coherence tomography: the first quantitative imaging biomarker for scleroderma. Ann Rheum Dis 2013;72(11):1845–51.
32. Liu CH, Assassi S, Theodore S, et al. Translational optical coherence elastography for assessment of systemic sclerosis. J Biophotonics 2019;12(12). e201900236.
33. Fleischmajer R, Gay S, Meigel WN, et al. Collagen in the cellular and fibrotic stages of scleroderma. Arthritis Rheum 1978;21(4):418–28.
34. Herrick AL, Assassi S, Denton CP. Skin involvement in early diffuse cutaneous systemic sclerosis: an unmet clinical need. Nat Rev Rheumatol 2022;18(5):276–85.
35. Khanna D, Spino C, Johnson S, et al. Abatacept in Early Diffuse Cutaneous Systemic Sclerosis: Results of a Phase II Investigator-Initiated, Multicenter, Double-Blind, Randomized, Placebo-Controlled Trial. Arthritis Rheum 2020;72(1):125–36.
36. Khanna D, Lin CJF, Furst DE, et al. Tocilizumab in systemic sclerosis: a randomised, double-blind, placebo-controlled, phase 3 trial. Lancet Respir Med 2020;8(10):963–74.
37. Distler O, Highland KB, Gahlemann M, et al. Nintedanib for Systemic Sclerosis-Associated Interstitial Lung Disease. N Engl J Med 2019;380(26):2518–28.
38. Khanna D, Allanore Y, Denton CP, et al. Riociguat in patients with early diffuse cutaneous systemic sclerosis (RISE-SSc): randomised, double-blind, placebo-controlled multicentre trial. Ann Rheum Dis 2020;79(5):618–25.
39. Mihai C, Dobrota R, Assassi S, et al. Enrichment Strategy for Systemic Sclerosis Clinical Trials Targeting Skin Fibrosis: A Prospective, Multiethnic Cohort Study. ACR Open Rheumatology 2020;2(8):496–502.

40. Steen VD. Autoantibodies in systemic sclerosis. Semin Arthritis Rheum 2005; 35(1):35–42.
41. Herrick AL, Peytrignet S, Lunt M, et al. Patterns and predictors of skin score change in early diffuse systemic sclerosis from the European Scleroderma Observational Study. Ann Rheum Dis 2018;77(4):563–70.
42. Zanatta E, Huscher D, Ortolan A, et al. Phenotype of limited cutaneous systemic sclerosis patients with positive anti-topoisomerase I antibodies: data from the EUSTAR cohort. Rheumatology 2022;61(12):4786–96.
43. Dobrota R, Maurer B, Graf N, et al. Prediction of improvement in skin fibrosis in diffuse cutaneous systemic sclerosis: a EUSTAR analysis. Ann Rheum Dis 2016;75(10):1743–8.
44. Domsic RT, Gao S, Laffoon M, et al. Defining the optimal disease duration of early diffuse systemic sclerosis for clinical trial design. Rheumatology 2021;60(10):4662–70.
45. Kuwana M, Hasegawa M, Fukue R, et al. Initial predictors of skin thickness progression in patients with diffuse cutaneous systemic sclerosis: Results from a multicentre prospective cohort in Japan. Mod Rheumatol 2021;31(2):386–93.
46. Whitfield ML, Finlay DR, Murray JI, et al. Systemic and cell type-specific gene expression patterns in scleroderma skin. Proc Natl Acad Sci U S A 2003; 100(21):12319–24.
47. Assassi S, Swindell WR, Wu M, et al. Dissecting the heterogeneity of skin gene expression patterns in systemic sclerosis. Arthritis Rheum 2015;67(11):3016–26.
48. Asano Y, Ihn H, Yamane K, et al. Clinical significance of surfactant protein D as a serum marker for evaluating pulmonary fibrosis in patients with systemic sclerosis. Arthritis Rheum 2001;44(6):1363–9.
49. Skaug B, Khanna D, Swindell WR, et al. Global skin gene expression analysis of early diffuse cutaneous systemic sclerosis shows a prominent innate and adaptive inflammatory profile. Ann Rheum Dis 2020;79(3):379–86.
50. Skaug B, Lyons MA, Swindell WR, et al. Large-scale analysis of longitudinal skin gene expression in systemic sclerosis reveals relationships of immune cell and fibroblast activity with skin thickness and a trend towards normalisation over time. Ann Rheum Dis 2022;81(4):516–23.
51. Moon SJ, Bae JM, Park KS, et al. Compendium of skin molecular signatures identifies key pathological features associated with fibrosis in systemic sclerosis. Ann Rheum Dis 2019;78(6):817–25.
52. Stifano G, Sornasse T, Rice LM, et al. Skin Gene Expression Is Prognostic for the Trajectory of Skin Disease in Patients With Diffuse Cutaneous Systemic Sclerosis. Arthritis Rheum 2018;70(6):912–9.
53. Franks JM, Martyanov V, Cai G, et al. A Machine Learning Classifier for Assigning Individual Patients with Systemic Sclerosis to Intrinsic Molecular Subsets. Arthritis Rheum 2019;71(10):1701–10.
54. Khanna D, Spino C, Johnson S, et al. Abatacept in Early Diffuse Cutaneous Systemic Sclerosis: Results of a Phase II Investigator-Initiated, Multicenter, Double-Blind, Randomized, Placebo-Controlled Trial. Arthritis Rheum 2020;72(1):125–36.
55. Rice LM, Ziemek J, Stratton EA, et al. A Longitudinal Biomarker for the Extent of Skin Disease in Patients with Diffuse Cutaneous Systemic Sclerosis. Arthritis Rheum 2015;67(11):3004–15.
56. Lafyatis R. Transforming growth factor beta–at the centre of systemic sclerosis. Nat Rev Rheumatol 2014;10(12):706–19.

57. Tabib T, Huang M, Morse N, et al. Myofibroblast transcriptome indicates SFRP2(hi) fibroblast progenitors in systemic sclerosis skin. Nat Commun 2021; 12(1):4384.

58. Farina G, Lafyatis D, Lemaire R, et al. A four-gene biomarker predicts skin disease in patients with diffuse cutaneous systemic sclerosis. Arthritis Rheum 2010;62(2):580–8.

59. Rice LM, Padilla CM, McLaughlin SR, et al. Fresolimumab treatment decreases biomarkers and improves clinical symptoms in systemic sclerosis patients. J Clin Invest 2015;125(7):2795–807.

60. Mantero JC, Kishore N, Ziemek J, et al. Randomised, double-blind, placebo-controlled trial of IL1-trap, rilonacept, in systemic sclerosis. A phase I/II biomarker trial. Clin Exp Rheumatol 2018;36(Suppl 113):146–9.

61. Lafyatis R, Mantero JC, Gordon J, et al. Inhibition of beta-Catenin Signaling in the Skin Rescues Cutaneous Adipogenesis in Systemic Sclerosis: A Randomized, Double-Blind, Placebo-Controlled Trial of C-82. J Invest Dermatol 2017;137(12): 2473–83.

62. Farutin V, Kurtagic E, Pradines JR, et al. Multiomic study of skin, peripheral blood, and serum: is serum proteome a reflection of disease process at the end-organ level in systemic sclerosis? Arthritis Res Ther 2021;23(1):259.

63. Bellocchi C, Ying J, Goldmuntz EA, et al. Large-scale characterization of systemic sclerosis serum protein profile: Comparison to peripheral blood cell transcriptome and correlations with skin/lung fibrosis. Arthritis Rheum 2020;73(4): 660–70.

64. Rice LM, Mantero JC, Stifano G, et al. A Proteome-Derived Longitudinal Pharmacodynamic Biomarker for Diffuse Systemic Sclerosis Skin. J Invest Dermatol 2017;137(1):62–70.

65. VandenHoogen FHJ, Boerbooms AMT, Swaak AJG, et al. Comparison of methotrexate with placebo in the treatment of systemic sclerosis: A 24 week randomized double-blind trial, followed by a 24 week observational trial. Br J Rheumatol 1996;35(4):364–72.

66. Pope JE, Bellamy N, Seibold JR, et al. A randomized, controlled trial of methotrexate versus placebo in early diffuse scleroderma. Arthritis Rheum 2001; 44(6):1351–8.

67. Tashkin DP, Elashoff R, Clements PJ, et al. Effects of 1-year treatment with cyclophosphamide on outcomes at 2 years in scleroderma lung disease2. Am J Respir Crit Care Med 2007;176(10):1026–34.

68. Tashkin DP, Roth MD, Clements PJ, et al. Mycophenolate mofetil versus oral cyclophosphamide in scleroderma-related interstitial lung disease (SLS II): a randomised controlled, double-blind, parallel group trial. Lancet Respir Med 2016;4(9):708–19.

69. van Laar JM, Farge D, Sont JK, et al. Autologous hematopoietic stem cell transplantation vs intravenous pulse cyclophosphamide in diffuse cutaneous systemic sclerosis: a randomized clinical trial. JAMA 2014;311(24):2490–8.

70. Sullivan KM, Goldmuntz EA, Keyes-Elstein L, et al. Myeloablative Autologous Stem-Cell Transplantation for Severe Scleroderma. N Engl J Med 2018;378(1): 35–47.

71. van Bijnen S, de Vries-Bouwstra J, van den Ende CH, et al. Predictive factors for treatment-related mortality and major adverse events after autologous haematopoietic stem cell transplantation for systemic sclerosis: results of a long-term follow-up multicentre study. Ann Rheum Dis 2020;79(8):1084–9.

72. Allanore Y, Wung P, Soubrane C, et al. A randomised, double-blind, placebo-controlled, 24-week, phase II, proof-of-concept study of romilkimab (SAR156597) in early diffuse cutaneous systemic sclerosis. Ann Rheum Dis 2020;79(12):1600–7.
73. Distler O, Gahlemann M, Maher TM. Nintedanib for Systemic Sclerosis-Associated Interstitial Lung Disease. N Engl J Med 2019;381(16):1596–7.
74. Spiera R, Hummers L, Chung L, et al. Safety and Efficacy of Lenabasum in a Phase II, Randomized, Placebo-Controlled Trial in Adults With Systemic Sclerosis. Arthritis Rheum 2020;72(8):1350–60.

Treatment of Vascular Complications in Systemic Sclerosis

What Is the Best Approach to Diagnosis and Management of Renal Crisis and Digital Ulcers?

Michael Hughes, BSc (Hons), MBBS, MSc, MRCP (UK) (Rheumatology), PhD[a,b,]*,
Ariane L. Herrick, MD, FRCP[b,c], Marie Hudson, MD, MPH, FRCPC[d,e,f]

KEYWORDS

- Systemic sclerosis • Scleroderma • Scleroderma renal crisis • Digital ulcers
- Vasculopathy

KEY POINTS

- Vascular disease is a cardinal feature of the complex pathobiology of SSc.
- SSc-related vasculopathy is associated with significant disease-related morbidity and mortality.
- There have been major advancements in the understanding and treatment of vasculopathy in SSc, including scleroderma renal crisis and digital ulcers.
- A multidisciplinary approach is required for the management of vasculopathy in SSc.
- There remain a number of unmet needs to optimise the therapeutic approach for scleroderma renal crisis and digital ulcers in SSc.

INTRODUCTION

Vascular disease is a cardinal feature within the complex pathobiology of systemic sclerosis (SSc).[1–3] Scleroderma renal crisis (SRC) and digital ulcers (DUs) share common pathophysiological processes, for example, fibroproliferative vasculopathy (**Figs.**

[a] Department of Rheumatology, Tameside and Glossop Integrated Care NHS Foundation Trust, Ashton-under-Lyne, UK; [b] Division of Musculoskeletal and Dermatological Sciences, The University of Manchester, Manchester, UK; [c] Northern Care Alliance NHS Foundation Trust, Manchester Academic Health Science Centre, Manchester, UK; [d] Department of Medicine, McGill University, Canada; [e] Division of Rheumatology, Jewish General Hospital, Canada; [f] Lady Davis Institute for Medical Research, Jewish General Hospital, Montreal, Quebec, Canada
* Corresponding author. Department of Rheumatology, Salford Care Organisation, Northern Care Alliance NHS Foundation Trust, Salford, M6 8HD, UK.
E-mail address: Michael.hughes-6@postgrad.manchester.ac.uk

Rheum Dis Clin N Am 49 (2023) 263–277
https://doi.org/10.1016/j.rdc.2023.01.004
0889-857X/23/© 2023 Elsevier Inc. All rights reserved.

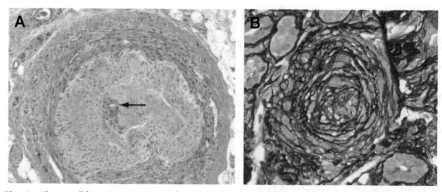

Fig. 1. Fibroproliferative vasculopathy in SSc. (*A*) Histological hematoxylin and eosin staining (magnification: 100×) of a digital artery from a patient with limited cutaneous SSc, showing intimal thickening. The lumen is occluded with visible recanalization (*arrow*).[86] (*B*): Concentric fibromucoid obliteration, small renal artery ("onion skin" lesion), PAMS silver stain (magnification: 20×). (*Courtesy of* [A] M Jeziorska, MD, PhD, Manchester, UK; and [B] C Bernard, Quebec, Canada.)

1 and **2**). SSc-related vasculopathy is associated with significant disease-related morbidity and mortality including in patients with early disease. In fact, SRC most commonly occurs in the first few years from disease onset in patients with the diffuse cutaneous subset,[4] and approximately 75% of patients with SSc who develop DUs do so within the first 5 years.[5] There have been major advancements in understanding the pathogenesis and management of vascular disease in SSc. SRC is now largely survivable including through early recognition and aggressive blood pressure control,[6,7] and there are now a wide range of drug treatments to prevent and heal DUs.[8]

Against this background, our aim was to provide a practical overview of the diagnosis and management of SRC and DUs in SSc, and to highlight unmet needs for future research.

SCLERODERMA RENAL CRISIS

The classic pathogenic triad of vasculopathy, inflammation, and fibrosis affects the kidneys of most patients with SSc. This is generally subclinical and rarely progressive.

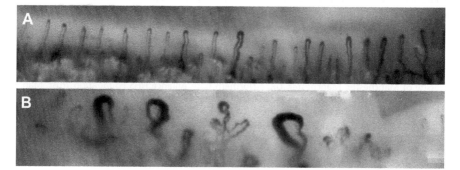

Fig. 2. Structural microvascular disease in SSc. The microangiopathy of SSc is very well demonstrated non-invasively by nailfold capillaroscopy. (*A*) Regularly shaped capillaries in a healthy control subject. (*B*) Enlarged capillary loops and avascularity in a patient with SSc.

However, a small subset of patients with SSc, in the range of 5% to 10%, develop SRC. SRC is characterized by acute hypertension and kidney injury. Historically, SRC was the leading cause of death in SSc, with 1-year survival rates of only 15%.[6,9] The discovery, in the late 1970s, that ACE inhibitors effectively controlled the hypertension and mitigated the effects of SRC on kidney function led to a dramatic improvement in survival.[10] Nevertheless, outcomes have not improved much since then,[7,11,12] and there is still much room to improve our understanding of SRC and identify novel, additional therapies.

Etiopathogenesis

The traditional conceptual framework for the pathophysiology of SRC proposed by Steen consists of a series of insults to the kidneys.[4,13] An initial injury to endothelial cells results in intimal thickening and proliferation of renal interlobular and arcuate arteries. Super-imposed platelet adhesion and aggregation leads to narrowing or total obliteration of vessel lumen, decreased renal perfusion, particularly in cortical blood flow, and tissue ischemia. In turn, this leads to hyperplasia of the juxtaglomerular apparatus and increased renin production. Activation of the renin-angiotensin system (RAS) results in the production of angiotensin II and elevation in blood pressure. This contributes to further vasoconstriction and sets up a vicious cycle of hypoperfusion and ischemia that feeds back into the pathogenic loop. Although the upstream mechanisms remain theoretical, the dramatic effect of ACE inhibitors in abrogating SRC supports the role of the RAS as a final common pathway to renal injury in SRC.

Complement activation is increasingly recognized as a possible mediator of renal damage in SRC.[14] Some experts have in fact recently proposed stratifying SRC into narrowly defined SRC or SSc-thrombotic microangiopathy (TMA), depending on whether elevation in blood pressure and kidney dysfunction appear before or after the onset of thrombocytopenia.[15]

Some triggers of SRC have been proposed, including episodic vasospasm, referred to as "renal Raynaud's," although the evidence to support this is sparse.[16] Anti-RNA polymerase III antibodies are strongly associated with SRC occurrence, but there is no evidence for direct pathogenicity.[17] Although high circulating levels of endothelin-1 have been reported at the time of SRC and endothelin ligand and receptor expression are increased in renal biopsies,[18] the inciting cause remains unknown.

There is some evidence to support genetic susceptibility for SRC, including associations with distinct MHC class I haplotypes, namely HLA-DRB1*0407 and *1304.[19] More recently, associations with GPATCH2L gene and CTNND2 have been identified.[20] Although the role of these genes in SRC remains to be clarified, it is interesting to note that they have also been associated with essential hypertension in the general population and pulmonary arterial hypertension in SSc.[21,22] Finally, of interest, polymorphisms in the endothelin ligand-receptor axis,[23] but not the ACE axis have been associated with SSc.[24]

Clinical Presentation

Presenting signs and symptoms of SRC are often nonspecific and include fatigue, malaise, headache, and visual disturbances. Regular home blood pressure monitoring thus plays a critical role in prompt detection. However, although most patients with SRC have striking elevations in their blood pressure, more modest elevations and at times normotensive presentations in up to 10% of cases can occur. Other common clinical features include encephalopathy, heart failure, and pericardial disease. Standardized definitions of hypertension, acute kidney injury, and target organ involvement in SRC are currently being validated prospectively (**Box 1**).[25]

Box 1
Proposed definitions for hypertension, AKI, and target organ involvement in SRC

Acute rise in blood pressure defined as any one of:
  Systolic blood pressure > 140 mm Hg
  Diastolic blood pressure > 90 mm Hg
  Rise in systolic blood pressure > 30 mm Hg above normal
  Rise in diastolic blood pressure > 20 mm Hg above normal

Acute kidney injury[a] defined as any one of:
  Increase in serum creatinine by > 26.5 μmol/L (>0.3 mg/dL) within 48 h
  Increase in serum creatinine to >1.5 times baseline, which is known or presumed to have occurred within the prior 7 days
  Urine volume < 0.5 mL/kg/h for 6 h

Microangiopathic hemolytic anemic defined as:
  New or worsening anemia not due to other causes
  Schistocytes or other red blood cell fragments on blood smear
  Thrombocytopenia < 100,000, confirmed by manual smear. Laboratory evidence of hemolysis, including elevated lactate dehydrogenase, reticulocytosis, and/or low/absent haptoglobin
  A negative direct anti-globulin test

Target organ dysfunction
  Hypertensive retinopathy
  Acute heart failure
  Acute pericarditis

[a]This is the definition of acute kidney injury from the Kidney Disease Improving Global Outcomes (KDIGO) guidelines.[31]

Risk factors for SRC include early (less than 5 years) rapidly progressive diffuse skin disease, male sex, and African American race.[26] The presence of anti-RNA polymerase III antibodies is a strong risk factor for SRC. In a recent study from the large European Scleroderma Trials and Research (EUSTAR) registry involving over 2800 SSc subjects, anti-RNA polymerase antibodies were independently associated with SRC (odds ratio 5.86, 95% confidence interval 2.6, 13.2).[27] Preexisting hypertension, proteinuria, and chronic kidney disease have also recently been reported as risk factors for SRC.[27,28] Exposure to glucocorticoids is commonly reported as a risk factor,[29] although whether the association is causal or instead represents confounding by disease severity remains uncertain.[30] Nevertheless, glucocorticoids, especially at moderate to high doses, should be used cautiously (ie, lowest dose for the shortest time possible) in patients with SSc and with risk factors for SRC, and patients should be carefully followed for the emergence of possible SRC.

Diagnostic Approach

All patients with new onset SSc should be educated about SRC and encouraged to seek medical care promptly should they develop signs and symptoms of SRC. Assessment of renal function is key, to distinguish essential hypertension from SRC. SSc experts have adopted the Kidney Disease Improving Global Outcomes (KDIGO) definition of AKI to define SRC (see **Box 1**).[31]

A patient presenting with SRC should undergo hematologic and cardiac investigations to identify target organ involvement. Ophthalmologic assessment, preferably by a trained expert, may be useful to stage the severity of the hypertensive crisis.

Urine microscopy is essential to rule out alternative explanations for new-onset hypertension and AKI. In particular, hematuria, dysmorphic red blood cells, and casts could suggest vasculitis or glomerulonephritis. Lupus serologies and ANCA antibodies are useful when considering the differential diagnosis of AKI in a patient with SSc.[4,32]

Kidney biopsies for SRC may be useful prognostically.[33] However, kidney biopsies are not routine in classic SRC, especially given the risks of bleeding in the setting of hypertension, anemia, and/or thrombocytopenia. Unexplained AKI in a normotensive SSc patient or in a patient with SSc with findings suggestive of alternative causes of AKI (eg, vasculitis or glomerulonephritis) are indications for kidney biopsy. A standardized definition of abnormalities on kidney biopsy in SRC is presently being prospectively validated.[25]

Management

Guidelines for the management of SRC have been proposed.[34] First-line management of SRC is rapid blood pressure control with ACE inhibition. Restoring the patient's baseline blood pressure over 2 to 3 days to preserve renal function should be the goal. The preferred initial drug for SRC is captopril, which has the advantage of rapid-onset and short-duration which facilitates rapid dose titration. Captopril is usually begun at a dose of 6.25 to 12.5 mg and increased in 12.5 to 25 mg increments every 4 to 8 h until baseline blood pressure is achieved. The maximum dose is 300 to 450 mg/d.

Experts recommend *adding* calcium channel blockers, angiotensin receptor blockers (ARBs), and alpha-blockers as second-, third-, and fourth-line treatments.[35] Combination therapy with intravenous nicardipine is particularly helpful to control blood pressure as the dose of oral ACE inhibitor is titrated to the maximal tolerated dose. Alternatively, oral nifedipine is also recommended by experts,[35] with short-acting preparations having the theoretical advantage of easier dose titration over extended-release forms. Although ARBs are recommended, they should not replace ACE inhibitors because, unlike ACE inhibitors, they do not inhibit the degradation of bradykinin, which is a potent vasodilator. There are theoretical advantages to using direct renin antagonists, but the published evidence remains sparse.[36,37] Beta blockers are generally avoided because of the risk of reducing cardiac output and contributing to "renal" as well as systemic Raynaud's. Although endothelin receptor antagonists (ERAs) represent an interesting approach, two small open-label studies of bosentan, an ERA,[18,38] for SRC have been published with generally inconclusive results. Additional anti-hypertensive medications, including iloprost, have been recommended in refractory cases.[34]

Although tight blood pressure control is the only proven treatment of SRC, there are reports on the use of plasmapheresis and complement inhibitors.[39,40] More data will be needed to understand the role of these other therapies in SRC, although presumably they would be used as add-on therapy to ACE inhibitors in patients with signs of thrombotic microangiopathy.

Inflammatory infiltrates have been described in SRC renal biopsies.[33] To date, though, there is no firm evidence to support a role for immunosuppression, including biologics, in this setting.

The rate of permanent dialysis after SRC in the post-ACE inhibitor era ranges from 19% to 40%, and 3% to 17% of SSc patients undergo renal transplants.[12] As opposed to other more common types of end-stage kidney disease such as diabetes mellitus and other manifestations of SSc that are generally irreversible, one of the remarkable aspects of SRC is that renal recovery can continue up to 18 months after SRC. Thus, in practice, decisions to proceed to renal transplant are often deferred for 1 to 2 years. Survival has been reported to be better in patients post-renal transplant (54% to 91%) compared with those who remain on dialysis (31% to 56%).[12] Graft survival has also improved over time and appears similar to that of patients with other types of ESRD.

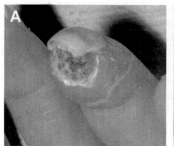
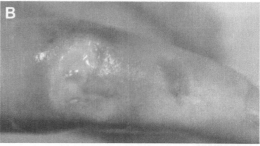

Fig. 3. Digital ulcers in SSc. A necrotic fingertip DU (*A*) and extensor aspect ulcer (*B*) with signs of infection.

Autologous hematopoietic stem cell transplant (AHSCT) is increasingly used to treat a subset of patients with severe SSc. "Renal insufficiency related to SSc", which would presumably include prior SRC, is included among the indications for AHSCT.[41,42] In general, though, renal dysfunction from chronic pre-transplant SRC is not expected to improve after AHSCT. In fact, creatinine clearance was significantly worse in the AHSCT arm of the ASTIS trial compared with the cyclophosphamide arm (−12.1 (29.7) vs −1.2 (24.1) mL/min, difference 10.9 (95% CI 1.5 to 20.3) mL/min, $p = 0.02$).[41] Rather, renal dysfunction is considered a marker of high risk to disease progression in other organs and thereby provides rationale for AHSCT in SSc.

DIGITAL ULCERS

Around half of the patients with SSc will develop DUs (**Fig. 3**) during their disease course.[8,43,44] DUs commonly occur on the fingertips, and also overlying the extensor (dorsal) aspects of the hands, particularly over the small joints.[45] DUs can also occur elsewhere including through the extrusion of underlying subcutaneous calcinosis through the skin. Prompt assessment and intervention are required because this can significantly modify the clinical course and minimize tissue loss.[46]

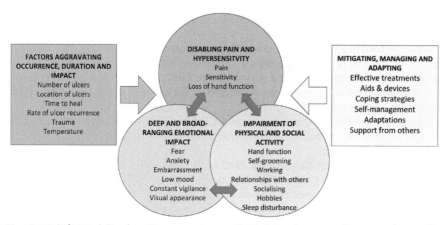

Fig. 4. Multifaceted lived patient experience of SSc-DUs. Conceptual map exploring the themes (and subthemes) of DUs in patients with SSc, which are closely inter-related. (*From* Hughes M, Pauling JD, Jones J, et al. A Multi-Centre Qualitative Study Exploring the Patient Experience of Digital Ulcers in Systemic Sclerosis. Arthritis Care Res (Hoboken) 2020;72:723-733.)

Etiopathogenesis

In general, ischemia is believed to drive DU pathogenesis and evolution, particularly ulcers occurring on the fingertips.[47] Whereas, DUs overlying the extensor aspects of the hands may be more related to recurrent microtrauma and skin fibrosis.[5,48] A range of associations with DUs has been reported including potential circulating and microvascular imaging biomarkers to predict DUs.[49]

Impact and Burden

Pain is a cardinal feature of DUs and can be severe. DUs significantly impact on patients' quality of life and function including occupation, and many patients live with great fear and uncertainty (**Fig. 4**).[50,51] DUs are associated with significant healthcare utilization including the need for hospitalisation.[44,52]

Complications

Ulcer complications (eg, infection and gangrene) significantly delay healing. DUs are commonly infected, particularly by *Staphylococcus aureus*, and not uncommonly by enteric organisms, highlighting the need for meticulous ulcer and hand hygiene.[53,54] Plain radiographic features of osteomyelitis may take several weeks to become apparent, and therefore clinicians need to maintain a high index of suspicion.[55,56] Increasingly, magnetic resonance imaging is being used to facilitate the early diagnosis of osteomyelitis (eg, through the detection of bone marrow edema).[55,56]

Ulcer Assessment

DUs can be very challenging to assess based on clinical examination, which is heavily reliant upon visual inspection (**Fig. 5**). Potential challenges include their small size and overlying material (eg, eschar) that limits assessment of the wound base. In a pilot study using high-frequency ultrasound, the average width and depth was approximately 6 mm and 1 mm, respectively.[57] Recently there have been significant advancements in DU assessment relevant to clinical practice and trial design. The composite

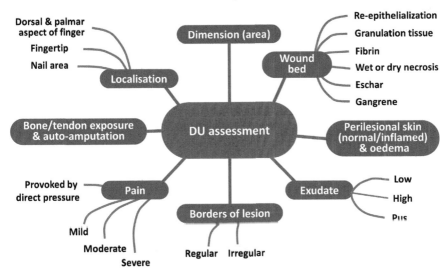

Fig. 5. Structured approach to DU wound bed assessment. (*Adapted from* Hughes M, Allanore Y, El Aoufy K, et al. A Practical Approach to the Management of Digital Ulcers in Patients With Systemic Sclerosis: A Narrative Review. JAMA Dermatol 2021;157:851–8.)

DU Clinical Assessment Score (DUCAS) has undergone preliminary validation with encouraging face, content, and construct validity, and warrants further evaluation.[58] The Hand Disability in Systemic Sclerosis-Digital Ulcers (HDISS-DU) patient-reported outcome measure has reliability, validity, discriminating ability, and responsiveness to change, based on psychometric analysis of SSc-DU patients from two large US-based studies.[59] DU photographs including those taken by smartphones could allow measurement of lesion size, bringing the possibility of remote monitoring.[60,61]

Definition
DU definitions have been developed by the World Scleroderma Foundation (WSF) and the UK Scleroderma Study Group (UKSSG).[62,63] Both recognize that DUs are characterized by loss of epithelization and have a discernible depth. Although intra-rater reliability was high for both definitions (0.90 and 0.71, respectively), inter-rater reliability was lower (0.51 and 0.15, respectively).[62,63]

Classification
Classification of individual DUs has been largely based on proposed DU etiopathogenesis and this has significant implications for management.[5,45] This includes optimizing the use of vascular-acting therapies for "ischemic" ulcers, whereas non-medical management (eg, avoiding trauma) should be prioritized for "mechanical" DUs. Surgical intervention is often required for calcinosis-related ulcers. Amanzi and colleagues[45] also recognized DUs secondary to digital pitting scars (DPS). A recent study from the EUSTAR cohort ($n = 9671$) observed that DPS were significantly associated with DUs (odds ratio of 22.03).[64]

A study from the Digital Ulcer Outcomes Registry identified four DU occurrence categories based on patients with SSc-DUs with ≥ 2 years follow-up: "no-DU" (33.2%), "episodic" (9.4%), "recurrent" (46.2%), and "chronic" (11.2%).[52] Patients with the "chronic" category had the highest rate of complications (eg, infection) and burden of DU disease (eg, occupational impairment).[52] Furthermore, a recent DeSScipher/EUSTAR survey found that 80% of centers preferred the categorization of DU into "episodic, recurrent and chronic" compared with the dichotomy of either "recurrent" or "not recurrent."[65]

Digital Ulcer Management

All DUs must be actively managed (including regular monitoring) by a specialist multidisciplinary team. Local (nonpharmacological) and systemic (pharmacological) treatments are often combined.

Nonpharmacological intervention
Patients require education about DU prevention and management, including the need to seek early health care advice for new ulcers. Dedicated nurse-led clinics improve access to timely DU care.[66] Optimal wound care management is essential including the appropriate choice of dressings. The ulcer should be kept slightly moist as this promotes wound healing, although excessive moisture can foster infection and damage the perilesional skin. Some clinicians undertake DU debridement which can be performed at the clinic using a "sharp" technique (eg, with a scalpel or curette) or through the application of autolytic dressings working over the course of several days.[67,68] DU infection should be promptly treated with appropriate antibiotic therapy and the analgesic regimen regularly should be reviewed and optimized.

Pharmacological intervention

Vasodilator therapy (eg, calcium channel blockers) has been reported to delay or prevent DUs, although this has been little studied to date.[5,69] For example, nifedipine (and intravenous iloprost) were both associated with a reduced number of ulcers at 16 weeks in a randomized controlled trial of SSc-associated Raynaud's phenomenon.[70] Intravenous prostanoids (ie, iloprost) are helpful for DU prevention and healing,[69,71,72] but require hospitalization and can be poorly tolerated due to systemic side effects. Overall, there is evidence to support the use of phosphodiesterase type-5 inhibitors (PDE5i) for DU prevention and healing.[71] Two large randomized controlled trials showed that treatment with the ERA bosentan reduced new DU occurrence, but had no impact on healing.[73,74] However, a similar treatment effect was not observed with macitentan.[75] In a recent prospective, multicenter, observational cohort study from Korea, the time to healing of the cardinal ulcer was comparable for both ERA and PDE5i.[69] However, ERAs were more effective in reducing new DU compared with PDE5i (hazard ratio of 0.39).[69] A multicenter randomized, double-blind, placebo-controlled pilot study of riociguat (a selective soluble guanylate cyclase stimulator) did not reduce the number of DU net burden (the primary end point) at 16 weeks.[76]

Surgical intervention and botulinum toxin injections

Surgical debridement may be required for the removal of necrotic tissue and/or pus, and when local debridement is not feasible or ineffective. Indications for surgery include infection (eg, osteomyelitis), ulcer-related calcinosis, and gangrene. There is increasing experience internationally using botulinum toxin injections for SSc-DUs: this approach has been reported to be safe and efficacious with improved ulcer healing and reduction in pain[77,78] although controlled clinical trials are required. Periarterial sympathectomy has been reported to be associated with ulcer healing and improved pain.[79,80] Arterial bypass or reconstruction should be considered for significant macrovascular involvement (where amenable to intervention).[80]

UNMET NEEDS/RESEARCH AGENDA
Scleroderma Renal Crisis

The absence of a gold standard for classifying SRC represents an important challenge for research in this condition. In an effort to overcome this challenge, the Scleroderma Clinical Trials Consortium (SCTC) Working Group on SRC has undertaken to develop and validate classification criteria for SRC.[81] Data on an inception SRC cohort and controls with other thrombotic microangiopathies have been collected and are being analyzed. This project will generate the first validated classification criteria for SRC which are expected to become the international standard to be used in future randomized trials and epidemiologic research of SSc.

Studies have suggested that prophylactic use of ACE inhibitors may be harmful in SSc, although confounding bias could not be entirely ruled out.[11] Studies replicating these findings are ongoing and mechanisms explaining a possible paradoxical effect of ACE inhibitors in the prevention as opposed to the treatment of SRC remain to be elucidated. Until more evidence if available, prophylactic use of ACE inhibitors is not recommended.

Which aspects of vascular, glomerular, and tubular function have the potential to improve after SRC remains to be elucidated. This could provide useful insights into other potentially reversible processes in SRC.

Historically, SRC was the leading cause of death in SSc and ACE inhibitors unquestionably transformed outcomes. However, a systematic literature review showed that there has been no further improvement in survival since the introduction of ACE inhibitors.[12] SRC mortality rates also remain proportionally higher than mortality rates associated with other SSc organ involvement and the rate of permanent dialysis after SRC in the post-ACE inhibitor era still ranges from 19% to 40%. There is an urgent need to identify novel treatments to improve outcomes of SRC.

Digital Ulcers

International collaborative research is looking to develop improved outcome measures for DUs including by SCTC Vascular and WSF DU Working Groups.[82] This includes research into ulcer definition, composite measures (eg, DUCAS), understanding the lived patient-experience of DUs (with a goal to develop a novel patient-reported outcome measure), and an OMERACT-endorsed core set.[83]

The optimal approach to DU management remains to be completely elucidated including the local (wound) bed management. In particular, there is significant international variation in DU debridement and a strong need for controlled trials to confirm the safety and efficacy of the technique.[67,68] The concept of a unified endovascular phenotype in SSc has been proposed in which vascular therapies could potentially be deployed as a putative form of *systemic* disease modification including for structural digital vascular disease and prevention of DUs.[84,85]

SUMMARY

In conclusion, a structured approach to the assessment and management of both SRC and SSc-DUs is required. Treatment outcomes have significantly improved for these vasculopathic complications including targeted pharmacological therapies and through multidisciplinary working. However, the management of SRC and DUs still remains challenging and ongoing collaborative international research should facilitate further advancements relevant to clinical care.

CLINICS CARE POINTS

- Systemic vasculopathy is a major driver of disease-related morbidity and mortality in systemic sclerosis (SSc), including in patients with early disease.
- Although angiotensin-converting enzyme (ACE) inhibitors improve survival in patients presenting with scleroderma renal crisis (SRC), there is a need to identify new avenues of therapy to further improve prognosis.
- Unexplained acute kidney injury in a normotensive patient with SSc should prompt consideration of etiologies other than SRC (and of the need for renal biopsy)
- Prophylactic use of ACE inhibitors to prevent SRC is not currently recommended
- Ulcer complications (eg, infection and gangrene) can significantly delay ulcer healing.
- A multidisciplinary approach is required for the management of SRC and digital ulcers (DUs).
- DUs require active management including regular monitoring and a structured approach to assessment.
- Local wound bed management is often combined with systemic (pharmacological) treatment.
- Surgical intervention for DUs is sometimes required and there is increasing international experience in botulinum toxin injection and periarterial sympathectomy.

DISCLOSURE

M. Hughes reports speaking fees from Actelion Pharmaceuticals, Eli Lilly, and Pfizer, outside of the submitted work (all <$10,000). He is a member of a Data and Safety Monitoring Board for Certa Therapeutics. A.L. Herrick–reports consultancy fees from Arena, Boehringer-Ingelheim, Camurus, CSL Behring, and Gesynta, research funding from Gesynta, and speaker's fees from Janssen. M. Hudson reports consulting fees from Boehringer Ingelheim, Alexion, and Mallinckrodt, outside of the submitted work (all <$10,000) and unrestricted research grants from Bristol-Myers Squibb and Boehringer Ingelheim.

REFERENCES

1. Allanore Y, Simms R, Distler O, et al. Systemic sclerosis. Nat Rev Dis Prim 2015;1: 15002.
2. Denton CP, Khanna DK. Systemic sclerosis. Lancet 2017;390:1685–99.
3. Hughes M, Herrick AL. Systemic sclerosis. Br J Hosp Med 2019;80:530–6.
4. Bruni C, Cuomo G, Rossi FW, et al. Kidney involvement in systemic sclerosis: From pathogenesis to treatment. J Scleroderma Relat Disord 2018;3(1):43–52.
5. Hachulla E, Clerson P, Launay D, et al. Natural history of ischemic digital ulcers in systemic sclerosis: Single-center retrospective longitudinal study. J Rheumatol 2007;34:2423–30.
6. Steen VD, Medsger TA. Changes in causes of death in systemic sclerosis, 1972-2002. Ann Rheum Dis 2007;66:940–4.
7. Hughes M, Zanatta E, Sandler RD, et al. Improvement with time of vascular outcomes in systemic sclerosis: a systematic review and meta-analysis study. Rheumatology (Oxford) 2021. https://doi.org/10.1093/rheumatology/keab850.
8. Hughes M, Herrick AL. Digital ulcers in systemic sclerosis. Rheumatology 2017; 56:14–25.
9. Steen VD, Costantino JP, Shapiro AP, et al. Outcome of renal crisis in systemic sclerosis: relation to availability of angiotensin converting enzyme (ACE) inhibitors. Ann Intern Med 1990;113:352–7.
10. Hickman RJ. The History of ACE inhibitors in Scleroderma Renal Crisis. In: The Rheumatologist 2021. Available at: https://www.the-rheumatologist.org/article/the-history-of-ace-inhibitors-in-scleroderma-renal-crisis/. Accessed May 01, 2022.
11. Hudson M, Baron M, Tatibouet S, et al. Exposure to ACE inhibitors prior to the onset of scleroderma renal crisis-results from the International Scleroderma Renal Crisis Survey. Semin Arthritis Rheum 2014;43:666–72.
12. Kim H, Lefebvre F, Hoa S, et al. Mortality and morbidity in scleroderma renal crisis: a systematic literature review. J Scleroderma Relat Disord 2020;6:21–36.
13. Steen VD. Scleroderma renal crisis. Rheum Dis Clin North Am 2003;29:315–33.
14. Okrój M, Johansson M, Saxne T, et al. Analysis of complement biomarkers in systemic sclerosis indicates a distinct pattern in scleroderma renal crisis. Arthritis Res Ther 2016;18:267.
15. Yamashita H, Kamei R, Kaneko H. Classifications of scleroderma renal crisis and reconsideration of its pathophysiology. Rheumatology 2019;58:2099–106.
16. Cannon PJ, Hassar M, Case DB, et al. The relationship of hypertension and renal failure in scleroderma (progressive systemic sclerosis) to structural and functional abnormalities of the renal cortical circulation. Medicine (Baltim) 1974; 53:1–46.
17. Nihtyanova SI, Parker JC, Black CM, et al. A longitudinal study of anti-RNA polymerase III antibody levels in systemic sclerosis. Rheumatology 2009;48:1218–21.

18. Penn H, Quillinan N, Khan K, et al. Targeting the endothelin axis in scleroderma renal crisis: rationale and feasibility. QJM 2013;106:839–48.

19. Nguyen B, Mayes MD, Arnett FC, et al. HLA-DRB1*0407 and *1304 are risk factors for scleroderma renal crisis. Arthritis Rheum 2011;63:530–4.

20. Stern EP, Guerra SG, Chinque H, et al. Analysis of Anti-RNA Polymerase III Antibody-positive Systemic Sclerosis and Altered GPATCH2L and CTNND2 Expression in Scleroderma Renal Crisis. J Rheumatol 2020;47:1668–77.

21. Levy D, Larson MG, Benjamin EJ, et al. Framingham Heart Study 100K Project: genome-wide associations for blood pressure and arterial stiffness. BMC Med Genet 2007;8(Suppl):S3.

22. Gao L, Emond MJ, Louie T, et al. Identification of rare variants in ATP8B4 as a risk factor for systemic sclerosis by whole-exome sequencing. Arthritis Rheumatol 2016;68:191–200.

23. Fonseca C, Lindahl GE, Ponticos M, et al. A polymorphism in the CTGF promoter region associated with systemic sclerosis. N Engl J Med 2007;357:1210–20.

24. Wipff J, Gallier G, Dieude P, et al. Angiotensin-converting enzyme gene does not contribute to genetic susceptibility to systemic sclerosis in European Caucasians. J Rheumatol 2009;36:337–40.

25. Butler E-A, Baron M, Fogo AB, et al. Generation of a Core Set of Items to Develop Classification Criteria for Scleroderma Renal Crisis Using Consensus Methodology. Arthritis Rheumatol 2019;71:964–71.

26. Morgan ND, Shah AA, Mayes MD, et al. Clinical and serological features of systemic sclerosis in a multicenter African American cohort: analysis of the genome research in african american scleroderma patients clinical database. Medicine (Baltim) 2017;96:e8980.

27. Moinzadeh P, Kuhr K, Siegert E, et al. Scleroderma renal crisis (SRC): risk factors for an increasingly rare organ complication. J Rheumatol 2020;47:241–8.

28. Gordon SM, Stitt RS, Nee R, et al. Risk factors for future scleroderma renal crisis at systemic sclerosis diagnosis. J Rheumatol 2019;46:85–92.

29. DeMarco PJ, Weisman MH, Seibold JR, et al. Predictors and outcomes of scleroderma renal crisis: the high-dose versus low-dose D-penicillamine in early diffuse systemic sclerosis trial. Arthritis Rheum 2002;46:2983–9.

30. Trang G, Steele R, Baron M, et al. Corticosteroids and the risk of scleroderma renal crisis: a systematic review. Rheumatol Int 2012;32:645–53.

31. Kellum J, Lameire N, Aspelin P, et al. KDIGO clinical practice guideline for acute kidney injury. Kidney Int Suppl 2012;2:1–138.

32. Hughes M, Kahaleh B, Denton CP, et al. ANCA in systemic sclerosis, when vasculitis overlaps with vasculopathy: a devastating combination of pathologies. Rheumatology 2021;60:5509–16.

33. Batal I, Domsic RT, Shafer A, et al. Renal biopsy findings predicting outcome in scleroderma renal crisis. Hum Pathol 2009;40:332–40.

34. Lynch BM, Stern EP, Ong V, et al. UK Scleroderma Study Group (UKSSG) guidelines on the diagnosis and management of scleroderma renal crisis. Clin Exp Rheumatol 2016;34(Suppl 1):106–9.

35. Fernández-Codina A, Walker KM, Pope JE, Scleroderma Algorithm Group. Treatment algorithms for systemic sclerosis according to experts. Arthritis Rheumatol 2018;70:1820–8.

36. Dhaun N, MacIntyre IM, Bellamy COC, et al. Endothelin receptor antagonism and renin inhibition as treatment options for scleroderma kidney. Am J Kidney Dis 2009;54:726–31.

37. Bütikofer L, Varisco PA, Distler O, et al. ACE inhibitors in SSc patients display a risk factor for scleroderma renal crisis-a EUSTAR analysis. Arthritis Res Ther 2020;22:59.
38. Berezné A, Abdoul H, Karras A, et al. Bosentan in scleroderma renal crisis: a national open label prospective study. Arthritis Rheumatol 2017;69(suppl 10). Abstract 2671. Available at: https://acrabstracts.org/abstract/bosentan-in-scleroderma-renal-crisis-a-national-open-label-prospective-study/.
39. Gouin A, Ribes D, Colombat M, et al. Role of C5 inhibition in Idiopathic Inflammatory Myopathies and Scleroderma Renal Crisis-Induced Thrombotic Microangiopathies. Kidney Int reports 2021;6:1015–21.
40. Cozzi F, Marson P, Cardarelli S, et al. Prognosis of scleroderma renal crisis: a long-term observational study. Nephrol Dial Transplant 2012;27:4398–403.
41. van Laar JM, Farge D, Sont JK, et al. Autologous hematopoietic stem cell transplantation vs intravenous pulse cyclophosphamide in diffuse cutaneous systemic sclerosis: a randomized clinical trial. JAMA 2014;311:2490–8.
42. Sullivan KM, Goldmuntz EA, Keyes-Elstein L, et al. Myeloablative autologous stem-cell transplantation for severe scleroderma. N Engl J Med 2018;378(1):35–47.
43. Mouthon L, Carpentier PH, Lok C, et al. Ischemic digital ulcers affect hand disability and pain in systemic sclerosis. J Rheumatol 2014;41:1317–23.
44. Morrisroe K, Stevens W, Sahhar J, et al. Digital ulcers in systemic sclerosis: their epidemiology, clinical characteristics, and associated clinical and economic burden. Arthritis Res Ther 2019;21:1–12.
45. Amanzi L, Braschi F, Fiori G, et al. Digital ulcers in scleroderma: staging, characteristics and sub-setting through observation of 1614 digital lesions. Rheumatology 2010;49:1374–82.
46. Hughes M, Allanore Y, El Aoufy K, et al. a practical approach to the management of digital ulcers in patients with systemic sclerosis: a narrative review. JAMA Dermatol 2021;157:851–8.
47. Hughes M, Allanore Y, Chung L, et al. Raynaud's phenomenon and digital ulcers in systemic sclerosis. Nat Rev Rheumatol 2020;4:208–21.
48. Hughes M, Murray A, Denton C, et al. Should all digital ulcers be included in future clinical trials of systemic sclerosis-related digital vasculopathy? Med Hypotheses 2018;116:101–4.
49. Silva I, Almeida J, Vasconcelos C. A PRISMA-driven systematic review for predictive risk factors of digital ulcers in systemic sclerosis patients. Autoimmun Rev 2015;14:140–52.
50. Guillevin L, Hunsche E, Denton CP, et al. Functional impairment of systemic scleroderma patients with digital ulcerations: results from the DUO Registry. Clin Exp Rheumatol 2013;31(2 Suppl 76):71–80.
51. Hughes M, Pauling JD, Jones J, et al. a multi-centre qualitative study exploring the patient experience of digital ulcers in systemic sclerosis. Arthritis Care Res 2020;72:723–33.
52. Matucci-Cerinic M, Krieg T, et al. Elucidating the burden of recurrent and chronic digital ulcers in systemic sclerosis: long-term results from the DUO Registry. Ann Rheum Dis 2016;75:1770–6.
53. Giuggioli D, Magnani L, Spinella A, et al. Infections of scleroderma digital ulcers: a single center cohort retrospective study. Dermatol reports 2021;13:9075.
54. Giuggioli D, Manfredi A, Colaci M, et al. Scleroderma digital ulcers complicated by infection with fecal pathogens. Arthritis Care Res 2012;64:295–7.

55. Haque A, Wyman M, Dargan D, et al. Hand osteomyelitis in patients with secondary raynaud phenomenon. J Clin Rheumatol 2021;27:S342–5.
56. Zhou AY, Muir L, Harris J, et al. The impact of magnetic resonance imaging in early diagnosis of hand osteomyelitis in patients with systemic sclerosis. Clin Exp Rheumatol 2014;32:S-232.
57. Hughes M, Moore T, Manning J, et al. A pilot study using high-frequency ultrasound to measure digital ulcers: a possible outcome measure in systemic sclerosis clinical trials? Clin Exp Rheumatol 2017;35(Suppl 1):218–9.
58. Bruni C, Ngcozana T, Braschi F, et al. Preliminary validation of the digital ulcer clinical assessment score in systemic sclerosis. J Rheumatol 2019;46:603–8.
59. Mouthon L, Poiraudeau S, Vernon M, et al. Psychometric validation of the Hand Disability in Systemic Sclerosis-Digital Ulcers (HDISS-DU®) patient-reported outcome instrument. Arthritis Res Ther 2020;22(1):3.
60. Simpson V, Hughes M, Wilkinson J, et al. Quantifying digital ulcers in systemic sclerosis: Reliability of digital planimetry in measuring lesion size. Arthritis Care Res 2018;70(3):486–90.
61. Dinsdale G, Moore TL, Manning JB, et al. Tracking digital ulcers in systemic sclerosis: a feasibility study assessing lesion area in patient-recorded smartphone photographs. Ann Rheum Dis 2018;77:1382–4.
62. Suliman YA, Bruni C, Johnson SR, et al. Defining skin ulcers in systemic sclerosis: systematic literature review and proposed world scleroderma foundation (WSF) definition. J Scleroderma Relat Disord 2017;2:115–20.
63. Hughes M, Tracey A, Bhushan M, et al. Reliability of digital ulcer definitions as proposed by the UK Scleroderma Study Group: a challenge for clinical trial design. J Scleroderma Relat Disord 2018;3:170–4.
64. Hughes M, Heal C, Henes J, et al. Digital pitting scars are associated with a severe disease course and death in systemic sclerosis: a study from the EUSTAR cohort. Rheumatology 2022;61:1141–7.
65. Blagojevic J, Bellando-Randone S, Abignano G, et al. Classification, categorization and essential items for digital ulcer evaluation in systemic sclerosis: a DeSScipher/European Scleroderma Trials and Research group (EUSTAR) survey. Arthritis Res Ther 2019;21:35.
66. Ngcozana T, Ong VH, Denton CP. Improving access to digital ulcer care through nurse-led clinic: a service evaluation. Muscoskel Care 2020;18:92–7.
67. Hughes M, Alcacer-Pitarch B, Gheorghiu AM, et al. Digital ulcer debridement in systemic sclerosis: a systematic literature review. Clin Rheumatol 2020;39:805–11.
68. Hughes M, Alcacer-Pitarch B, Allanore Y, et al. Digital ulcers: should debridement be a standard of care in systemic sclerosis? Lancet Rheumatol 2020;2:e302–7.
69. Chang SH, Jun JB, Lee YJ, et al. A clinical comparison of an endothelin receptor antagonist and phosphodiesterase type 5 inhibitors for treating digital ulcers of systemic sclerosis. Rheumatology 2021;60:5814–9.
70. Rademaker M, Cooke ED, Almond NE, et al. Comparison of intravenous infusions of iloprost and oral nifedipine in treatment of Raynaud's phenomenon in patients with systemic sclerosis: a double blind randomised study. BMJ 1989;298(6673):561–4.
71. Tingey T, Shu J, Smuczek J, et al. Meta-analysis of healing and prevention of digital ulcers in systemic sclerosis. Arthritis Care Res 2013;65:1460–71.
72. Cruz JE, Ward A, Anthony S, et al. Evidence for the use of epoprostenol to treat raynaud's phenomenon with or without digital ulcers. Ann Pharmacother 2016;50:1060–7.

73. Korn JH, Mayes M, Matucci Cerinic M, et al. Digital ulcers in systemic sclerosis: prevention by treatment with bosentan, an oral endothelin receptor antagonist. Arthritis Rheum 2004;50:3985–93.
74. Matucci-Cerinic M, Denton CP, Furst DE, et al. Bosentan treatment of digital ulcers related to systemic sclerosis: results from the RAPIDS-2 randomised, double-blind, placebo-controlled trial. Ann Rheum Dis 2011;70:32–8.
75. Khanna D, Denton CP, Merkel PA, et al. Effect of macitentan on the development of new ischemic digital ulcers in patients with systemic sclerosis: Dual-1 and Dual-2 randomized clinical trials. JAMA 2016;315:1975–88.
76. Nagaraja V, Spino C, Bush E, et al. A multicenter randomized, double-blind, placebo-controlled pilot study to assess the efficacy and safety of riociguat in systemic sclerosis-associated digital ulcers. Arthritis Res Ther 2019;21:1–14.
77. Lautenbach G, Dobrota R, Mihai C, et al. Evaluation of botulinum toxin A injections for the treatment of refractory chronic digital ulcers in patients with systemic sclerosis. Clin Exp Rheumatol 2020;38(Suppl 1):154–60.
78. Shenavandeh S, Sepaskhah M, Dehghani S, et al. A 4-week comparison of capillaroscopy changes, healing effect, and cost-effectiveness of botulinum toxin-A vs prostaglandin analog infusion in refractory digital ulcers in systemic sclerosis. Clin Rheumatol 2022;41:95–104.
79. Momeni A, Sorice SC, Valenzuela A, et al. Surgical treatment of systemic sclerosis-is it justified to offer peripheral sympathectomy earlier in the disease process? Microsurgery 2015;35:441–6.
80. Satteson ES, Chung MP, Chung LS, et al. Microvascular hand surgery for digital ischemia in scleroderma. J Scleroderma Relat Disord 2020;5:130–6.
81. SCTC Working Groups. Available at: https://sclerodermaclinicaltrialsconsortium. org/working-groups. Accessed May 01, 2022.
82. Pauling JD, Frech TM, Hughes M, et al. Patient-reported outcome instruments for assessing Raynaud's phenomenon in systemic sclerosis: A SCTC vascular working group report. J Scleroderma Relat Disord 2018;3:249–52.
83. Maltez N, Hughes M, Brown E, et al. Developing a core set of outcome measure domains to study Raynaud's phenomenon and digital ulcers in systemic sclerosis: Report from OMERACT 2020. Semin Arthritis Rheum 2021;51:640–3.
84. Hughes M, Huang S, Pauling JD, et al. Factors Influencing Patient Decision-Making Concerning Treatment Escalation in Raynaud's Phenomenon Secondary to Systemic Sclerosis. Arthritis Care Res 2021;73:1845–52.
85. Hughes M, Khanna DK, Pauling JD. Drug initiation and escalation strategies of vasodilator therapies for Raynaud's phenomenon: can we treat to target? Rheumatology 2019;59:464–6.
86. Herrick AL. The pathogenesis, diagnosis and treatment of Raynaud phenomenon. Nat Rev Rheumatol 2012;8:469–79.

Interstitial Lung Disease
How Should Therapeutics Be Implemented?

Cosimo Bruni, MD, PhD[a,b,*,1], Corrado Campochiaro, MD[c,1],
Jeska K. de Vries-Bouwstra, MD, PhD[d]

KEYWORDS

- Systemic sclerosis • Interstitial lung disease • Combination therapy
- Targeted therapies • Treatment

KEY POINTS

- Interstitial lung disease (ILD) is highly prevalent in systemic sclerosis (SSc) and associated with morbidity and mortality.
- SSc-ILD course is highly variable and prediction at the individual patient level is challenging.
- Evidence-based guidelines on the definition of clinically relevant progression of SSc ILD, and on the content and timing of monitoring SSc-ILD patients are urgently awaited.
- Recently, important new treatment options have become available that contribute to improved treatment of SSc-ILD.
- How to best apply these drugs, in terms of timing, and mono versus combination, needs to be determined in the coming years.

INTRODUCTION

Interstitial lung disease (ILD) is a frequent organ manifestation in systemic sclerosis (SSc) and is associated with high morbidity and mortality. Reported prevalence varies between 35% and 75% of patients with SSc, depending on the patient selection and definitions applied.[1–3] Importantly, SSc-ILD is a leading cause of morbidity and mortality in SSc,[4,5] determining a mortality risk nearly three times greater than in SSc patients without ILD,[6] particularly in youngers and in males.

[a] Department of Rheumatology, University Hospital Zurich, University of Zurich, Schmelzbergstrasse 24, Zurich 8006, Switzerland; [b] Division of Rheumatology, Department of Experimental Medicine, Careggi University Hospital - University of Florence, Florence, Italy; [c] Unit of Immunology, Rheumatology, Allergy and Rare Diseases (UnIRAR), IRCCS San Raffaele Hospital, Vita-Salute San Raffaele University, Via Olgettina 60, Milan, Italy; [d] Department of Rheumatology, Leiden University Hospital, Postal Zone C1-R, PO Box 9600, Leiden 2300 RC, the Netherlands
[1] Equal contribution as first author.
* Corresponding author.
E-mail address: cosimo.bruni@usz.ch
Twitter: @CosimoBruni (C.B.); @CampochiaroCor (C.C.)

Rheum Dis Clin N Am 49 (2023) 279–293
https://doi.org/10.1016/j.rdc.2023.01.005
0889-857X/23/© 2023 Elsevier Inc. All rights reserved.

rheumatic.theclinics.com

High-resolution computed tomography (HRCT) is to date the gold standard for ILD diagnosis.[7] HRCT has been shown to be superior to pulmonary function testing (PFT) in detecting SSc-ILD.[8] Of all SSc patients with typical ILD changes on HRCT, only a minority will show a clear restrictive pattern with PFT.[1] Given the high prevalence and its association with worse prognosis it is recommended to screen each SSc patient by HRCT for ILD at SSc diagnosis, also in the absence of specific respiratory symptoms.

The severity and course of SSc-ILD varies widely, from mild and stable to severe and rapidly progressing.[9] Overall, 20% to 30% of SSc-ILD patients will show the progression of ILD over time, whereas approximately 50% of patients will show a stable disease course and some even show improvement in lung function over time (**Fig. 1**).

Paramount to identify ILD progression and characterizing clinical phenotypes of progressive SSc-ILD is reaching a consensus on how to define progression, considering the various definitions currently available.[10–12] Probably, a multidimensional definition including symptoms, functional assessments, and imaging might best capture clinically relevant progression.

When a patient is diagnosed with SSc-ILD, starting immunomodulatory therapy should be considered based on functional impairment, complaints, and extent of ILD on HRCT.[13]

Although increasing, the number of possible drugs that have proven efficacy in the treatment of SSc-ILD is still limited. Efficacy of cyclophosphamide (CYC) has been shown in two high-quality randomized controlled trials (RCTs) and, therefore, CYC is included in current recommendations for the treatment of SSc-ILD.[14–17] A third high-quality RCT evaluated the efficacy of mycophenolate mofetil (MMF) with oral CYC as a comparator and showed comparable efficacy of MMF and CYC in improving pulmonary function (reflected by Forced Vital Capacity; FVC), complaints, and extent of ILD on HRCT.[18] Use of MMF for SSc-ILD was further substantiated by a post hoc study comparing SSc-ILD patients on placebo that participated in the RCT evaluating CYC (SLS I) with those treated with MMF in the trial comparing CYC and MMF (SLS II). Here, treatment with MMF resulted in significant improvement in lung volumes and dyspnea as compared with placebo.[19] For a selected subgroup of patients with SSc-ILD, hematopoietic stem cell transplantation (HSCT) could be considered. Three RCTs have confirmed the superior efficacy of HSCT in improving FVC as compared with intravenous CYC.[20–22] In addition, few data suggest that treatment with HSCT might even

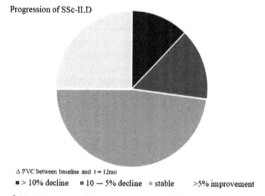

Progression of SSc-ILD

Δ FVC between baseline and t = 12mo

■ > 10% decline   ■ 10 — 5% decline   ▨ stable   >5% improvement

Fig. 1. Progression of SSc-ILD over 12 months in the EUSTAR cohort (9). FVC, forced vital capacity; ILD, interstitial lung disease; SSc, systemic sclerosis.

decrease fibrosis extent on HRCT.[20,23] In view of the risks associated with this strategy, not all SSc-ILD patients are candidates for HSCT, which could be considered in a subgroup of patients with diffuse skin disease and rapid disease progression. Recently, tocilizumab and nintedanib have been added to the treatment arsenal for SSc-ILD based on RCT evidence[24,25]: these will be addressed in the section below, together with a discussion on the positioning of the different drugs available for the treatment of SSc-ILD. As a last option, when the situation is deteriorating despite maximum pharmacological and non-pharmacological efforts, lung transplantation should be considered, and patients should be referred to a transplantation center.[26]

The variable course of SSc-ILD, the complexity in determining and predicting the progression of SSc-ILD, and the limited but highly diverse treatment options for SSc-ILD, pose many challenges for everyday clinical practice (**Fig. 2**). In this review, we discuss the currently available evidence for treatment together with areas where additional evidence is highly warranted. In the meantime, multidisciplinary team care involving experts from rheumatology, pulmonology, and radiology is recommended to offer SSc-ILD patients high-quality care following the most recent insights.[27]

DISCUSSION
Selection of Patients

Risk factors for the presence of systemic sclerosis-interstitial lung disease
First challenge in clinical practice is to identify the patients with SSc-ILD. Given the high prevalence and its association with a worse prognosis, it is recommended to screen each SSc patient by HRCT for ILD at the time of SSc diagnosis, also in the absence of specific respiratory symptoms. In support, to determine the urgency and timing of performing the HRCT, several clinical characteristics have been associated with presence of SSc-ILD (**Fig. 2**). Impaired lung function at the time of SSc diagnosis and respiratory symptoms like cough and dyspnea are associated with ILD presence. Also male gender, presence of anti-topoisomerase antibodies (ATA), the diffuse skin type as well as the higher extent of skin involvement evaluated by the modified Rodnan Skin score (mRSS) have been associated with presence of

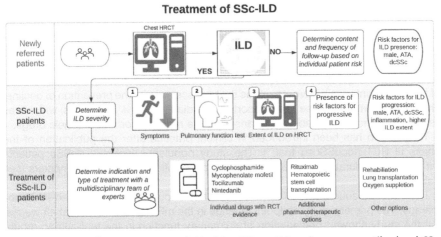

Fig. 2. Overview of the treatment of SSc-ILD. ATA, anti-topoisomerase antibody; dcSSc, diffuse cutaneous SSc; HRCT, high-resolution computed tomography; ILD, interstitial lung disease; SSc, systemic sclerosis.

ILD.[28–33] In addition, other organ manifestations such as gastroesophageal reflux disease, digital ulcers, and pulmonary hypertension (PH) have been linked to the presence of ILD.[34,35] ILD has also been described to be associated with non-Caucasian and African American race.[36] In contrast, presence of anti-centromere antibodies (ACA) is associated with a lower risk for presence of ILD. Nonetheless, It is important to realize that also lcSSc patients and ACA can have ILD.[1,37]

Risk factors for the progression of systemic sclerosis-interstitial lung disease

Once presence of SSc-ILD is confirmed, the next challenge is to determine the content and frequency of monitoring for possible progression (**Fig. 2**). Among patients who do experience ILD progression, the rate of progression can be either rapid or slow.[9] Only a small subgroup of patients, about 8%, will show rapid progression of ILD. It is however paramount to identify this subgroup early as these patients typically experience rapidly increasing parenchymal lung changes leading to a substantial loss of lung function early in their disease course.[9] Clinical risk factors for rapid progression of SSc-ILD include diffuse skin involvement, presence of ATA, increased CRP, worse PFT at baseline, and higher ILD extent on HRCT.[38] These clinical factors can help to customize adequate and timely follow-up of SSc-ILD. In addition, in patients with SSc-ILD and clinical worsening with symptoms like dyspnea and cough, re-evaluation of SSc-ILD is warranted.

Selection of Medications

Thanks to the results of two recent phase III randomized placebo-controlled trials[24,25] showing the efficacy of tocilizumab and nintedanib, the therapeutic armamentarium now available for SSc-ILD has significantly increased. In fact, nintedanib has been approved by the FDA and the EMA for the treatment of SSc-ILD, while tocilizumab by FDA for the same indication.

Nintedanib, a multi-tyrosine kinase inhibitor that blocks FGF receptor-1, VEGF receptor-2, and PDGF receptor-α and β52,[39] was approved for the treatment of idiopathic pulmonary fibrosis in 2014[40] and has become the first treatment approved for the treatment of SSc-ILD after the publication of the largest phase III RCT in SSc-ILD.[24] The SENSCIS trial randomized SSc-ILD patients with a disease duration < 7 years, regardless of their cutaneous disease subset, but with an SSc-ILD extent >10% on HRCT, to receive oral nintedanib 150 mg twice daily or placebo (**Table 1**). This protocol allowed concomitant immunosuppression and 48% of patients were on stable MMF therapy at baseline. Over the study period, the adjusted annual rate of change in FVC was significantly lower in the nintedanib compared with the placebo group (-52 mL/year versus -93 mL/year, $p = 0.04$). The combination of MMF plus nintedanib gave signals as the best scenario for the prevention of decline. The most common adverse event reported was diarrhea (76% of patients) which was usually mild and manageable with transient dose reduction or anti-diarrheic drugs.

Tocilizumab has been introduced in clinical practice after the publication of the phase III RCT (focuSSced trial[25]). The study population included dcSSc patients with a disease duration $\leq$ 5 years and with raised inflammatory serum markers (see **Table 1**).

The subcutaneous formulation (162 mg subcutenous weekly) was used in monotherapy. The primary study endpoint (change in the mRSS) was not met at 48 weeks, but the study showed preservation of pulmonary function in the tocilizumab group, whereas the placebo group showed a slight decrease. The cumulative distribution of change in %predicted FVC favored tocilizumab compared with placebo (-3.9 versus -0.6, $p = 0.0015$) and the mean difference in FVC change from baseline

Table 1
Characteristics of phase 3 studies

Trial Drug	Mechanism of Action	Inclusion Criteria	Treatment	IS	Endpoints	Duration	Results
Nintedanib (NTD) SENSCIS	Tyrosine kinase inhibition (FGF, VEGF, and PDGF)	SSc-ILD HRCT ≥10% Early (≤7 years)	150 mg oral BID	Yes[a]	(1) Annual ΔFVC. (2) mRSS, SGRQ	52 weeks	↓ FVC decline in NTD ($p = 0.04$) No change in mRSS or SGRQ
Tocilizumab (TCZ) focuSSced	IL-6 receptor blockage	Early (≤5 years) dcSSc (mRSS≥10) Inflammation[b]	162 mg sc weekly	No	(1) mRSS. (2) Δ%pFVC	48 weeks	No significant mRSS change ($p = 0.098$) FVC change favored TCZ ($p = 0.0015$)

Abbreviations: %pFVC, % predicted forced vital capacity; BID, bis in die; HRCT, high-resolution computed tomography; ILD, interstitial lung disease; IS, immunosuppressive treatment; mRSS, modified Rodnan skin score; sc, subcutaneous; SGRQ, St. George's Respiratory Questionnaire; SSc, systemic sclerosis.
[a] Stable IS therapy for at least 6 months before study enrollment with prednisone ≤ 10 mg daily, methotrexate, or mycophenolate mofetil.
[b] At least one of the following: C-reactive protein ≥6 mg/L, ESR ≥28 mm/h, or platelet count ≥330 × 10⁹/L.

was 167 mL in favor of tocilizumab. No significant increase in adverse events and serious adverse events was observed in the trial. Subsequent subanalyses[41] showed that SSc-ILD patients included in the trial and receiving tocilizumab had preservation of %predicted FVC over 48 weeks compared with placebo (−0.1% versus −6.3%) and this was particularly pronounced in patients with severe SSc-ILD patients as defined by lung involvement at HRCT >20% extent at baseline.

Other targeted treatments, including the anti-CD20 monoclonal antibody rituximab, have also been studied.[42] Unfortunately, the nature of the studies prevents drawing clear conclusions about its effectiveness and positioning for SSc-ILD, as most retrospective or uncontrolled prospective studies are so far available.[43–45] The results of the RECITAL study, a clinical trial comparing the efficacy of rituximab with CYC as first-line treatment in connective tissue disease (CTD)-related ILD have been recently published, with 40% of patients being represented by SSc-ILD cases. In this trial, Rituximab was not superior to CYC, as both drugs showed comparable improvement FVC% and patient-reported outcomes. Despite this, rituximab determined fewer side effects than CYC, as well as lower exposure to corticosteroids.[46] In this light, rituximab might be taken into consideration in specific populations, given the positive results observed in these studies, and it could also be considered in combination with nintedanib ± MMF.

Although the management of SSc-ILD patients has changed since the introduction of nintedanib and tocilizumab, many open questions on how to implement the full potential of these drugs are still unanswered. First, besides the many differences in the two study populations (including cutaneous subtype, enrichment in inflammatory patients, disease duration, see **Table 1**), the possibility of combining therapies—that is, with MMF, which is considered the "anchor drug" in SSc—was only allowed in the SENSCIS trial. This fundamental difference opens the possibility that the use of such a strategy even for tocilizumab might further increase the efficacy of the drug, as already observed for the nintedanib. This fascinating scenario should though be carefully investigated, given the possible synergistic effect in the beneficial side as well as in the rate and grade of adverse events. Moreover, even though the combination therapy of nintedanib plus MMF and/or methotrexate was allowed in the SENSCIS trial, other possible combinations have potential additional benefits, as recently reported in a multi-center real-life retrospective study of ninedanib in Italy.[47] Currently, while waiting for stronger prospective evidence, we advocate to start with immunomodulatory therapy in SSc patients with new onset or first detection ILD as these treatments have been shown to stabilize or even improve pulmonary function. The choice of drug, either MMF, TCZ, or their combination, should depend on a careful evaluation of extra-pulmonary manifestations (eg, skin, cardiac, and musculoskeletal involvement) and of specific disease features (eg, disease duration and elevation of inflammatory markers). In SSc-ILD patients with ongoing progression of ILD despite immunosuppressive treatment and in patients with rapidly declining FVC (>10% within 12 months) and >10% of ILD extent on HRCT additional treatment with nintedanib in combination with MMF could be considered.

Another matter of debate is whether a combination therapy should be advocated since the very beginning of SSc-ILD treatment, even in subclinical ILD (with the risk of potential adverse events in patients who may not progress) or whether an "add-on strategy" (ie, starting with MMF, then adding nintedanib) should be considered only for progressive patients (with the risk of irreversibly losing lung functionality). Both strategies might have pros and cons. In the first scenario, the need to wait for patients' lung deterioration and the occurrence of irreversible damage might be avoided. However, with the relatively low numbers of SSc-ILD patients that will actually show progression, this scenario might also result in important overtreatment, urging the need to validate risk factors to accurately identify progressors.[38,48]

Following this line, a possible upfront combination therapy including nintedanib plus tocilizumab has been hypothesized by some authors as an alternative to HSCT, as it might offer the possibility of achieving beneficial effects on multiple domains including skin, musculoskeletal system and quality of life (QoL).[20,49] This is similar to what is currently recommended for SSc-PAH,[50] a field in which studies have identified combination therapies as the best therapeutic option, as they can significantly impact mortality and QoL.[51]

A clinical distinction should also be made for SSc-ILD patients with concomitant PH, who represent a group of patients at high risk of poor outcomes and who have been neglected or poorly represented in the studies published so far.[5,52] The possibility that these new treatments might be effective also in this subpopulation and that they could positively impact the evolution of PH is yet to be determined and offers exciting opportunities for the whole scleroderma community.

On this background, SSc-ILD experts have suggested that baseline HRCT-defined (sub)clinical ILD involvement[53] together with a complete evaluation of at-risk features for ILD progression should be taken into consideration to decide which is the most suitable strategy.[49] Despite this, it is crucial to remember that the best strategy should always meet patients' demands and preferences regarding the route of administration and the potential side effects should carefully be discussed, as they might limit patients' compliance.[54] Therefore, stratification for the occurrence of severe or intolerable side effects should also be implemented for a more comprehensive therapeutic algorithm.[55]

Follow-up Assessment

Despite the availability of therapeutic recommendations and additional options, we are currently lacking robust data-supported guidance for the specific follow-up of SSc-ILD patients, after therapy initiation. This reflects in different areas in the management of SSc-ILD cases, which require standardization and optimization.

Monitoring efficacy

Current data derived from RCTs and observational studies targeting SSc-ILD support the evaluation of treatment efficacy after average 12 months from drug initiation. Although this might follow regulatory requirements for the registration of drugs in the approved therapeutic armamentarium, this timespan may not represent the clinical approach of most physicians treating SSc-ILD.[48] As reported in a recent expert opinion article, patients may be assessed at least every 6 months with various tests which may capture different domains of SSc-ILD progression.[56] This timepoint, or even a shorter one, may reflect the need to verify the efficacy of the medication in stopping the progression and might be indirectly in line with the RCT data. In fact, protocols in which background medications were allowed at the beginning of the treatment phase, such as the case of methotrexate and mycophenolic acid in the SENSCIS trial,[24] required a stable medication status for at least six months. This reflects the fact that both tolerability and efficacy of the drugs might have reached a "steady state" after six months of administration and, therefore, start showing both beneficial effect and safety concerns. Moreover, data from both the SLS I, SLS II, SENSCIS, and FocuSSced have shown that curves presenting FVC decline over time show separation between placebo and treatment arms at 6 months.[16,18,24,25] In line with this, although one might feel urgency to evaluate 3 months after initiation of treatment, in particular in symptomatically progressive patients, the treating physician should realize that the efficacy of available drugs mostly takes >3 months to become functionally and clinically apparent. In addition, the limited number of available drugs should be kept in mind when deciding that treatment is not efficacious.

Agreeing on 6-monthly evaluations, in particular after the initiation of new treatments, better guidance is desirable on which assessments should be performed, ideally reflecting a clinically meaningful improvement of SSc-ILD. The definition of "ILD progression" from Goh and colleagues[10] included FVC relative decline over 12 months ≥10% or FVC relative decline between 5-9% associated with a DLco relative decline≥15% and it was identified as a surrogate biomarker for mortality. Subsequently, a more heterogeneous definition of ILD progressive phenotype was used as inclusion criteria for the INBUILD study, considering various combinations of FVC, ILD extent, and symptoms worsening.[12] A joined initiative from the American Thoracic Society, European Respiratory Society, Japanese Respiratory Society, and Asociaciòn Latinoamericana the Tòrax has recently released guidelines for the diagnosis and treatment of pulmonary progressive fibrosis (PPF) in fibrotic ILDs. These combine previous data from RCTs and observational studies and consider an ILD patient as PPF in case of at least 2 of worsening of respiratory symptoms, functional or radiological progression.[11] This more recent and multi-domain definition requires, therefore, multiple evaluations to be performed, and association with for example mortality, has not been fully addressed yet in SSc-ILD.

Pulmonary function testing. PFT is an effective follow-up assessment of SSc-ILD.[57] In particular, FVC represents the endorsed instrument for use in both RCTs and observational studies, contrary to DLco which was mostly used as a secondary outcome and not always showing positive results. Although DLco is less specific than FVC in identifying pure parenchymal disease changes and it is still part of both definitions of "ILD progression", it might reflect other concomitant changes such as anemia, vasculopathy, or emphysema. In this context, DLco decline in a patient with worsening respiratory symptoms but stable FVC/ILD extent on HRCT may guide the physician to investigate concomitant PH. Different definitions regarding progression based on PFT are available. In comparison to Goh and colleagues, Raghu and colleagues[11] have defined "functional progression" as FVC absolute decline ≥5% or DLco corrected absolute decline ≥10% over 12 months, the latter requiring a thorough exclusion of other possible causes. Both definitions have pros and cons: although only the former has been validated in SSc-ILD, the second ensures ILD is a relevant cause by the simultaneous presence of symptoms worsening or HRCT progression. Specific validation of the most recent functional definition of progression and comparison with the previous one in terms of prognostic impact in SSc-ILD is awaited.

High-resolution computed tomography. The extent of SSc-ILD on HRCT has been associated with both functional decline and mortality.[58] Nevertheless, only few studies showed numerical and probably not clinically meaningful changes in ILD extent detected on HRCT during treatment, although associated with functional changes.[25,38,59] In addition to identifying treatment effects, the increase of total ILD extent ≥ 2% over 12-24 months has been recently identified as an independent predictor of mortality, therefore representing another candidate surrogate biomarker. The recent guidelines include HRCT progression as one of the possible features of a PPF patient: in this context, not only the extent of ILD, but also the appearance of new ILD areas or transition from one ILD pattern to the other is considered ILD progression, despite no SSc-ILD specific data are available.[11] In addition, whether this evaluation may rely on visual or also on computerized quantitative evaluation is not yet established. When moving from RCTs to clinical practice, the application of HRCTs in the follow-up of SSc-ILD patients is not standardized. A recent EUSTAR-SCTC survey has shown that almost one-third of the 205 responders regularly perform HRCTs in the follow-up of SSc-ILD cases, whereas the majority prescribe it only according to clinical judgment.[60] This included mostly cases with functional decline, new onset or worsening of dyspnea, or of crackles on auscultation. This is also in line with that derived from the European Consensus, in which there was disagreement on repeating HRCT annually after SSc-ILD diagnosis.[48] If applying the new definition of PPF, HRCT might be considered in all patients presenting functional decline or a worsening of respiratory symptoms. As for DLco, also HRCT is pivotal in the differential diagnosis of respiratory symptoms. Infections, thrombo-embolic events, and emphysema can be detected on HRCT and would then guide to a different therapeutic approach. These concomitant conditions might be missed if considering only functional tests during the follow-up evaluation. As this approach might lead to a high number of tests, algorithms suggesting when to scan the patients during the follow-up are eagerly awaited.

Other assessments. Additional evaluations, such as the 6-minute walking test and patients reported outcomes (including QoL and symptoms) also carry positive and negative aspects. When both have been used in RCT as secondary outcomes, no significant efficacy was detected for most of the evaluations performed.[61] This might reflect the multi-domain nature of these evaluations and the lack of specificity for SSc-ILD changes. Observational studies identified oxygen desaturation at the six minutes walking test, together with presence/history of arthritis, as a predictor for future functional worsening of SSc-ILD.[62] With a similar attitude, change in QoL or symptoms is something to always consider at a patient level, being the real target of the treatment. Lower performance in exercise test and increase in patients' complaints are indeed non-specific for SSc-ILD, but both should trigger further assessment to detect either ILD progression or concomitant extra-pulmonary complications.

Safety and additional considerations
Although SSc-ILD studies mostly target mortality or SSc-ILD progression, other events also represent important outcomes at patient level. The safety profile of the treatments is of pivotal importance, in particular for medications determining more stability than clinically meaningful improvement.[63] Although the adverse events profile of the medications is well known and strategies are available for the management of some of them (such as gastrointestinal and liver toxicities), the increased risk of infections using immunosuppressants remains a major concern. In this light, scientific societies' advice should be followed regarding vaccinations when using immunosuppressive agents.[64,65] In addition, guidance regarding prophylactic antibiotics to prevent opportunistic infections might be considered in the context of both ILD and immunosuppression.

The overall follow-up assessment of a patient with SSc-ILD should go beyond the control of lung functionality and drug toxicities: it should consider a multi-disciplinary team evaluation, in collaboration with other specialists, including pulmonologists and radiologists.[27] Both specialists are pivotal in the close collaboration with the rheumatologists, to identify clinically meaningful progression, rule out other causes for the clinical worsening of a patient, and to choose the optimal drug strategy. Bronchoalveolar lavage, for example, represents a useful instrument to rule out infections and other concomitant lung pathologies, requiring pulmonologist experience and expertise.

Evidence regarding the additional beneficial effect of non-pharmacological interventions is scarce. These include pulmonary rehabilitation, as a very safe procedure

---

Box 1
Research agenda regarding the treatment of SSc-ILD

Initiation: when to start treatment?

To treat at diagnosis (primary prevention of progression) versus at progression (secondary prevention), identifying high-risk patient profiles.

Combination: is an upfront combination superior to an add-on treatment strategy?

Upfront versus sequential use of immunosuppressants and/or antifibrotics, taking also into account extra-pulmonary disease features.

Supportive measures: which supportive measurements are most effective for patient's symptoms?

Identify interventions most effective on patients' perception, such as dyspnea, QoL, cough, fatigue, depression, also including medications indirectly targeting ILD.

Continuation: how long should SSc-ILD treatment be continued?

Lack of data on long-term efficacy and treatment tapering/withdrawal.

Monitoring: how often and according to which definition should we evaluate the efficacy of initiated treatment?

Validation of SSc-ILD multi-domain definition of progression, and timing of assessments.

---

to expose SSc-ILD patients to,[66] as well as oxygen supplementation. The latter is mostly seen as a treatment failure outcome and usually started when hypoxia presents at rest. In reality, SSc-ILD patients might present with desaturation and hypoxia during exercise while not being hypoxic at rest. A recent prospective RCT administered oxygen supplementation to patients with ILD secondary to different causes and hypoxemia after the 6MWT showed a beneficial effect on QoL and dyspnea.[67] In this light, oxygen supplementation could be offered earlier to SSc-ILD patients, to preserve QoL. Finally, referral to lung transplantation should be considered when the situation is deteriorating despite maximum pharmacological and non-pharmacological efforts. Although the possible simultaneous involvement of the cardiac and gastrointestinal systems has been regarded as a possible contraindication, more recent data showed comparable outcomes in SSc-ILD patients after lung transplantation as compared with other transplanted patients, despite the high prevalence of severe esophageal dysfunction in this group.[26]

SUMMARY

The body of evidence on how to treat SSc-ILD is definitely growing. However, several major knowledge gaps have been identified.[68] In our opinion, future research should focus on the practical use of the available drugs to answer specific unmet needs in the therapeutic approach. This would allow us to move beyond expert opinions and compensate for the lack of real evidence on different points with specific strategies, including initiation, combination, and continuation of treatment and monitoring (**Box 1**).

CLINICS CARE POINTS

- Interstitial lung disease (ILD) is highly prevalent in systemic sclerosis (SSc) and associated with high mortality
- All SSc patients need to be screened for ILD with high-resolution computed tomography

- SSc-ILD course is highly variable, and prediction at the individual patient level is challenging
- Next to cyclophosphamide, mycophenolate mofetil and hematopoietic stem cell transplantation, nintedanib, and tocilizumab have proven efficacy in the treatment of SSc-ILD
- Different profiles of concomitant medications and patients' characteristics make the efficacy data of randomized controlled trials not directly comparable.
- Follow-up evaluation of SSc-ILD may include a combination of functional, radiologic, and clinical assessment, to identify progressive patients.
- Timing and indication of the specific assessment parameters for follow-up of SSc-ILD are not clearly indicated.

DISCLOSURE

C. Bruni received consulting fees and/or honoraria from Actelion, Eli-Lilly, Boehringer Ingelheim. Research grants from Foundation for research in Rheumatology (FOREUM), Gruppo Italiano Lotta alla Sclerodermia (GILS), European Scleroderma Trials and Research Group (EUSTAR), Scleroderma Clinical Trials Consortium (SCTC). Educational grants from AbbVie. C. Campochiaro, received consulting fees and/or honoraria from SOBI, Novartis, Pfizer, Roche, Jannsen Boehringer Ingelheim. J.K. de Vries-Bouwstra, received consulting fees from Abbvie, Janssen and Boehringer Ingelheim, and received research grants from Roche, Galapagos, Janssen, ReumaNederland, NVLE (Dutch society for patients with lupus, scleroderma, MCTD and APS).

REFERENCES

1. Hoffmann-Vold AM, Fretheim H, Halse AK, et al. Tracking impact of interstitial lung disease in systemic sclerosis in a complete nationwide cohort. Am J Respir Crit Care Med 2019;200(10):1258–66.
2. Vonk MC, Broers B, Heijdra YF, et al. Systemic sclerosis and its pulmonary complications in The Netherlands: an epidemiological study. Ann Rheum Dis 2009; 68(6):961–5.
3. Walker UA, Tyndall A, Czirjak L, et al. Clinical risk assessment of organ manifestations in systemic sclerosis: a report from the EULAR Scleroderma Trials And Research group database. Ann Rheum Dis 2007;66(6):754–63.
4. Elhai M, Meune C, Boubaya M, et al. Mapping and predicting mortality from systemic sclerosis. Ann Rheum Dis 2017;76(11):1897–905.
5. Young A, Vummidi D, Visovatti S, et al. Prevalence, treatment, and outcomes of coexistent pulmonary hypertension and interstitial lung disease in systemic sclerosis. Arthritis Rheumatol 2019;71(8):1339–49.
6. Rubio-Rivas M, Royo C, Simeon CP, et al. Mortality and survival in systemic sclerosis: systematic review and meta-analysis. Semin Arthritis Rheum 2014;44(2): 208–19.
7. Elicker BM, Kallianos KG, Henry TS. The role of high-resolution computed tomography in the follow-up of diffuse lung disease: Number 2 in the Series "Radiology" Edited by Nicola Sverzellati and Sujal Desai. Eur Respir Rev 2017;26(144). https://doi.org/10.1183/16000617.0008-2017.
8. Suliman YA, Dobrota R, Huscher D, et al. Brief report: pulmonary function tests: high rate of false-negative results in the early detection and screening of scleroderma-related interstitial lung disease. Arthritis Rheumatol 2015;67(12): 3256–61.

9. Hoffmann-Vold AM, Allanore Y, Alves M, et al. Progressive interstitial lung disease in patients with systemic sclerosis-associated interstitial lung disease in the EU-STAR database. Ann Rheum Dis 2021;80(2):219–27.

10. Goh NS, Hoyles RK, Denton CP, et al. Short-term pulmonary function trends are predictive of mortality in interstitial lung disease associated with systemic sclerosis. Arthritis Rheumatol 2017;69(8):1670–8.

11. Raghu G, Remy-Jardin M, Richeldi L, et al. Idiopathic pulmonary fibrosis (an update) and progressive pulmonary fibrosis in adults: an official ATS/ERS/JRS/ALAT clinical practice guideline. Am J Respir Crit Care Med 2022;205(9):e18–47.

12. Flaherty KR, Wells AU, Cottin V, et al. Nintedanib in progressive interstitial lung diseases: data from the whole INBUILD trial. Eur Respir J 2022;59(3). https://doi.org/10.1183/13993003.04538-2020.

13. Ruaro B, Confalonieri M, Matucci-Cerinic M, et al. The treatment of lung involvement in systemic sclerosis. Pharmaceuticals 2021;14(2). https://doi.org/10.3390/ph14020154.

14. Kowal-Bielecka O, Fransen J, Avouac J, et al. Update of EULAR recommendations for the treatment of systemic sclerosis. Ann Rheum Dis 2017;76(8):1327–39.

15. Hoyles RK, Ellis RW, Wellsbury J, et al. A multicenter, prospective, randomized, double-blind, placebo-controlled trial of corticosteroids and intravenous cyclophosphamide followed by oral azathioprine for the treatment of pulmonary fibrosis in scleroderma. Arthritis Rheum 2006;54(12):3962–70.

16. Tashkin DP, Elashoff R, Clements PJ, et al. Cyclophosphamide versus placebo in scleroderma lung disease. N Engl J Med 2006;354(25):2655–66.

17. Bruni C, Tashkin DP, Steen V, et al. Intravenous versus oral cyclophosphamide for lung and/or skin fibrosis in systemic sclerosis: an indirect comparison from EU-STAR and randomised controlled trials. Clin Exp Rheumatol 2020;38(Suppl 125 3):161–8.

18. Tashkin DP, Roth MD, Clements PJ, et al. Mycophenolate mofetil versus oral cyclophosphamide in scleroderma-related interstitial lung disease (SLS II): a randomised controlled, double-blind, parallel group trial. Lancet Respir Med 2016;4(9):708–19.

19. Volkmann ER, Tashkin DP, Li N, et al. Mycophenolate mofetil versus placebo for systemic sclerosis-related interstitial lung disease: an analysis of scleroderma lung studies I and II. Arthritis Rheumatol 2017;69(7):1451–60.

20. Sullivan KM, Goldmuntz EA, Keyes-Elstein L, et al. Myeloablative Autologous Stem-Cell Transplantation for Severe Scleroderma. N Engl J Med 2018;378(1): 35–47.

21. Burt RK, Shah SJ, Dill K, et al. Autologous non-myeloablative haemopoietic stem-cell transplantation compared with pulse cyclophosphamide once per month for systemic sclerosis (ASSIST): an open-label, randomised phase 2 trial. Lancet 2011;378(9790):498–506.

22. van Laar JM, Farge D, Sont JK, et al. Autologous hematopoietic stem cell transplantation vs intravenous pulse cyclophosphamide in diffuse cutaneous systemic sclerosis: a randomized clinical trial. JAMA 2014;311(24):2490–8.

23. Ciaffi J, van Leeuwen NM, Boonstra M, et al. Evolution of systemic sclerosis-associated interstitial lung disease one year after hematopoietic stem cell transplantation or cyclophosphamide. Arthritis Care Res 2022;74(3):433–41.

24. Distler O, Highland KB, Gahlemann M, et al. Nintedanib for systemic sclerosis-associated interstitial lung disease. N Engl J Med 2019;380(26):2518–28.

25. Khanna D, Lin CJF, Furst DE, et al. Tocilizumab in systemic sclerosis: a randomised, double-blind, placebo-controlled, phase 3 trial. Lancet Respir Med 2020;8(10):963–74.

26. Miele CH, Schwab K, Saggar R, et al. Lung transplant outcomes in systemic sclerosis with significant esophageal dysfunction. A comprehensive single-center experience. Ann Am Thorac Soc 2016;13(6):793–802.

27. Farina N, Benanti G, De Luca G, et al. The role of the multidisciplinary health care team in the management of patients with systemic sclerosis. J Multidiscip Healthc 2022;15:815–24.

28. Assassi S, Sharif R, Lasky RE, et al. Predictors of interstitial lung disease in early systemic sclerosis: a prospective longitudinal study of the GENISOS cohort. Arthritis Res Ther 2010;12(5):R166.

29. Becker M, Graf N, Sauter R, et al. Predictors of disease worsening defined by progression of organ damage in diffuse systemic sclerosis: a European Scleroderma Trials and Research (EUSTAR) analysis. Ann Rheum Dis 2019;78(9):1242–8.

30. Hoffmann-Vold AM, Aalokken TM, Lund MB, et al. Predictive value of serial high-resolution computed tomography analyses and concurrent lung function tests in systemic sclerosis. Arthritis Rheumatol 2015;67(8):2205–12.

31. Khanna D, Tashkin DP, Denton CP, et al. Etiology, risk factors, and biomarkers in systemic sclerosis with interstitial lung disease. Am J Respir Crit Care Med 2020;201(6):650–60.

32. Nihtyanova SI, Denton CP. Scleroderma lung involvement, autoantibodies, and outcome prediction: the confounding effect of time. J Rheumatol 2017;44(4):404–6.

33. Nihtyanova SI, Schreiber BE, Ong VH, et al. Prediction of pulmonary complications and long-term survival in systemic sclerosis. Arthritis Rheumatol 2014;66(6):1625–35.

34. Allanore Y, Simms R, Distler O, et al. Systemic sclerosis. Nat Rev Dis Prim 2015;1:15002.

35. Denton CP, Khanna D. Systemic sclerosis. Lancet 2017;390(10103):1685–99.

36. McNearney TA, Reveille JD, Fischbach M, et al. Pulmonary involvement in systemic sclerosis: associations with genetic, serologic, sociodemographic, and behavioral factors. Arthritis Rheum 2007;57(2):318–26.

37. Hudson M, Pope J, Mahler M, et al. Clinical significance of antibodies to Ro52/TRIM21 in systemic sclerosis. Arthritis Res Ther 2012;14(2):R50.

38. Distler O, Assassi S, Cottin V, et al. Predictors of progression in systemic sclerosis patients with interstitial lung disease. Eur Respir J 2020;55(5). https://doi.org/10.1183/13993003.02026-2019.

39. Huang J, Maier C, Zhang Y, et al. Nintedanib inhibits macrophage activation and ameliorates vascular and fibrotic manifestations in the Fra2 mouse model of systemic sclerosis. Ann Rheum Dis 2017;76(11):1941–8.

40. Richeldi L, du Bois RM, Raghu G, et al. Efficacy and safety of nintedanib in idiopathic pulmonary fibrosis. N Engl J Med 2014;370(22):2071–82.

41. Roofeh D, Lin CJF, Goldin J, et al. Tocilizumab prevents progression of early systemic sclerosis-associated interstitial lung disease. Arthritis Rheumatol 2021;73(7):1301–10.

42. Campochiaro C, Allanore Y. An update on targeted therapies in systemic sclerosis based on a systematic review from the last 3 years. Arthritis Res Ther 2021;23(1):155.

43. Goswami RP, Ray A, Chatterjee M, et al. Rituximab in the treatment of systemic sclerosis-related interstitial lung disease: a systematic review and meta-analysis. Rheumatology 2021;60(2):557-67.

44. Campochiaro C, De Luca G, Lazzaroni MG, et al. Safety and efficacy of rituximab biosimilar (CT-P10) in systemic sclerosis: an Italian multicentre study. Rheumatology 2020;59(12):3731-6.

45. Elhai M, Boubaya M, Distler O, et al. Outcomes of patients with systemic sclerosis treated with rituximab in contemporary practice: a prospective cohort study. Ann Rheum Dis 2019;78(7):979-87.

46. Maher TM, Tudor VA, Saunders P, et al. Rituximab versus intravenous cyclophosphamide in patients with connective tissue disease-associated interstitial lung disease in the UK (RECITAL): a double-blind, double-dummy, randomised, controlled, phase 2b trial. Lancet Respir Med 2023;11(1):45-54.

47. Campochiaro C, De Luca G, Lazzaroni MG, et al. POS0890 nintedanib real-life efficacy and safety in systemic sclerosis (SSc)-interstitial lung disease (ILD): an italian multicentre preliminary study. Ann Rheum Dis 2022;81(Suppl 1):741-2.

48. Hoffmann-Vold AM, Maher TM, Philpot EE, et al. The identification and management of interstitial lung disease in systemic sclerosis: evidence-based European consensus statements. Lancet Rheumatology 2020;2(2):E71-83.

49. Khanna D, Denton CP. Integrating new therapies for systemic sclerosis-associated lung fibrosis in clinical practice. Lancet Respir Med. Jun 2021;9(6):560-2.

50. Hassoun PM, Zamanian RT, Damico R, et al. Ambrisentan and tadalafil up-front combination therapy in scleroderma-associated pulmonary arterial hypertension. Am J Respir Crit Care Med 2015;192(9):1102-10.

51. Coghlan JG, Galie N, Barbera JA, et al. Initial combination therapy with ambrisentan and tadalafil in connective tissue disease-associated pulmonary arterial hypertension (CTD-PAH): subgroup analysis from the AMBITION trial. Ann Rheum Dis 2017;76(7):1219-27.

52. Bruni C, Guignabert C, Manetti M, et al. The multifaceted problem of pulmonary arterial hypertension in systemic sclerosis. The Lancet Rheumatology 2021;3(2):e149-59.

53. Roofeh D, Jaafar S, Vummidi D, et al. Management of systemic sclerosis-associated interstitial lung disease. Curr Opin Rheumatol 2019;31(3):241-9.

54. El Aoufy K, Bruni C, Rasero L, et al. Patient preferences for systemic sclerosis treatment: a descriptive study within an Italian cohort. J Scleroderma Relat Disord 2021;6(2):165-9.

55. Bruni C, Heidenreich S, Duenas A, et al. Patient preferences for the treatment of systemic sclerosis-associated interstitial lung disease: a discrete choice experiment. Rheumatology 2022. https://doi.org/10.1093/rheumatology/keac126.

56. Khanna D, Lescoat A, Roofeh D, et al. Systemic sclerosis-associated interstitial lung disease: how to incorporate two food and drug administration-approved therapies in clinical practice. Arthritis Rheumatol 2022;74(1):13-27.

57. Roofeh D, Barratt SL, Wells AU, et al. Outcome measurement instrument selection for lung physiology in systemic sclerosis associated interstitial lung disease: A systematic review using the OMERACT filter 2.1 process. Semin Arthritis Rheum 2021;51(6):1331-41.

58. Landini N, Orlandi M, Bruni C, et al. Computed tomography predictors of mortality or disease progression in systemic sclerosis-interstitial lung disease: a systematic review. Front Med 2021;8:807982.

59. Goldin J, Elashoff R, Kim HJ, et al. Treatment of scleroderma-interstitial lung dis-ease with cyclophosphamide is associated with less progressive fibrosis on serial thoracic high-resolution CT scan than placebo: findings from the scleroderma lung study. Chest 2009;136(5):1333–40.
60. Bruni C, Chung L, Hoffmann-Vold AM, et al. High-resolution computed tomogra-phy of the chest for the screening, re-screening and follow-up of systemic sclerosis-associated interstitial lung disease: a EUSTAR-SCTC survey. Clin Exp Rheumatol 2022. https://doi.org/10.55563/clinexprheumatol/7ry6zz.
61. Hoffmann-Vold AM, Allanore Y, Bendstrup E, et al. The need for a holistic approach for SSc-ILD - achievements and ambiguity in a devastating disease. Respir Res 2020;21(1):197.
62. Wu W, Jordan S, Becker MO, et al. Prediction of progression of interstitial lung disease in patients with systemic sclerosis: the SPAR model. Ann Rheum Dis 2018;77(9):1326–32.
63. Kafaja S, Clements PJ, Wilhalme H, et al. Reliability and minimal clinically impor-tant differences of forced vital capacity: results from the Scleroderma Lung Studies (SLS-I and SLS-II). Am J Respir Crit Care Med 2018;197(5):644–52.
64. Furer V, Rondaan C, Heijstek MW, et al. 2019 update of EULAR recommendations for vaccination in adult patients with autoimmune inflammatory rheumatic dis-eases. Ann Rheum Dis 2020;79(1):39–52.
65. Curtis JR, Johnson SR, Anthony DD, et al. American College of Rheumatology Guidance for COVID-19 Vaccination in Patients With Rheumatic and Musculo-skeletal Diseases: Version 4. Arthritis Rheumatol 2022;74(5):e21–36.
66. Liem SIE, Vliet Vlieland TPM, Schoones JW, et al. The effect and safety of exer-cise therapy in patients with systemic sclerosis: a systematic review. Rheumatol Adv Pract 2019;3(2):rkz044.
67. Visca D, Mori L, Tsipouri V, et al. Effect of ambulatory oxygen on quality of life for patients with fibrotic lung disease (AmbOx): a prospective, open-label, mixed-method, crossover randomised controlled trial. Lancet Respir Med 2018;6(10):759–70.
68. Campochiaro C, Lazzaroni MG, Bruni C, et al. Open questions on the manage-ment of targeted therapies for the treatment of systemic sclerosis-interstitial lung disease: results of a EUSTAR survey based on a systemic literature review. Ther Adv Musculoskelet Dis 2022;14. 1759720X221116408.

Gastrointestinal Tract Considerations Part I

How Should a Rheumatologist Best Manage Common Upper Gastrointestinal Tract Complaints in Systemic Sclerosis?

Alannah Quinlivan, MBBS[a,b], Zsuzsanna H. McMahan, MD, MHS[c],
Eun Bong Lee, MD, PhD[d], Mandana Nikpour, MBBS, PhD[a,b],*

KEYWORDS

- Systemic sclerosis • Upper gastrointestinal tract • Dysphagia • Reflux

KEY POINTS

- Gastrointestinal symptoms (GI) are common in systemic sclerosis (SSc, affecting up to 90% of patients, yet there are few guidelines for investigation or treatment of GI complications.
- There is no evidence that immunomodulatory agents prevent or treat GI complications but promotility agents may have a role.
- In this review, we present an integrated approach to investigating and treating upper GI symptoms in SSc and highlight knowledge gaps that require further research.

INTRODUCTION

Systemic sclerosis (ie, scleroderma) is an autoimmune connective tissue disease with a heterogenous clinical presentation. It is characterized by autoimmunity, inflammation, vasculopathy and/or fibrosis of affected organs.[1] The gastrointestinal tract (GIT) is the most commonly involved internal organ system, affecting up to 90% of patients, and GIT manifestations vary broadly in terms of site and severity.[2] GIT complications have a significant impact on a variety of factors, including quality of life, physical function, mood, fatigue and sleep.[3-10] In its most severe form, GIT dysfunction significantly

[a] Department of Rheumatology, St Vincent's Hospital, 41 Victoria Parade, Fitzroy, Victoria 3065, Australia; [b] Department of Medicine, The University of Melbourne at St Vincent's Hospital, 41 Victoria Parade, Fitzroy, Victoria, Australia; [c] Division of Rheumatology, Johns Hopkins University, 5200 Eastern Avenue, Suite 5200, Mason F. Lord Building, Center Tower, Baltimore, MD, 21224, USA; [d] Division of Rheumatology, Seoul National University College of Medicine, 103 Daehak-ro, Jongno-gu, Seoul, Republic of Korea
* Corresponding author.
E-mail address: m.nikpour@unimelb.edu.au

Rheum Dis Clin N Am 49 (2023) 295–318
https://doi.org/10.1016/j.rdc.2023.01.006
0889-857X/23/© 2023 Elsevier Inc. All rights reserved.

impacts survival with an estimated 85% mortality at 9 years.[11–13] Although there are some data to suggest that intravenous immunoglobulins (IVIG) may have a positive effect on GI motility in SSc, there is no strong evidence that immunosuppressive agents are able to prevent or treat GI involvement in SSc.[14–16]

GI disease begins early in the disease process although patients may be asymptomatic at this stage.[17–19] When present, GIT symptoms are nonspecific and can be attributed to numerous sites within the GIT, yet complaints are often treated symptomatically without further investigation.[20] This may in part be due to the lack of guidelines with regard to screening and investigation of GIT symptoms, and/or a limited awareness of the possible diagnostic tests available.

The aim of this review is to provide an overview of how to assess, investigate, and treat specific GIT symptoms, and to provide details to clinicians about how to integrate investigations into clinical care. As there are few guidelines for investigation and management of GIT symptoms in SSc, the advice provided in this article is collated from the available studies in SSc, general gastroenterological guidelines and the authors' clinical experience. This review is presented in two parts. The first part focuses on assessment and management of common upper GIT symptoms including oral symptoms, dysphagia, reflux, and bloating.

Pathogenesis

The pathogenesis of GIT disease in SSc is thought to reflect systemic disease, with evidence to support the presence of autoimmunity and antibody formation, vasculopathy and increased production of profibrotic growth factors.[21,22] The precise etiology however remains unclear. The sera of patients with SSc have been shown to contain functional type 3 muscarinic receptors antibodies (M_3R) which block the cholinergic neural pathways and antivinculin antibodies, whose presence is inversely associated with interstitial cells of Cajal (ICC) or pacemaker cells in the GIT.[3,23–26] The presence of these autoantibodies has also been correlated with more severe symptoms of GIT dysmotility in patients with SSc.[3,23–26] Autoantibodies against nicotinic acetylcholine receptors (gAChR), found in the autonomic ganglia and associated with autoimmune autonomic dysfunction, have also been found in SSc patients with higher levels seen in those with GIT symptoms.[27,28] Evidence of vasculopathy can be seen in gastric antral vascular ectasia (GAVE) and capsule studies have shown vascular mucosal lesions and telangiectasias affecting the stomach, small bowel and duodenum in approximately 50% of patients with SSc.[29] Finally, autopsy studies show vascular intimal proliferation, loss of ICC in the esophagus and prominent smooth muscle atrophy with some fibrosis throughout the GIT from esophagus to colon.[22,30] Although the natural history of GI disease in SSc is presumed to progress from enteric neuron dysfunction to muscle atrophy, the exact pathologic mechanisms and how to prevent or treat these complications is yet to be fully elucidated.

Patient-Reported Outcomes

There exist several questionnaires to measure GIT symptoms and two have been validated for use in SSc (**Table 1**). The first is the University of California Los Angeles Scleroderma Clinical Trials Consortium Gastrointestinal Tract 2.0 Questionnaire (UCLA GIT). This survey is one of the most commonly used tools to measure GIT symptoms in SSc, and has been validated across many languages.[31,39] The UCLA GIT 2.0 assesses the severity of GIT symptoms experienced over the previous seven days. This questionnaire provides a total score as well as scores in five symptom domains (reflux, distension, diarrhea, constipation, and fecal incontinence) and two quality of life domains (emotional and social wellbeing). The second is the Patient-

Table 1
Gastrointestinal questionnaires

Questionnaire	Focus	Key Features (eg, Vomiting, Abdominal Pain, etc.)	Scoring (Recall)	Validated?	Tested in SSc (Y/N)
UCLA SCTC GIT 2.0 (34 items)	Upper GI Lower GI QoL	Reflux Distension/bloating Diarrhea Constipation Fecal incontinence/soilage (1 question) Social functioning Emotional well-being	Higher score = worse GI symptoms (1 week)	Yes[31]	Yes[31]
PROMIS-GI (60 items)	Upper GI Lower GI QoL	Reflux/regurgitation Distension/bloating Dysphagia Diarrhea Constipation Fecal incontinence/soilage Nausea and vomiting Abdominal pain	Higher score = worse GI symptoms (1 week)	Yes[32]	Yes[33]
MHISS (12 items)	Oral/mouth opening	Microstomia Oral Dryness Dentition Aesthetic concerns	Higher score = worse GI symptoms (indefinite)	Yes[34]	Yes[34]
GERD-Q (6 items)	GERD/upper GI	Reflux/regurgitation Upper abdominal pain Nausea Sleep interference Medication	Total score = Likelihood of GERD 0 to 2 = 0% 3 to 7 = 50% 8 to 10 = 79% 11 to 18 = 89% (1 week)	Yes[35]	Yes, shown to correlate with esophagitis in SSc[36]

(continued on next page)

Table 1 (continued)					
Questionnaire	Focus	Key Features (eg, Vomiting, Abdominal Pain, etc.)	Scoring (Recall)	Validated?	Tested in SSc (Y/N)
PAGI-SYM (20 items)	GERD/upper GI Gastroparesis GERD	Reflux/regurgitation* Nausea/vomiting Post-prandial fullness/early satiety Bloating Upper abdominal pain Lower abdominal pain	higher scores with worsening QOL with responses ranging from scale of 0 to 5 (2 weeks)	Yes[37]	No
QOLRAD (25 items)	QoL GERD/upper GI	Emotional distress sleep disturbance Vitality Food/drink problems Physical/social functioning	A low score indicates low quality of life, whereas a high score indicates better quality of life (1 week)	Yes[38]	Yes[39]
PAGI-QoL (30 items)	QoL Mood	Daily activities Clothing Diet/food habits Relationship Psychological well-being distress	0 (lowest QoL) to 5 (highest QoL) (2 weeks)	Yes[40]	No

Abbreviations: GERD, gastroesophageal reflux disease; GI, gastrointestinal; MHISS, mouth handicap in systemic sclerosis; PAGI-QoL, patient assessment of upper gastrointestinal disorders-quality of life; PAGI-SYM, patient assessment of upper gastrointestinal symptoms; PROMIS-GI, patient-reported outcomes measurement information system -gastrointestinal symptom scales; QoL, quality of life; QOLRAD, quality of life in reflux and dyspepsia; SSc, systemic sclerosis; UCLA SCTC GIT, University of California Scleroderma Clinical Trial Consortium Gastrointestinal Tract.
Data from Refs.[31–40]

Reported Outcomes Measurement Information System -Gastrointestinal Symptom Scales (PROMIS-GI), which consists of eight symptom domains including gastro-esophageal reflux, disrupted swallowing, diarrhea, bowel incontinence/soilage, nausea and vomiting, constipation, belly pain, and gas/bloat/flatulence.[39,41] Despite the fact that both surveys provide a valid means of measuring GIT symptoms in SSc, results do not always correlate with objective findings of GI dysfunction; howev-er, this may be due to the timing of administration of questionnaires in relation to investigations.[42]

Upper gastrointestinal complaints (oral, esophageal, and gastric)
Oral symptoms. Oral manifestations are common in SSc. Patients may report dry mouth/xerostomia (occurring in 60% to 80% of patients), poor dental hygiene, diffi-culty opening their mouth/microstomia (present in 60% to 91% of patients with SSc) or pain in their jaw.[43–45]

Assessment of oral symptoms Symptoms can be assessed using the Mouth Hand-icap in Systemic Sclerosis Score (MHISS), a validated questionnaire assessing oral manifestations in SSc (see **Table 1**).[46] As autoantibodies do not correlate with SICCA symptom severity and do not affect management, it is not recommended to test for them unless there is clinical concern for Sjogren's syndrome overlap.[47]

Treatment of oral symptoms General advice regarding avoidance of sugar-rich foods and medications that worsen dry mouth, hydration, use of sugar free gums to stimulate saliva production and regular dental review is recommended.[43,48,49] Pilocar-pine (a nonselective muscarinic receptor agonist) is often used in Sjogren's syndrome to increase saliva production. Another oral agent shown to be effective for the treat-ment of dry mouth in Sjogren's syndrome is cevimeline, a muscarinic receptor agonist with a stronger affinity to M3 receptors.[50] Although their use in SSc-related dry mouth has not yet been studied, given the lack of alternative treatments, and their beneficial effect on symptoms of dry mouth in other conditions such as Sjogren's syndrome,[51] both pilocarpine and cevimeline may be considered in SSc. Rehabilitation with daily facial exercises has been shown to increase mouth opening but is limited in long-term use due to compliance issues.[43,52]

Oropharyngeal Dysphagia

Dysphagia in SSc can be due to oropharyngeal or esophageal pathologies (**Fig. 1**). Symptoms associated with oropharyngeal dysphagia can include complaints of food "sticking" in the throat, a sensation of "fullness" in the neck, pain when swallow-ing, and/or coughing during or immediately after eating or drinking.[53] Oral manifesta-tions in SSc can also contribute to dysphagia and are important to identify and manage.

Assessment of oropharyngeal dysphagia
Symptoms can be assessed with SSc-specific GI questionnaires (such as UCLA and PROMIS GI) and use of the MHISS (see above) is recommended to identify and manage contributing oral manifestations. Red flag symptoms which should prompt immediate investigation with imaging (see recommended investigations below) or gastroscopy include rapidly progressive dysphagia, unexplained weight loss and dysphagia to solids only.

Lifestyle measures for oropharyngeal dysphagia
In absence of red flag symptoms, recommendations should be made to modify eating behaviors. Advising patients to sit upright when eating, decrease the size of the food

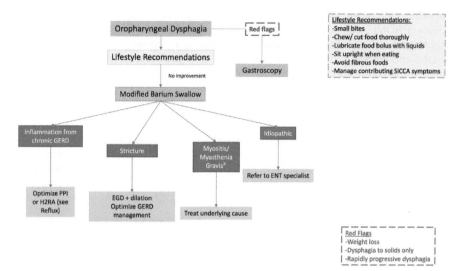

Fig. 1. Oropharyngeal dysphagia. [a]confirm with CK aldolase, myositis Ab (myositis) and anti-AChR, MuSK or LRP4 Ab (MG).

bolus by taking small bites, cutting and chewing their food well, avoiding fibrous foods and using water, sauce or gravy to lubricate the food bolus may improve symptoms.[54,55]

Recommended investigations for oropharyngeal dysphagia

Modified Barium Swallow Study (MBSS) is considered as one of the gold-standard tests in the diagnosis of pharyngeal dysphagia and can be useful as a first line tool for assessing the site of pathology in dysphagia.[56] MBSS otherwise known as Video fluoroscopic swallowing study (VFSS) evaluates the oropharyngeal part of swallowing and is used to assess swallowing impairments, airway protection (safety of oral intake) and efficiency (clearance of food) through administration of boluses of various consistencies (soft, thick, etc.) and volumes.[53] This study does involve radiation exposure; however, it would be considered a low-dose radiation study, less than that of a mammogram.[53] MBSS is contraindicated in patients who have a reduced conscious state, are unable to follow instructions, or have an allergy to the contrast material used (most commonly barium).[53] If the MBSS reveals a structural cause of dysphagia, such as stricture, referral should be made to a gastroenterologist for consideration of dilatation. Evidence of pharyngeal dysphagia should prompt consideration of myositis/ overlap syndromes or myasthenia gravis.[57,58] Depending on the clinical picture, a finding of pharyngeal dysphagia may warrant investigation of myositis with clinical assessment of muscle weakness and measurement of serum CK and/or aldolase.[59] Autoantibodies associated with clinical myositis in SSc include PM/Scl (75 or 100), U1RNP and anti-Ku; however, a third of these patients may be autoantibody negative.[60–62] Alternatively, if there are clinical features suggestive of Myasthenia Gravis (MG), such as fatigability, autoantibodies such as anti-acetylcholine receptor (AChR), anti–muscle-specific tyrosine kinase (anti-MuSK) or anti-low-density lipoprotein receptor-related protein 4 (LRP4) should be tested.[63]

Treatment of oropharyngeal dysphagia

Management of oropharyngeal dysphagia involves the identification and treatment of underlying causes and minimization of aspiration risk.[59] If a myositis overlap syndrome is diagnosed, treatment would consist of immune suppression that can have a positive effect on both symptoms and objective findings in dysphagia secondary to Idiopathic Inflammatory Myopathies.[64]

Esophageal Dysphagia

Esophageal dysmotility can present with dysphagia to both solids and liquids, regurgitation or vomiting, sensation of food getting stuck or chest pain.[65] There is evidence that esophageal dysmotility is present in up to 85% of early SSc although it may be asymptomatic.[17,66]

Assessment of esophageal dysphagia

Symptoms, when present, can be assessed with SSc-specific GI questionnaires (such as UCLA GIT 2.0 and PROMIS GI). Although PROMIS-GI offers more in-depth questions as to the cause of dysphagia, UCLA GIT reflux and total scores have been shown to be associated with esophageal dysmotility on high-resolution manometry (HRM).[67,68] Red flag symptoms are the same as for oropharyngeal dysphagia.

Lifestyle measures for esophageal dysphagia

In the absence of red flag symptoms, recommendations should be made to modify eating behaviors as recommended in the previous section regarding oropharyngeal dysphagia as well as maintaining an upright posture following meals or elevating the head of the bed.[54,55]

Investigation of esophageal dysphagia

HRM is currently the gold standard for diagnosing esophageal motility disorders.[69] It involves insertion of a catheter extending from the hypopharynx to the stomach with pressure sensors spaced 1 to 2 cm apart (in contrast to standard manometry where sensors are 3 to 5 cm apart). The pressures generated by the esophagus are measured and allow insight into the function of sphincters and peristaltic waves of the esophagus.[69] Measurements are taken at rest and after swallowing in upright and supine positions. In SSc the most common findings are that of absent contractility, ineffective esophageal motility (IEM) and/or a hypotensive lower esophageal sphincter (LES).[70]

When HRM is unavailable or not tolerated by the patient, high-resolution computed tomography (CT) (HRCT) of the chest may also be useful for predicting esophageal pathology. Esophageal dilatation on CT (width >10 mm) is associated with HRM findings of esophageal dysmotility (OR 14.67, $p = 0.002$) and "scleroderma esophagus" (ie, absent contractility and hypotensive LES), whereas food in the esophagus observed on upper endoscopy is also associated with esophageal dysmotility on HRM (OR 6.85, $p = 0.05$).[71,72]

Novel investigations

Multiple rapid swallows (MRS) can be performed during HRM and may have a role in predicting which patients will respond to prokinetics. This test involves multiple small water swallows less than 3 s apart while the patient is in the supine position. In normal individuals the intense contractions/peristalsis provoked after the final swallow (deglutitive excitation) involve both cholinergic and non-cholinergic mechanisms.[73] Approximately 25% of SSc patients with IEM may respond normally to MRS,[74] indicating their muscles are still able to respond when given appropriate stimulus and these patients may respond best to prokinetics.[73]

Treatment of esophageal dysphagia

With regards to esophageal dysmotility, international guidelines recommend the use of promotility agents for the management of symptoms of esophageal dysmotility although there is minimal evidence from clinical trials to support this practice.[75,76] There is evidence that agents such as cisapride, metoclopramide, erythromycin, buspirone, and domperidone increase LES pressure and promote esophageal motility (refer to **Table 2** for dosages and adverse effects).[77–81] Unfortunately, there are no large randomized controlled trials to support their therapeutic benefit in SSc or long-term data as to the efficacy of these agents in managing symptoms of esophageal dysmotility. In addition, there are major safety concerns regarding cisapride and domperidone particularly with regards to arrhythmias; therefore their availability internationally is variable.[82] Although data to support the use of prokinetics in SSc esophageal disease are limited, in patients with severe symptoms treatment options can also be limited. Therefore, a trial of prokinetic agents should be considered to improve QoL after careful consideration of risks associated with treatment.

Table 2
Management

Medication	Common Doses	Uses	Serious Adverse Effects
Prokinetics	Prucalopride 2 mg daily	Constipation ↓ gastroparesis sx	
	Metoclopramide 5 to 10 mg (up to 4x daily)	↑LES pressure ↑ esophageal motility ↑gastric emptying	Tremors Tardive dyskinesia Anxiety
	Erythromycin (IV 2 mg/kg/h)	↑gastric emptying	Arrhythmias and sudden death
	Buspirone 20 mg daily	↑LES pressure ↑ esophageal motility	
	Domperidone 10 mg (up to 3x daily)	↓GERD symptoms	Arrhythmias and sudden death
PPI	Esomeprazole 40 mg daily/twice daily Lansoprazole 30 mg daily/twice daily Pantoprazole 40 mg daily/twice daily Omeprazole 20 mg daily/twice daily Rabeprazole 20 mg daily/twice daily	GERD Gastritis Gastric ulcer	Electrolyte abnormalities (hypocalcemia, hypomagnesemia, hypokalemia) SIBO
H2RA	Cimetidine 400 mg twice daily Famotidine 20 mg twice daily Nizatidine 150 mg twice daily Ranitidine 150 mg twice daily	GERD Gastritis Reflux hypersensitivity	Hepatotoxicity
Potassium-competitive acid blocker	Vonoprazan 20 mg daily	GERD Gastritis Gastric ulcer	

Abbreviations: GERD, gastroesophageal reflux disease; IV, intravenous; LES, lower esophageal sphincter.

Heartburn or Acid Reflux

Gastroesophageal reflux disease (GERD) (**Fig. 2**) is commonly encountered in SSc patients with up to 76% to 79% complaining of heartburn (burning sensation rising from epigastrium to neck), acid reflux (a sensation of bitter or sour fluid coming up from stomach into mouth) or regurgitation (reflux of food into esophagus).[83,84] Other extra-esophageal symptoms include cough, voice hoarseness and laryngitis.

Assessment of gastroesophageal reflux disease

The utility SSc-specific questionnaires (such as UCLA GIT and PROMIS-GI) for prediction of esophagitis is variable, in part due to the diverse esophageal complications seen in SSc.[42,85] GERD-Q is a validated reflux questionnaire which, while not SSc-specific, has been found to have a sensitivity and specificity of 96.9% and 50% respectively in predicting GERD in SSc as assessed by pH-metry.[36] In the event of atypical or red flag symptoms (such as weight loss, suspected GI bleeding, anemia, or dysphagia) gastroscopy is recommended as a first-line investigation before initiation of lifestyle measures or gastric acid suppression.[86] In addition, if there is clinical concern for alternative diagnoses such as eosinophilic esophagitis (EoE) (in the context of prolonged steroid use) or Barrett's esophagus (in patients with longstanding, poorly controlled GERD symptoms) gastroscopy is recommended.

Initial management and lifestyle measures for gastroesophageal reflux disease

First line treatment consists of lifestyle modification and dietary intervention. Patients should be advised to eat smaller meals, ensure adequate time between eating dinner and bed (at least 2 to 3 h), elevate the head of the bed and avoid precipitant foods (caffeine, alcohol, chocolate).[87] Post-prandial diaphragmatic breathing or "deep belly breathing" (discussed here[88]) may also help decrease symptoms of GERD.[89]

If lifestyle measures are insufficient to manage symptoms, gastric acid suppression using daily proton pump inhibitor (PPI) or H2 receptor antagonists (H2RA) is the next recommended step. The American College of Gastroenterology (ACG) recommends commencing treatment with 8 weeks of daily PPI (taken before meals) if typical

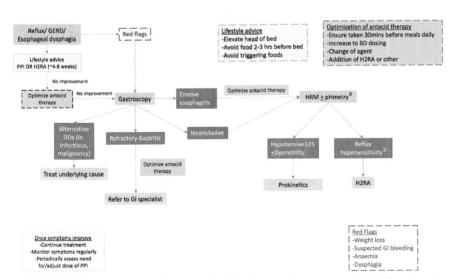

Fig. 2. Reflux/GERD/esophageal dysphagia. [a]High-resolution manometry with pH-metry. [b]Non-acid reflux that triggers symptoms.

symptoms (heartburn, regurgitation) are present without the need for further investigation.[86] If prescribing a PPI, ensuring it is taken correctly (ie, 30 to 60 min before meals) and increasing to twice daily dosing may improve symptoms.[86,90] PPIs are recommended in the general population first line as they have superior healing of erosive esophagitis (EE) and faster relief of symptoms compared with H2 receptor antagonists (H2RA).[91,92] However, there have been no head-to-head trials in SSc. H2RA have been shown to reduce esophageal acid sensitivity and so are also recommended in the management of reflux hypersensitivity (non-acid reflux that precipitates symptoms of heartburn/acid reflux), which may account for GERD symptoms in up to in 43% of patients with SSc.[93,94] H2RA agents (such as ranitidine, nizatidine, famotidine, and cimetidine) may also have some benefit in managing nocturnal acid secretion, which largely depends on histamine release,[95] although there are limited data to support this clinically in SSc.

Recommended investigations for gastroesophageal reflux disease symptoms

Esophagogastroduodenoscopy or gastroscopy (EGD) is recommended by the ACG as a tool for the assessment of refractory GERD (those who have failed a trial of PPI) or as a first line investigation in patients with red flag/atypical symptoms.[86] EGD is used to assess gastric/and esophageal mucosa with findings of EE or Barrett's esophagus considered diagnostic for GERD. It can also be helpful in assessing for diagnostic differentials including Candida esophagus, EoE, hiatal hernias as well as complications of GERD, including strictures.[96] Ideally, it is recommended to perform EGD when the patient is off PPI treatment for 2 to 4 weeks prior as it may disguise endoscopic and histologic features of underlying EE and EoE. However, this may not be feasible in patients with SSc with severe symptoms.[86] If a patient is unable to tolerate withdrawal of PPI due to severity of symptoms or continues to suffer reflux in absence of findings on EGD, pH-metry with impedance could be considered.

Multichannel intraluminal impedance monitoring combined with pH-metry (MII-pH) would be recommended in patients with symptomatic reflux despite PPI therapy. The procedure involves insertion of a catheter transnasally after a 4 to 6 h fast, which is left *in situ* for 24 h and connected to a monitor typically worn on the patient's belt. The patient is also required to keep a diary of the timing of meals and symptoms. There can be some discomfort and complications with regards to the insertion of the catheter (throat discomfort and occasionally epistaxis); however, it is mostly reported to be well tolerated. MII-pH uses paired sensors spaced throughout the esophagus (with placing determined by manometry) which are able to detect a bolus passing between them. The sensors are triggered by a change in the resistance to current flow which provides information on the site (proximal or distal), volume and composition (gas, liquid, acidity) of the refluxate as well as its relation to symptoms. One of the advantages of this test is its ability to relate symptoms with reflux episodes. MII-pH is considered abnormal if either the number of reflux episodes is abnormal or there is found to be a positive association between reflux episodes and patient symptoms.[97–100] The results of MII-pH may show failure of acid suppression despite PPI use (with pathologic acid exposure/PAE), non-acid reflux due to dysmotility or LES hypotension, or it could reveal no correlation between reflux episodes and symptoms. Ensuring adequate acid suppression is important given that the extent of esophageal acid exposure has been associated with increased risk of ILD in patients with SSc.[101,102] The data from MII-pH provides guidance as to whether enhancement of acid suppression would benefit the patient's symptom control. It is therefore an important study that helps to avoid excessive acid suppression and reduces long-term consequences of PPI use such as small intestinal bacterial overgrowth. Although there are newer methods involving wireless telemetry capsules, these are only available for pH monitoring (not impedance) and have not yet been tested in SSc.

Additional treatments for gastroesophageal reflux disease

Vonoprazan, a novel potassium-competitive acid blocker, works through inhibition of proton pump potassium–exchange. In SSc, vonoprazan effectively facilitated the healing of EE, significantly improved symptoms of reflux in treatment refractory GERD, and was well-tolerated by patients.[103–105] Unfortunately, vonoprazan is not widely available at this time.

Esophageal dysmotility and hypotensive LES can both contribute to refractory reflux symptoms in SSc. Therefore, prokinetics which may improve both of these parameters, may be indicated for symptom control.[93,106–108] A recent meta-analysis of 2400 patients evaluated the addition of prokinetics to PPI-refractory GERD in the general population. The investigators found that, compared with PPI alone, combination therapy was associated with some improvement in QoL and reduction in reflux episodes although this approach did not decrease acid exposure time or complications of EE.[109] Baclofen has been shown to decrease transient LES relaxation and reduce acid exposure time as well as the number and length of reflux episodes.[110,111] However, there have been no studies to date evaluating the efficacy of baclofen in SSc-GI disease. Baclofen may also result in more adverse events than 5HT agonists including dizziness, drowsiness and headaches, which may limit its use in patients.[96,109]

More recently, two small studies examined the efficacy and safety of buspirone (a 5-HT1A receptor agonist)[81] and prucalopride (a 5HT4 receptor agonist)[112] on upper GI symptoms in SSc over a 4 week period. Buspirone 20 mg daily (open label) increased LES pressures and decreased symptoms of heartburn and regurgitation in consecutive SSc patients with upper GI symptoms on PPI treatment.[81] Reflux (as measured by UCLA GIT) was also improved in a crossover study of 40 SSc patients treated with prucalopride 2 mg/day for chronic constipation.[112]

Probiotics

There is some evidence to support the use of daily probiotics alone to improve reflux symptoms in SSc although results are mixed. One open label study of 10 patients with SSc showed daily use of either Bifidobacterium or lactobacillus containing probiotics significantly reduced symptoms of reflux (as measured by UCLA GIT).[113] However, this effect was not seen in an 8-week randomized placebo controlled study of 73 patients taking a multi-strain probiotic (containing Bifidobacterium and lactobacillus), which did not significantly improve symptoms of reflux compared with placebo.[114] This result was again seen in a double blind, randomized controlled trial of multi-strain probiotic (containing *Bifidobacterium*, *Lactobacillus*, and *Streptococcus*) for 60 days.[115] However, in this trial patients who received 120 days of the same probiotic did show reduced reflux symptoms.[115] Importantly there were minimal side effects reported in all studies.

Bloating and Early Satiety

Bloating can be due to gastric, small or large bowel causes and is not always easy to distinguish on history alone (**Fig. 3**). If diarrhea is also a prominent feature, differentials such as small intestinal bacterial overgrowth (SIBO), fructose and lactose malabsorption should be considered, whereas significant abdominal pain and constipation may indicate pseudo-obstruction[116,117] (discussed below). Gastroparesis can present with abdominal bloating in 75% of cases as well as nausea (92%), vomiting (84%), and

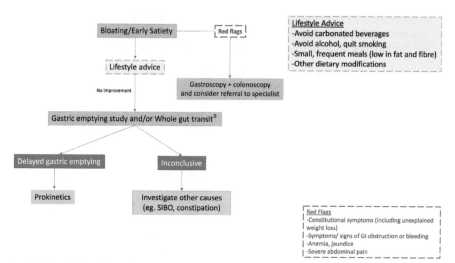

Fig. 3. Bloating/early satiety. [a]Using Whole gut transit scintigraphy or Wireless motility capsule (smart pill).

early satiety (60%) although symptoms do not always correlate with objective findings.[118–120] Gastroparesis occurs in approximately 50% of patients with SSc and associations with SSc clinical phenotype are conflicting.[119–123]

Assessment of gastroparesis and delayed gastric emptying
The UCLA reflux and distension domains show a modest association with delayed gastric emptying in patients with SSc.[119,124] Patient Assessment of Gastrointestinal Symptoms (PAGI-SYM) (**Table 3**) is validated for use in gastroparesis in patients without SSc and includes the Gastroparesis Cardinal Symptom Index (GCSI) which is commonly used to characterize symptoms of gastroparesis in the broader gastroenterology literature.[125] If red flag symptoms such as constitutional symptoms, unexplained weight loss, signs or symptoms of GI bleeding, anemia, jaundice or severe abdominal pain are present, then investigation with upper and lower GI endoscopy should be considered. Symptoms or signs of pseudo obstruction should prompt referral for abdominal imaging which might include (X-ray or CT scan).

Lifestyle measures for gastroparesis
Lifestyle measures include partaking in multiple, small meals low in fat and fiber and avoidance of carbonated beverages, smoking and alcohol.[126,127] If concern regarding malnutrition arises, nutritious high calorie drinks and careful monitoring of electrolytes should be considered.[128]

Recommended investigations for gastroparesis
The gold standard diagnosis of delayed gastric emptying requires either scintigraphy (which can be done with a solid, liquid or combined meal, with combined meal found to be more sensitive in SSc), or stable isotope breath test, both of which involve ingestion of a radio-labelled meal after an overnight fast; testing generally takes approximately 4 h.[119,127] Gastric emptying scintigraphy then requires images taken at baseline and 1, 2, and 4 h in a standing position with abnormalities at 2 and/or 4 h diagnostic for gastroparesis. During breath testing (using *Spirulina platensis* or octanoic acid as a substrate) the radiolabeled carbon is released during digestion into expired

Table 3
Assessment of upper gastrointestinal tract symptoms

Symptoms/ Indication for Study	Differential	Red Flags	Possible Investigations
Upper dysphagia/ oropharyngeal dysphagia/Globus sensation	Proximal esophageal Dysmotility Sicca syndrome Pharyngeal myositis Myasthenia gravis	Weight loss Muscle weakness Coughing after meals/recurrent aspiration pneumonia	*Bloods* CK and aldolase *Autoantibodies* Myositis (PM-Scl, Ku/ U1RNP) MG (AChR, anti-MuSK, anti-LRP4 *Imaging* Modified Barium swallow/VFSS
Lower dysphagia/ regurgitation/ coughing	*Motility* Esophageal dysmotility LES dysfunction *Structural* Esophageal strictures Hiatal hernia Malignancy *Infection* Eosinophilic esophagitis Esophageal candidiasis and/or other infection	Weight loss Problems with solids only History of poorly controlled reflux	*Imaging* HRM Barium swallow HRCT (food in esophagus, esophageal dilatation) *Procedures* EGD
Acid reflux	GERD Hiatus hernia		*Procedure* EGD HRM/pH-metry
Nausea/early satiety/ vomiting /bloating	*Upper GI* Abnormal gastric Accommodation delayed gastric emptying/ gastroparesis Esophageal dysmotility Peptic ulcer disease *Lower GI* SIBO Coeliac disease Lactose intolerance Fructose malabsorption Pseudo-obstruction CIPO PCI	Constipation Weight loss Overflow diarrhea	*Imaging* AXR Gastric emptying scintigraphy or breath test Whole gut transit study *Procedure* EGD *Bloods* Autoantibodies (anti-endomysial and tissue transglutaminase) *Breath tests* Glucose/lactulose Lactose/fructose *Imaging* Gastric emptying study AXR

(continued on next page)

Table 3 (continued)			
Symptoms/ Indication for Study	Differential	Red Flags	Possible Investigations
			Whole gut transit study *Procedures* EGD/gastric and duodenal biopsy

Abbreviations: AChR, anti-acetylcholine receptor; anti-LRP4, anti-low-density lipoprotein receptor-related protein 4; anti-MuSK, anti–muscle-specific tyrosine kinase; AXR, abdominal x-ray; CIPO, chronic intestinal pseudo-obstruction; CK, creatinine kinase; EGD, esophagogastroduodenoscopy; FBE, full blood exam; FOBT, fecal occult blood test; GERD, gastroesophageal reflux disease; GI, gastrointestinal; HRCT, high resolution computed tomography; HRM, high-resolution manometry (HRM) with impedance monitoring; LES, lower esophageal sphincter; PCI, Pneumatosis cystoides intestinalis; PCR, polymerase chain reaction; SIBO, small intestinal bacterial overgrowth; VFSS, video fluoroscopic swallow study.

air and measured 4 to 6 h later.[126,129] Barium studies are of limited diagnostic value even in moderate to severe symptoms.[129] Whole gut transit/WGT scintigraphy may also be used to measure gastric emptying times. Although the test takes up to 72 h to complete, it is able to investigate slow transit in other areas of the bowel, which is a common finding in SSc patients with gastroparesis.[119,126,129] Novel methods of investigation include magnetic tracking system (MTS), wireless motility capsule (SmartPill)[130] and gastric ultrasound[131]; however, these are not readily accessible in most centers. Gastric ultrasound is also operator-dependent and only reliable for liquid emptying rates.[127]

Additional management of gastroparesis

Prokinetic medications can be used to increase both tone and amplitude of gastric contractions and relax the pyloric sphincter. Although metoclopramide, erythromycin and domperidone have been shown to improve gastric emptying in SSc and general populations, their toxicities limit their use.[79,123,132,133] Mirtazapine improves symptoms of gastroparesis in the general population and may have a role in patients with associated nausea and/or weight loss.[134] Due to potential cardiac side effects, monitoring with regular ECGs may be indicated. Buspirone enhances post-prandial gastric accommodation in the general population.[135] In SSc, ghrelin infusions have been shown to improve symptoms and gastric emptying times.[136] Prucalopride improves symptoms of gastroparesis in the general population and may have a particular role in patients with gastroparesis and associated slow colonic transit.[112,137]

Miscellaneous

Although GAVE does not present with GI symptoms, it is an important complication affecting 1-5% of patients with SSc and should be considered in patients presenting with iron deficiency anaemia.[138,139] It is more common among patients with anti-RNA-polymerase 3 antibodies.[138,140,141] Diagnosis is made via upper GI endoscopy which shows the characteristic "watermelon stomach" consisting of multiple longitudinal columns of blood vessels. Conservative management, for chronic non-life-threatening bleeds, would be iron replacement (with caution to prevent constipation) and volume repletion (with blood or IV fluids).[139] Endoscopic management can consist of argon plasma coagulation (APC), laser photocoagulation or endoscopic band ligation and may require multiple treatments.[21,142] Radiofrequency ablation (RFA) has also been shown to be effective in the event of APC failure and multiple case reports show cyclo-phosphamide to be useful in patient's refractory to endoscopic management.[21,143-145]

Conclusion and Recommendations

The upper GI tract is frequently involved in SSc and may impact quality of life, physical function and survival. Although we are currently very proactive in terms of screening for heart and lung involvement, patients with SSc are not routinely screened for GI involvement. This review has detailed the available investigations for common upper GI symptoms in SSc, including dysphagia, reflux and bloating and provided advice as to how to integrate these investigations into current clinical care. Identifying SSc patient subgroups who are at high risk of GI progression, determining whether base-line screening studies of GI function should be completed in asymptomatic patients, and determining the optimal utilization of these investigations longitudinally in the monitoring of GI progression, are all important areas of future study.

CLINICS CARE POINTS

Prokinetic/promotility agent practice points
- Promotility agents may have some effect early in disease; however, they are ineffective in late disease due to smooth muscle atrophy and do not prevent disease progression.[146,147]
- In the absence of literature and guidelines, the authors recommend consideration of a trial in patients (subject to availability) with caution regarding toxicities. As many of these medications are also not without risk, the authors advise proof and documentation of dysmotility where feasible, before starting prokinetics.
- Further studies regarding the efficacy of newer agents with less toxicities (such as prucalopride) in SSc is recommended.

Dysphagia practice points
- Modified barium/video fluoroscopy swallow study (MBSS/VFSS) is a noninvasive test that can be undertaken to investigate oropharyngeal dysphagia and risk of aspiration
- Red flags on history are weight loss, rapidly progressive dysphagia or dysphagia to solids only, and history of poorly controlled reflux. Red flag symptoms should prompt investigation with gastroscopy.
- Treatment of oropharyngeal dysphagia consists of minimizing aspiration risk and treatment of underlying cause
- Prokinetics should be considered for treatment of esophageal dysphagia, particularly when symptoms are bothersome to the patient.

Reflux practice points
- Typical symptoms of reflux (such as heartburn and acid reflux) should be treated empirically with lifestyle measures and a trial of PPI.
- Red flag symptoms (weight loss, suspected gastrointestinal [GI] bleeding, anemia or dysphagia) should be investigated immediately with esophagogastroduodenoscopy or gastroscopy (EGD).
- EGD and pH-metry are not required for diagnosis and should not be undertaken unless there is failure to respond to proton pump inhibitor (PPI) or red flag symptoms are present.
- In refractory reflux, PPI can be increased and additional agents added, though data in SSc are limited.

Bloating practice points
- Bloating can be due to several pathologies and careful history can help direct investigations
- Gastroparesis occurs in up to 50% of patients with SSc and is associated with slowed transit in other areas of the GI tract
- Mirtazapine, buspirone, and prucalopride may provide some relief of symptoms of gastroparesis if lifestyles measures prove ineffective

---

FUNDING

NIH, United States/NIAMS, United States K23 AR071473, Rheumatology Research Foundation, Scleroderma Research Foundation, and Jerome L. Greene Foundation to Z.H. McMahan.

REFERENCES

1. Gu YS, Kong J, Cheema GS, et al. The immunobiology of systemic sclerosis. Semin Arthritis Rheum 2008;38(2):132–60.
2. Sjogren RW. Gastrointestinal motility disorders in scleroderma. Review. Arthritis Rheum 1994;37(9):1265–82.
3. Ebert E. Gastric and enteric involvement in progressive systemic sclerosis. J Clin Gastroenterol 2008;42(1):5–12.
4. Faezi ST, Paragomi P, Shahali A, et al. Prevalence and severity of depression and anxiety in patients with systemic sclerosis: an epidemiologic survey and investigation of clinical correlates. J Clin Rheumatol 2017;23(2):80–6.
5. Bodukam V, Hays RD, Maranian P, et al. Association of gastrointestinal involvement and depressive symptoms in patients with systemic sclerosis. Research Support, N.I.H., Extramural. Rheumatology 2011;50(2):330–4.
6. Frantz C, Avouac J, Distler O, et al. Impaired quality of life in systemic sclerosis and patient perception of the disease: a large international survey. Elsevier; 2016. p. 115–23.
7. Franck-Larsson K, Graf W, Rönnblom A. Lower gastrointestinal symptoms and quality of life in patients with systemic sclerosis: a population-based study. Eur J Gastroenterol Hepatol 2009;21(2):176–82.
8. Sharif R, Mayes MD, Nicassio PM, et al. Determinants of work disability in patients with systemic sclerosis: a longitudinal study of the GENISOS cohort. Elsevier; 2011. p. 38–47.
9. Basta F, Afeltra A, Margiotta DPE. Fatigue in systemic sclerosis: a systematic review. Systematic Review. Clin Exp Rheumatol 2018;36(Suppl 113 4):150–60.
10. Horsley-Silva JL, Umar SB, Vela MF, et al. The impact of gastroesophageal reflux disease symptoms in scleroderma: effects on sleep quality. Dis Esophagus 2019;32(5):doy136.
11. Steen VD, Medsger TA Jr. Severe organ involvement in systemic sclerosis with diffuse scleroderma. Arthritis Rheum 2000;43(11):2437–44.
12. Hoffmann-Vold A-M, Volkmann ER. Gastrointestinal involvement in systemic sclerosis: Effects on morbidity and mortality and new therapeutic approaches. Journal of Scleroderma and Related Disorders 2019;6(1):37–43.
13. Richard N, Hudson M, Wang M, et al. Severe gastrointestinal disease in very early systemic sclerosis is associated with early mortality. Rheumatology 2019;58(4):636–44.
14. Richard N, Gyger G, Hoa S, et al. Immunosuppression does not prevent severe gastrointestinal tract involvement in systemic sclerosis. Clin Exp Rheumatol 2021;39(4):S142–8.
15. Raja J, Nihtyanova SI, Murray CD, et al. Sustained benefit from intravenous immunoglobulin therapy for gastrointestinal involvement in systemic sclerosis. Rheumatology 2016;55(1):115–9.
16. Kumar S, Singh J, Kedika R, et al. Role of muscarinic-3 receptor antibody in systemic sclerosis: correlation with disease duration and effects of IVIG. Am J Physiol Gastrointest Liver Physiol 2016;310(11):G1052–60.

17. Vettori S, Tolone S, Capocotta D, et al. Esophageal high-resolution impedance manometry alterations in asymptomatic patients with systemic sclerosis: prevalence, associations with disease features, and prognostic value. Clin Rheumatol 2018;37(5):1239–47.
18. Luciano L, Granel B, Bernit E, et al. Esophageal and anorectal involvement in systemic sclerosis: a systematic assessment with high resolution manometry. Clin Exp Rheumatol 2016;34(Suppl 100 5):63–9.
19. Lepri G, Guiducci S, Bellando-Randone S, et al. Evidence for oesophageal and anorectal involvement in very early systemic sclerosis (VEDOSS): report from a single VEDOSS/EUSTAR centre. Ann Rheum Dis 2015;74(1):124–8.
20. Kumar S, Singh J, Rattan S, et al. pathogenesis and clinical manifestations of gastrointestinal involvement in systemic sclerosis. Aliment Pharmacol Ther 2017;45(7):883–98.
21. McFarlane IM, Bhamra MS, Kreps A, et al. Gastrointestinal manifestations of systemic sclerosis. Rheumatology 2018;8(1):235.
22. D'Angelo WA, Fries JF, Masi AT, et al. Pathologic observations in systemic sclerosis (scleroderma): a study of fifty-eight autopsy cases and fifty-eight matched controls. Am J Med 1969;46(3):428–40.
23. Goldblatt F, Gordon TP, Waterman SA. Antibody-mediated gastrointestinal dysmotility in scleroderma. Gastroenterology 2002;123(4):1144–50.
24. Kawaguchi Y, Nakamura Y, Matsumoto I, et al. Muscarinic-3 acetylcholine receptor autoantibody in patients with systemic sclerosis: contribution to severe gastrointestinal tract dysmotility. Ann Rheum Dis 2009;68(5):710.
25. Suliman Y, Kafaja S, Oh SJ, et al. Anti-vinculin antibodies in scleroderma (SSc): a potential link between autoimmunity and gastrointestinal system involvement in two SSc cohorts. Clin Rheumatol 2020. https://doi.org/10.1007/s10067-020-05479-5.
26. Singh J, Mehendiratta V, Del Galdo F, et al. Immunoglobulins from scleroderma patients inhibit the muscarinic receptor activation in internal anal sphincter smooth muscle cells. Am J Physiol Gastrointest Liver Physiol 2009;297(6): G1206–13.
27. Nakane S, Umeda M, Kawashiri S-y, et al. Detecting gastrointestinal manifestations in patients with systemic sclerosis using anti-gAChR antibodies. Arthritis Res Ther 2020;22(1):32.
28. Imamura M, Mukaino A, Takamatsu K, et al. Ganglionic acetylcholine receptor antibodies and autonomic dysfunction in autoimmune rheumatic diseases. Int J Mol Sci 2020;21(4):1332.
29. Marie I, Antonietti M, Houivet E, et al. Gastrointestinal mucosal abnormalities using videocapsule endoscopy in systemic sclerosis. Multicenter Study Research Support, Non-U.S. Gov't. Alimentary Pharmacology & Therapeutics 2014;40(2): 189–99.
30. Roberts CG, Hummers LK, Ravich WJ, et al. A case–control study of the pathology of oesophageal disease in systemic sclerosis (scleroderma). Gut 2006; 55(12):1697–703.
31. Khanna D, Hays R, Maranian P, et al. Reliability, validity, and minimally important differences of the UCLA scleroderma clinical trial consortium gastrointestinal tract (UCLA SCTC 2.0) instrument. Arthritis Rheum 2009;10:603.
32. Spiegel BMR, Hays RD, Bolus R, et al. Development of the NIH Patient-Reported Outcomes Measurement Information System (PROMIS) gastrointestinal symptom scales. Am J Gastroenterol 2014;109(11):1804–14.

33. Nagaraja V, Hays RD, Khanna PP, et al. Construct validity of the patient-reported outcomes measurement information system gastrointestinal symptom scales in systemic sclerosis. Arthritis Care Res 2014;66(11):1725–30.

34. Mouthon L, Rannou F, Berezne A, et al. Development and validation of a scale for mouth handicap in systemic sclerosis: the Mouth Handicap in Systemic Sclerosis scale. Validation Study. Ann Rheum Dis 2007;66(12):1651–5.

35. Jonasson C, Wernersson B, Hoff DA, et al. Validation of the GerdQ questionnaire for the diagnosis of gastro-oesophageal reflux disease. Aliment Pharmacol Ther 2013;37(5):564–72.

36. Chunlertrith K, Noiprasit A, Foocharoen C, et al. GERD questionnaire for diagnosis of gastroesophageal reflux disease in systemic sclerosis. Clin Exp Rheumatol 2014;32(Suppl 86):98–102.

37. Rentz AM, Kahrilas P, Stanghellini V, et al. Development and psychometric evaluation of the patient assessment of upper gastrointestinal symptom severity index (PAGI-SYM) in patients with upper gastrointestinal disorders. Qual Life Res 2004;13(10):1737–49.

38. Wiklund IK, Junghard O, Grace E, et al. Quality of Life in Reflux and Dyspepsia patients. Psychometric documentation of a new disease-specific questionnaire (QOLRAD). Eur J Surg Suppl 1998;(583):41–9.

39. McMahan ZH, Frech T, Berrocal V, et al. Longitudinal Assessment of Patient-reported Outcome Measures in Systemic Sclerosis Patients with Gastroesophageal Reflux Disease - Scleroderma Clinical Trials Consortium. Research Support, Non-U.S. Gov't. J Rheumatol 2019;46(1):78–84.

40. de la Loge C, Trudeau E, Marquis P, et al. Cross-cultural development and validation of a patient self-administered questionnaire to assess quality of life in upper gastrointestinal disorders: the PAGI-QOL. Qual Life Res 2004;13(10):1751–62.

41. Kwakkenbos L, Thombs BD, Khanna D, et al. Performance of the Patient-Reported Outcomes Measurement Information System-29 in scleroderma: a Scleroderma Patient-centered Intervention Network Cohort Study. Multicenter Study Validation Study. Rheumatology 2017;56(8):1302–11.

42. Zampatti N, Garaiman A, Jordan S, et al. Performance of the UCLA Scleroderma Clinical Trials Consortium Gastrointestinal Tract 2.0 instrument as a clinical decision aid in the routine clinical care of patients with systemic sclerosis. Arthritis Res Ther 2021;23(1):1–11.

43. Veale B, Jablonski R, Frech T, et al. Orofacial manifestations of systemic sclerosis. Br Dent J 2016;221(6):305–10.

44. Avouac J, Sordet C, Depinay C, et al. Systemic sclerosis–associated Sjögren's syndrome and relationship to the limited cutaneous subtype: Results of a prospective study of sicca syndrome in 133 consecutive patients. Arthritis Rheum 2006;54(7):2243–9.

45. Smirani R, Poursac N, Naveau A, et al. Orofacial consequences of systemic sclerosis: A systematic review. Journal of Scleroderma and Related Disorders 2018;3(1):81–90.

46. Abdouh I, Porter S, Fedele S, et al. Validity and reliability of the Mouth Handicap of Systemic Sclerosis questionnaire in a UK population. J Oral Pathol Med 2020;49(10):986–93.

47. Salliot C, Mouthon L, Ardizzone M, et al. Sjögren's syndrome is associated with and not secondary to systemic sclerosis. Rheumatology 2007;46(2):321–6.

48. Crincoli V, Fatone L, Fanelli M, et al. Orofacial manifestations and temporomandibular disorders of systemic scleroderma: an observational study. Int J Mol Sci 2016;17(7):1189.

49. Jung S, Martin T, Schmittbuhl M, et al. The spectrum of orofacial manifestations in systemic sclerosis: a challenging management. Oral Dis 2017;23(4):424–39.

50. Ramos-Casals M, Tzioufas AG, Stone JH, et al. Treatment of primary Sjögren syndrome: a systematic review. JAMA 2010;304(4):452–60.

51. Vivino FB, Al-Hashimi I, Khan Z, et al. Pilocarpine tablets for the treatment of dry mouth and dry eye symptoms in patients with Sjögren syndrome: a randomized, placebo-controlled, fixed-dose, multicenter trial. Arch Intern Med 1999;159(2): 174–81.

52. Alantar A, Cabane J, Hachulla E, et al. Recommendations for the care of oral involvement in patients with systemic sclerosis. Arthritis Care Res 2011;63(8): 1126–33.

53. Martin-Harris B, Bonilha HS, Brodsky MB, et al. The Modified Barium Swallow Study for Oropharyngeal Dysphagia: Recommendations From an Interdisciplinary Expert Panel. Perspectives of the ASHA Special Interest Groups 2021; 6(1):610–9.

54. Shreiner AB, Murray C, Denton C, et al. Gastrointestinal manifestations of systemic sclerosis. Journal of Scleroderma and Related Disorders 2016;1(3): 247–56.

55. Smout A, Fox M. Weak and absent peristalsis. Neuro Gastroenterol Motil 2012; 24:40–7.

56. Labeit B, Ahring S, Boehmer M, et al. Comparison of simultaneous swallowing endoscopy and videofluoroscopy in neurogenic dysphagia. J Am Med Dir Assoc 2021;23(8):1360–6.

57. Colton–Hudson A, Koopman WJ, Moosa T, et al. A prospective assessment of the characteristics of dysphagia in myasthenia gravis. Dysphagia 2002;17(2): 147–51.

58. Azola A, Mulheren R, McKeon G, et al. Dysphagia in myositis: a study of the structural and physiologic changes resulting in disordered swallowing. Am J Phys Med Rehabil 2020;99(5):404–8.

59. Cook IJ. Oropharyngeal dysphagia. Gastroenterol Clin 2009;38(3):411–31.

60. Leurs A, Dubucquoi S, Machuron F, et al. Extended myositis-specific and-associated antibodies profile in systemic sclerosis: a cross-sectional study. Joint Bone Spine 2021;88(1):105048.

61. Jung M, Bonner A, Hudson M, et al. Myopathy is a poor prognostic feature in systemic sclerosis: results from the Canadian Scleroderma Research Group (CSRG) cohort. Scand J Rheumatol 2014;43(3):217–20.

62. Casal-Dominguez M, Pinal-Fernandez I, Corse AM, et al. Muscular and extramuscular features of myositis patients with anti-U1-RNP autoantibodies. Neurology 2019;92(13):e1416–26.

63. Gilhus NE, Skeie GO, Romi F, et al. Myasthenia gravis — autoantibody characteristics and their implications for therapy. Nat Rev Neurol 2016;12(5):259–68.

64. Labeit B, Pawlitzki M, Ruck T, et al. The impact of dysphagia in myositis: a systematic review and meta-analysis. J Clin Med 2020;9(7):2150.

65. Frech TM, Mar D. Gastrointestinal and hepatic disease in systemic sclerosis. Rheum Dis Clin 2018;44(1):15–28.

66. Thonhofer R, Siegel C, Trummer M, et al. Early endoscopy in systemic sclerosis without gastrointestinal symptoms. Rheumatol Int 2012;32(1):165–8.

67. Abozaid HSM, Imam HMK, Abdelaziz MM, et al. High-resolution manometry compared with the University of California, Los Angeles Scleroderma Clinical Trials Consortium GIT 2.0 in Systemic Sclerosis. Semin Arthritis Rheum 2017; 47(3):403–8.

68. Crowell MD, Umar SB, Griffing WL, et al. Esophageal motor abnormalities in patients with scleroderma: heterogeneity, risk factors, and effects on quality of life. Clin Gastroenterol Hepatol 2017;15(2):207–13.e1.

69. Carlson DA, Pandolfino JE. High-Resolution Manometry in Clinical Practice. Gastroenterol Hepatol 2015;11(6):374–84.

70. Yadlapati R, Kahrilas PJ, Fox MR, et al. Esophageal motility disorders on high-resolution manometry: Chicago classification version 4.0. Neuro Gastroenterol Motil 2021;33(1):e14058.

71. de Carlan M, Lescoat A, Brochard C, et al. Association between clinical manifestations of systemic sclerosis and esophageal dysmotility assessed by high-resolution manometry. Journal of Scleroderma and Related Disorders 2017; 2(1):50–6.

72. Karamanolis GP, Denaxas K, Panopoulos S, et al. Severe oesophageal disease and its associations with systemic sclerosis. Clin Exp Rheumatol 2017; 35(4):82–5.

73. Fornari F, Bravi I, Penagini R, et al. Multiple rapid swallowing: a complementary test during standard oesophageal manometry. Neuro Gastroenterol Motil 2009; 21(7):718-e41.

74. Carlson DA, Crowell MD, Kimmel JN, et al. Loss of peristaltic reserve, determined by multiple rapid swallows, is the most frequent esophageal motility abnormality in patients with systemic sclerosis. Research Support, N.I.H. Extramural. Clinical Gastroenterology & Hepatology 2016;14(10):1502–6.

75. Kowal-Bielecka O, Fransen J, Avouac J, et al. Update of EULAR recommendations for the treatment of systemic sclerosis. Ann Rheum Dis 2017;76(8): 1327–39.

76. Hansi N, Thoua N, Carulli M, et al. Consensus best practice pathway of the UK scleroderma study group: gastrointestinal manifestations of systemic sclerosis. Clin Exp Rheumatol 2014;32(6 Suppl 86):214–21.

77. Horowitz M, Maddern GJ, Maddox A, et al. Effects of cisapride on gastric and esophageal emptying in progressive systemic sclerosis. Clinical Trial Controlled Clinical Trial Research Support, Non-U.S. Gov't. Gastroenterology 1987;93(2): 311–5.

78. Kahan A, Chaussade S, Gaudric M, et al. The effect of cisapride on gastro-oesophageal dysfunction in systemic sclerosis: a controlled manometric study. Clinical Trial Randomized Controlled Trial Research Support, Non-U.S. Gov't. Br J Clin Pharmacol 1991;31(6):683–7.

79. Johnson DA, Drane WE, Curran J, et al. Metoclopramide response in patients with progressive systemic sclerosis: effect on esophageal and gastric motility abnormalities. Arch Intern Med 1987;147(9):1597–601.

80. Ramirez-Mata M, Ibanez G, Alarcon-Segovia D. Stimulatory effect of metoclopramide on the esophagus and lower esophageal sphincter of patients of patients with PSS. Clinical Trial. Arthritis Rheum 1977;20(1):30–4.

81. Karamanolis GP, Panopoulos S, Denaxas K, et al. The 5-HT1A receptor agonist buspirone improves esophageal motor function and symptoms in systemic sclerosis: a 4-week, open-label trial. Clinical Trial. Arthritis Res Ther 2016;18:195.

82. Cubeddu LX. Iatrogenic QT abnormalities and fatal arrhythmias: mechanisms and clinical significance. Curr Cardiol Rev 2009;5(3):166–76.

83. Adarsh MB, Sharma SK, Sinha SK, et al. Gastrointestinal dysmotility and infections in systemic sclerosis- an indian scenario. observational study. Curr Rheumatol Rev 2018;14(2):172–6.
84. Abu-Shakra M, Guillemin F, Lee P. Gastrointestinal manifestations of systemic sclerosis. Review. Seminars in Arthritis & Rheumatism. 1994;24(1):29–39.
85. Bae S, Allanore Y, Furst DE, et al. Associations between a scleroderma-specific gastrointestinal instrument and objective tests of upper gastrointestinal involvements in systemic sclerosis. Clin Exp Rheumatol 2013;31(2 Suppl 76):57–63.
86. Katz PO, Dunbar KB, Schnoll-Sussman FH, et al. ACG Clinical Guideline for the Diagnosis and Management of Gastroesophageal Reflux Disease. Journal of the American College of Gastroenterology 2022;117(1):27–56.
87. Nagaraja V, McMahan ZH, Getzug T, et al. Management of gastrointestinal involvement in scleroderma. Current Treatment Options in Rheumatology 2015;1(1):82–105.
88. Chitkara DK, Van Tilburg M, Whitehead WE, et al. Teaching diaphragmatic breathing for rumination syndrome, *Journal of the American College of Gastroenterology*, 101(11), 2006. 2449-2452.
89. Halland M, Bharucha AE, Crowell MD, et al. Effects of diaphragmatic breathing on the pathophysiology and treatment of upright gastroesophageal reflux: a randomized controlled trial. Journal of the American College of Gastroenterology 2021;116(1):86–94.
90. Graham DY, Tansel A. Interchangeable use of proton pump inhibitors based on relative potency. Clin Gastroenterol Hepatol. Jun 2018;16(6):800–8.e7.
91. Wang WH, Huang JQ, Zheng GF, et al. Head-to-head comparison of H2-receptor antagonists and proton pump inhibitors in the treatment of erosive esophagitis: a meta-analysis. World J Gastroenterol 2005;11(26):4067–77.
92. Khan M, Santana J, Donnellan C, et al. Medical treatments in the short term management of reflux oesophagitis. Cochrane Database Syst Rev 2007;(2): Cd003244.
93. Lee JS, Kim H-S, Moon JR, et al. Esophageal involvement and determinants of perception of esophageal symptoms among south koreans with systemic sclerosis. Journal of Neurogastroenterology and Motility 2020;26(4):477–85.
94. Aggarwal P, Kamal AN. Reflux hypersensitivity: how to approach diagnosis and management. Curr Gastroenterol Rep 2020;22(9):42.
95. Rackoff A, Agrawal A, Hila A, et al. Histamine-2 receptor antagonists at night improve gastroesophageal reflux disease symptoms for patients on proton pump inhibitor therapy. Dis Esophagus 2005;18(6):370–3.
96. Patel A, Yadlapati R. Diagnosis and management of refractory gastroesophageal reflux disease. Gastroenterol Hepatol 2021;17(7):305–15.
97. Zerbib F, Roman S, Ropert A, et al. Esophageal pH-impedance monitoring and symptom analysis in GERD: a study in patients off and on therapy. Journal of the American College of Gastroenterology 2006;101(9):1956–63.
98. Shay S, Tutuian R, Sifrim D, et al. Twenty-four hour ambulatory simultaneous impedance and pH monitoring: a multicenter report of normal values from 60 healthy volunteers. LWW; 2004. p. 1037–43.
99. Kushnir V, Sathyamurthy A, Drapekin J, et al. Assessment of concordance of symptom reflux association tests in ambulatory pH monitoring. Aliment Pharmacol Ther 2012;35(9):1080–7.
100. Vela MF. Multichannel intraluminal impedance and pH monitoring in gastroesophageal reflux disease. Expet Rev Gastroenterol Hepatol 2008;2(5):665–72.

101. Savarino E, Bazzica M, Zentilin P, et al. Gastroesophageal reflux and pulmonary fibrosis in scleroderma: a study using pH-impedance monitoring. Am J Respir Crit Care Med 2009;179(5):408–13.

102. Schmulson MJ, Drossman DA. What Is New in Rome IV. J Neurogastroenterol Motil 2017;23(2):151–63.

103. Shirai Y, Kawami N, Iwakiri K, et al. Use of vonoprazan, a novel potassium-competitive acid blocker, for the treatment of proton pump inhibitor-refractory reflux esophagitis in patients with systemic sclerosis. Journal of Scleroderma and Related Disorders 2021;7(1):57–61.

104. Ashida K, Sakurai Y, Hori T, et al. Randomised clinical trial: vonoprazan, a novel potassium-competitive acid blocker, vs. lansoprazole for the healing of erosive oesophagitis. Aliment Pharmacol Ther 2016;43(2):240–51.

105. Tabuchi M, Minami H, Akazawa Y, et al. Use of vonoprazan for management of systemic sclerosis-related gastroesophageal reflux disease. Biomedical Reports 2021;14(2):1.

106. De Giorgi F, Palmiero M, Esposito I, et al. Pathophysiology of gastro-oesophageal reflux disease. Acta Otorhinolaryngol Ital 2006;26(5):241–6.

107. Lahcene M, Oumnia N, Matougui N, et al. Esophageal Involvement in Scleroderma: Clinical, Endoscopic, and Manometric Features. ISRN Rheumatology 2011;325826. https://doi.org/10.5402/2011/325826.

108. Aggarwal N, Lopez R, Gabbard S, et al. Spectrum of esophageal dysmotility in systemic sclerosis on high-resolution esophageal manometry as defined by Chicago classification. Article. Dis Esophagus 2017;30(12):1–6.

109. Ren L-H, Chen W-X, Qian L-J, et al. Addition of prokinetics to PPI therapy in gastroesophageal reflux disease: a meta-analysis. World J Gastroenterol 2014;20(9):2412–9.

110. Li S, Shi S, Chen F, et al. The effects of baclofen for the treatment of gastro-esophageal reflux disease: a meta-analysis of randomized controlled trials. Gastroenterology Research and Practice 2014;307805. https://doi.org/10.1155/2014/307805.

111. Vela MF, Tutuian R, Katz PO, et al. Baclofen decreases acid and non-acid post-prandial gastro-oesophageal reflux measured by combined multichannel intra-luminal impedance and pH. Aliment Pharmacol Ther 2003;17(2):243–51.

112. Vigone B, Caronni M, Severino A, et al. Preliminary safety and efficacy profile of prucalopride in the treatment of systemic sclerosis (SSc)-related intestinal involvement: results from the open label cross-over PROGASS study. Randomized Controlled Trial Research Support, Non-U.S. Gov't. Arthritis Res Ther 2017; 19(1):145.

113. Frech TM, Khanna D, Maranian P, et al. Probiotics for the treatment of systemic sclerosis-associated gastrointestinal bloating/distention. Clin Exp Rheumatol 2011;29(2 Suppl 65):S22–5.

114. Marighela TF, Arismendi MI, Marvulle V, et al. Effect of probiotics on gastrointestinal symptoms and immune parameters in systemic sclerosis: a randomized placebo-controlled trial. Randomized Controlled Trial Research Support, Non-U.S. Gov't. Rheumatology 2019;58(11):1985–90.

115. Low AHL, Teng GG, Pettersson S, et al. A double-blind randomized placebo-controlled trial of probiotics in systemic sclerosis associated gastrointestinal disease. Clinical Trial, Phase II Randomized Controlled Trial Research Support, Non-U.S. Gov't. Semin Arthritis Rheum 2019;49(3):411–9.

116. De Giorgio R, Knowles C. Acute colonic pseudo-obstruction. Journal of British Surgery 2009;96(3):229–39.

117. Antonucci A, Fronzoni L, Cogliandro L, et al. Chronic intestinal pseudo-obstruction. World J Gastroenterol 2008;14(19):2953–61. https://doi.org/10.3748/wjg.14.2953.
118. Soykan I, Sivri B, Sarosiek I, et al. Demography, clinical characteristics, psychological and abuse profiles, treatment, and long-term follow-up of patients with gastroparesis. Dig Dis Sci 1998;43(11):2398–404.
119. Adler B, Hummers LK, Pasricha PJ, et al. Gastroparesis in systemic sclerosis: a detailed analysis using whole-gut scintigraphy. Rheumatology 2022. https://doi.org/10.1093/rheumatology/keac074.
120. Franck-Larsson K, Hedenstrom H, Dahl R, et al. Delayed gastric emptying in patients with diffuse versus limited systemic sclerosis, unrelated to gastrointestinal symptoms and myoelectric gastric activity. Comparative Study. Scand J Rheumatol 2003;32(6):348–55.
121. Weston S, Thumshirn M, Wiste J, et al. Clinical and upper gastrointestinal motility features in systemic sclerosis and related disorders. Comparative Study Support and AuthorAnonymous, Research Support, Non-U.S. Gov'tResearch Support, U.S. Gov't, P.H.S. Am J Gastroenterol 1998;93(7):1085–9.
122. Marie I, Levesque H, Ducrotte P, et al. Gastric involvement in systemic sclerosis: a prospective study. Clinical Trial Controlled Clinical Trial. Am J Gastroenterol 2001;96(1):77–83.
123. Sridhar KR, Lange RC, Magyar L, et al. Prevalence of impaired gastric emptying of solids in systemic sclerosis: diagnostic and therapeutic implications. Clinical Trial. J Lab Clin Med 1998;132(6):541–6.
124. McMahan ZH, Tucker AE, Perin J, et al. The relationship between gastrointestinal transit, Medsger GI severity, and UCLA GIT 2.0 symptoms in patients with systemic sclerosis. Arthritis Care Res 2020;16:16.
125. Jehangir A, Parkman HP. Rome IV Diagnostic Questionnaire Complements Patient Assessment of Gastrointestinal Symptoms for Patients with Gastroparesis Symptoms. Dig Dis Sci 2018;63(9):2231–43.
126. Kumar M, Chapman A, Javed S, et al. The investigation and treatment of diabetic gastroparesis. Clin Therapeut 2018;40(6):850–61.
127. Parkman HP, Hasler WL, Fisher RS. American Gastroenterological Association technical review on the diagnosis and treatment of gastroparesis. Gastroenterology 2004;127(5):1592–622.
128. Domsic R, Fasanella K, Bielefeldt K. Gastrointestinal manifestations of systemic sclerosis. Dig Dis Sci 2008;53(5):1163–74.
129. Camilleri M, Sanders KM. Gastroparesis. Gastroenterology 2022;162(1):68–87.e1.
130. Fynne L, Worsoe J, Gregersen T, et al. Gastrointestinal transit in patients with systemic sclerosis. Scand J Gastroenterol 2011;46(10):1187–93.
131. Cozzi F, Parisi G, Ciprian L, et al. Gastric dysmotility after liquid bolus ingestion in systemic sclerosis: an ultrasonographic study. Rheumatol Int 2012;32(5):1219–23.
132. Fiorucci S, Distrutti E, Bassotti G, et al. Effect of erythromycin administration on upper gastrointestinal motility in scleroderma patients. Scand J Gastroenterol 1994;29(9):807–13.
133. Koch KL, Stern RM, Stewart WR, et al. Gastric emptying and gastric myoelectrical activity in patients with diabetic gastroparesis: effect of long-term domperidone treatment. Am J Gastroenterol 1989;84(9).
134. Malamood M, Roberts A, Kataria R, et al. Mirtazapine for symptom control in refractory gastroparesis. Drug Des Dev Ther 2017;11:1035–41.

135. Camilleri M, Atieh J. New Developments in Prokinetic Therapy for Gastric Motility Disorders. Front Pharmacol 2021;12:711500.
136. Ariyasu H, Iwakura H, Yukawa N, et al. Clinical effects of ghrelin on gastrointestinal involvement in patients with systemic sclerosis. Clinical Trial Randomized Controlled Trial Research Support, Non-U.S. Gov't. Endocr J 2014;61(7): 735–42.
137. Carbone F, Van den Houte K, Clevers E, et al. Prucalopride in Gastroparesis: A Randomized Placebo-Controlled Crossover Study. Journal of the American College of Gastroenterology 2019;114(8):1265–74.
138. Ghrenassia E, Avouac J, Khanna D, et al. Prevalence, correlates and outcomes of gastric antral vascular ectasia in systemic sclerosis: a EUSTAR case-control study. Research Support, N.I.H., Extramural. J Rheumatol 2014;41(1):99–105.
139. Marie I, Ducrotte P, Antonietti M, et al. Watermelon stomach in systemic sclerosis: its incidence and management. Aliment Pharmacol Ther 2008;28(4): 412–21.
140. Serling-Boyd N, Chung MP-S, Li S, et al. Gastric antral vascular ectasia in systemic sclerosis: Association with anti-RNA polymerase III and negative antinuclear antibodies. Semin Arthritis Rheum 2020;50(5):938–42.
141. Ingraham KM, O'BRIEN MS, Shenin M, et al. Gastric antral vascular ectasia in systemic sclerosis: demographics and disease predictors. J Rheumatol 2010; 37(3):603–7.
142. Emmanuel A. Current management of the gastrointestinal complications of systemic sclerosis. Review Research Support, Non-U.S. Gov't. Nat Rev Gastroenterol Hepatol 2016;13(8):461–72.
143. Schulz SW, O'brien M, Maqsood M, et al. Improvement of severe systemic sclerosis-associated gastric antral vascular ectasia following immunosuppressive treatment with intravenous cyclophosphamide. J Rheumatol 2009;36(8): 1653–6.
144. Lorenzi AR, Johnson AH, Davies G, et al. Gastric antral vascular ectasia in systemic sclerosis: complete resolution with methylprednisolone and cyclophosphamide. Case Reports Review. Annals of the Rheumatic Diseases. 2001; 60(8):796–8.
145. Matsumoto Y, Hayashi H, Tahara K, et al. Intravenous cyclophosphamide for gastric antral vascular ectasia associated with systemic sclerosis refractory to endoscopic treatment: a case report and review of the pertinent literature. Intern Med 2019;58(1):135–9.
146. Lock G, Holstege A, Lang B, et al. Gastrointestinal manifestations of progressive systemic sclerosis. Am J Gastroenterol 1997;92(5):763–71.
147. Clements PJ, Becvar R, Drosos AA, et al. Assessment of gastrointestinal involvement. Review. Clin Exp Rheumatol 2003;21(3 Suppl 29):S15–8.

Gastrointestinal Tract Considerations: Part II

How Should a Rheumatologist Best Manage Common Lower Gastrointestinal Tract Complaints in Systemic Sclerosis?

Alannah Quinlivan, MBBS[a,b], Zsuzsanna H. McMahan, MD, MHS[c],
Eun Bong Lee, MD, PhD[d], Mandana Nikpour, MBBS, PhD[a,b,*]

KEYWORDS

- Gastrointestinal symptoms • Systemic sclerosis • Lower gastrointestinal tract

KEY POINTS

- Gastrointestinal (GI) symptoms are common in systemic sclerosis (SSc), affecting up to 90% of patients, yet there are few guidelines for investigation or treatment of GI complications in SSc.
- There is no evidence that immunomodulatory agents prevent or treat GI complications, but promotility agents may have a role.
- In this review, the authors present an integrated approach to investigating and treating lower GI symptoms in SSc.

INTRODUCTION

Systemic sclerosis (SSc; ie, scleroderma) is an autoimmune connective tissue with pathogenic features of autoimmunity, inflammation, vasculopathy, and/or fibrosis of the skin and internal organs.[1] Gastrointestinal tract (GI) complications affect up to 90% of patients with SSc and negatively impact morbidity and mortality.[2–12]

In Part 1 of this 2-part review series, the authors focused on common upper GIT complaints encountered in patients with SSc. The aim of this review is to provide information on the assessment, investigation, and management of common lower

ᵃ Department of Rheumatology, St Vincent's Hospital, 41 Victoria Parade, Fitzroy, Victoria, 3065, Australia; ᵇ Department of Medicine, The University of Melbourne at St Vincent's Hospital, 41 Victoria Parade, Fitzroy, Victoria 3065, Australia; ᶜ Division of Rheumatology, Johns Hopkins University, 5200 Eastern Avenue, Suite 5200, Mason F. Lord Building, Center Tower, Baltimore, MD 21224, USA; ᵈ Division of Rheumatology, Seoul National University College of Medicine, 103 Daehak-ro, Jongno-gu, Seoul, Republic of Korea
* Corresponding author.
E-mail address: m.nikpour@unimelb.edu.au

Rheum Dis Clin N Am 49 (2023) 319–336
https://doi.org/10.1016/j.rdc.2023.01.007
0889-857X/23/© 2023 Elsevier Inc. All rights reserved.

GIT symptoms (**Table 1**), including diarrhea, constipation, and fecal incontinence. The recommendations provided in this review have been sourced from the available SSc literature, gastroenterologic guidelines, and the authors' clinical experience.

Lower Gastrointestinal Complaints (Small Bowel and Colon)

Diarrhea and weight loss

Diarrhea is a common symptom encountered in SSc, affecting up to 80% of patients (**Fig. 1**).[13,14] There exists a wide range of differentials, and a careful history can assist with directing investigations. Acute diarrhea (lasting <4 weeks) should prompt consideration of infectious sources.[15] In SSc, small bowel dysmotility predisposes to the development of small intestinal bacterial overgrowth or SIBO, present in a third of patients with SSc, manifesting as diarrhea, bloating, and sometimes weight loss.[12,16–18]

Assessment of diarrhea. GIT questionnaires, such as UCLA GIT 2.0 and PROMIS GI, are not particularly useful in differentiating between diarrheal causes and have not been shown to correlate with objective investigation findings.[19,20] Red flags on history, including weight loss, iron deficiency anemia, evidence of inflammation, or blood in bowel movements, should prompt consideration of inflammatory bowel disease (IBD), celiac disease (CD), or malignancy.[21] History of antibiotic use, frequent hospital

Table 1
Assessment of lower gastrointestinal tract symptoms

Symptoms/Indication For Study	Differential	Red Flags	Possible Investigations
Diarrhea	SIBO Celiac disease Lactose malabsorption Fructose malabsorption Infection IBD Microscopic colitis	Blood/mucous in bowel motions Weight loss Iron deficiency anemia Recent antibiotic use	*Blood* Autoantibodies (antiendomysial and tissue transglutaminase) Iron studies, FBE, albumin *Fecal* Calprotectin *C difficile* toxin/PCR *Breath tests* Glucose/lactulose Lactose/fructose *Procedures* EGD/duodenal biopsy Colonoscopy
Constipation	Colonic dysmotility ± fecal impaction Colon cancer Anorectal dysfunction	Weight loss Lack of flatus Blood/mucous in bowel motion Family history of GI malignancy Age >50 y	*Imaging* AXR/CT (rule out obstruction) Colonic transit Anorectal manometry *Fecal* FOBT
Fecal incontinence	Internal anal sphincter dysfunction diarrhea	Constipation Loose bowels	*Imaging* AXR/CT (rule out obstruction) Anorectal manometry

Abbreviations: AXR, abdominal radiograph; CT, computed tomography; EGD, esophagogastroduodenoscopy; FBE, full blood examination; FOBT, fecal occult blood test; PCI, pneumatosis cystoides intestinalis; PCR, polymerase chain reaction.

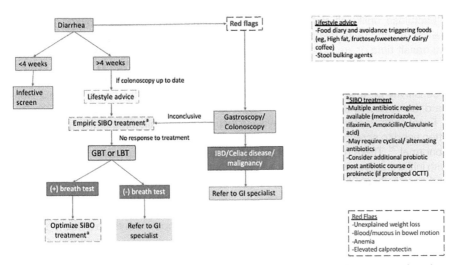

Fig. 1. Diarrhea. GBT, glucose breath test; IBD, inflammatory bowel disease; LBT, lactulose breath test; OCTT, orocecal transit time.

visits, or chronic proton-pump inhibitor (PPI) use should prompt consideration for *Clostridium difficile* testing.

Lifestyle advice for diarrhea. There are currently a number of dietary modifications available for the management of chronic diarrhea, including restriction of fats, fermentable carbohydrates (FODMAPs), or lactose-containing foods.[22,23] A food diary can be a useful tool to identify specific food or drink items that may play a role in worsening symptoms (such as high-fat foods, artificial sweeteners, fructose, and/or coffee) and may help target dietary interventions.[22,24] With the exception of proven lactose intolerance, fructose malabsorption, or CD, there is little evidence that dietary interventions are useful in SSc-related diarrhea.[25–27] Lactose intolerance and fructose malabsorption are present in 44% and 40% of patients with SSc, respectively, and can be further investigated using elimination diets or hydrogen breath testing with either lactose or fructose used as a substrate.[28–30]

Investigations for small intestinal bacterial overgrowth. The most common diagnostic tests used for SIBO in clinical practice and in research settings are breath tests, in which either glucose (GBT) or lactulose (LBT) is used as a substrate for gut bacteria to metabolize, resulting in the excretion of hydrogen (H_2) or methane (CH_4), which can be measured. Patients ingest a drink containing glucose or lactulose, and samples of expired air are collected every 15 to 20 minutes. Although the traditional gold-standard diagnosis is a bacterial count of greater than 10^5 colony forming units per milliliter obtained via jejunal aspirate, this test is rarely performed, as it requires endoscopy, an invasive procedure (with the risks of sedation and perforation), which is not always possible in SSc (owing to narrowing of the oral aperture).[31–34] Furthermore, contemporary laboratories seldom have the resources needed for such quantitative cultures. A recent meta-analysis found GBT to have a sensitivity of 54% and specificity of 83% for diagnosis of SIBO compared with jejunal aspirate. GBT had a higher sensitivity and specificity in patients with preexisting conditions predisposing to SIBO, such as SSc.[35–37] As glucose is rapidly metabolized within the first 3 feet of small bowel, it can be falsely negative in distal SIBO.[31]

Lactulose, unlike glucose, is poorly absorbed in the small bowel, allowing it to reach the cecum and be fermented by colonic bacteria, providing a measurement of orocecal transit time or small bowel transit time.[37] LBT is also used to diagnose SIBO but can be falsely positive in rapid transit times, as the early elevation in hydrogen excretion (produced by colonic fermentation) can be mistaken for an SIBO peak.[31] LBT has a sensitivity of 42% and specificity of 70% compared with the traditional gold standard; however, no studies have yet been done to validate these findings in SSc.[35]

Fecal calprotectin (Fc) is a noninvasive test measuring inflammation in the GIT and is often used to screen for and manage IBD, with levels greater than 50 μg/g considered abnormal.[21] There has been interest in the use of Fc as a diagnostic marker of SIBO with initial studies suggesting that a value greater than 275 μ/g has a sensitivity of 93% and specificity of 95% for the diagnosis of SIBO.[38,39] However, these patients did not undergo gastroscopy or colonoscopy, so other conditions, which can result in elevated calprotectin, such as IBD, could not be ruled out. If Fc is elevated, more invasive investigations, such as gastroscopy and colonoscopy, would be indicated to rule out CD or IBD.

If there is clinical concern for infection, with recent travel or factors that would predispose to C difficile colitis (ie, hospitalization or antibiotic use), fecal specimens can also be used for culture, parasite testing, and detection of C difficile toxin.

Novel investigations for bowel inflammation. Noninvasive imaging modalities, such as intestinal ultrasound (IUS) and magnetic resonance enterography (MRE), are being increasingly used in IBD to assess intestinal inflammation and motility.[40] IUS is a bedside investigation tool used for assisting in both diagnosis and monitoring of treatment response in patients with IBD.[41–43] MRE is another noninvasive diagnostic technique that does not require ionizing radiation and has the ability to obtain information about both intramural and extramural involvement of the small bowel in IBD.[40] As of yet, there are no studies of IUS or MRE in patients with SSc; however, these investigations may be useful in ruling out IBD and in providing a noninvasive means of assessing gastrointestinal (GI) disease in SSc.

Treatment of small intestinal bacterial overgrowth. With regards to treatment of SIBO in SSc, there is no current recommended standardized protocol. Antibiotics are the most commonly used treatment, and their use is associated with varying eradication rates. Antibiotics are often prescribed empirically based on a clinical suspicion for SIBO. Rifaximin, an antibiotic used commonly in traveler's diarrhea and hepatic encephalopathy, has been shown to have a 73% to 100% cure rate in SSc-SIBO,[38,44,45] although recurrence may be common. Other options include amoxicillin/clavulanic acid, ciprofloxacin, and metronidazole. There is evidence that in patients who produce methane on breath testing, combining neomycin with rifaximin may improve eradication rates.[46]

There are variable data to support the use of probiotics in SSc-SIBO. A meta-analysis of 18 SIBO trials in the general population demonstrated increased effectiveness of antibiotic treatments when used in combination with probiotics.[47] These findings were reflected in 1 study of 40 patients with SSc-SIBO treated with metronidazole, Saccharomyces boulardii, or a combination of both. Patients treated with probiotics (alone or in combination with metronidazole) reported decreased symptoms of bloating, abdominal pain, and diarrhea.[48] The addition of S boulardii to metronidazole therapy also reduced the frequency of side effects of reflux and constipation.

Prokinetics, which improve GI dysmotility, may also play a role in the treatment of SIBO. Such medications improve intestinal transit and have been shown to reduce

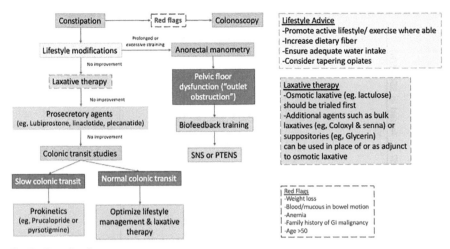

Fig. 2. Constipation.

the incidence of bacterial overgrowth in patients on PPI medication.[49] In a small study of 5 patients with SSc-SIBO, there was a 100% cure rate using octreotide.[50] In patients with hepatic cirrhosis, 6 months of cisapride was found to be noninferior to rotating antibiotics for treatment of SIBO.[51] As delayed small bowel transit time has been shown in SSc and the general population to be associated with SIBO,[45,52] prokinetics should be considered for treatment of SIBO.

Constipation

Constipation may present with symptoms of infrequent bowel motions (<3 weekly bowel motions) or difficulty passing stool (including straining, sensation of incomplete evacuation; **Fig. 2**).[53,54] Colonic involvement is common in SSc, affecting 20% to 50% of patients and occurs in the context of colonic dysmotility and subsequent smooth muscle atrophy in conjunction with an impaired gastrocolic reflex.[55]

Assessment of constipation. Both UCLA and PROMIS GI questionnaires include questions regarding constipation, although UCLA constipation scores have not been shown to correlate with objective findings of delayed colonic transit (**Table 2**).[56] It is important to note that the constipation domain of the UCLA questionnaire is not included in the calculation of the total score and should be looked at separately. Red flag symptoms, including weight loss, blood or mucous in bowel motion, a family history of GI malignancy, or age greater than 50 years, should prompt referral for colonoscopy. In addition, if symptoms such as prolonged or excessive straining before defecation are reported, a diagnosis of pelvic floor dysfunction (or "outlet obstruction") should be considered.[57]

Initial management and lifestyle modifications for constipation. Consensus guidelines recommend treatment based on symptoms before further investigation, unless red flag symptoms are present (**Table 1**).[53] Initial management should include encouragement of fluids (although there is no evidence to support this) and exercise, which has been shown in a large systematic review to have a beneficial effect on constipation.[58]

Osmotic laxatives (such as lactulose) and stimulant laxatives are both effective in increasing the number of bowel motions per week in chronic constipation, although

Table 2
Gastrointestinal questionnaires

Questionnaire	Focus	Key Features (eg, Vomiting, Abdominal Pain)	Scoring (Recall)	Validated?	Tested in SSc (Y/N)
UCLA SCTC GIT 2.0 (34 items)	Upper GI Lower GI QoL	Reflux Distension/bloating Diarrhea Constipation Fecal incontinence/soilage (1 question) Social functioning Emotional well-being	Higher score = worse GI symptoms (1 wk)	Yes[94]	Yes[94]
PROMIS-GI (60 items)	Upper GI Lower GI QoL	Reflux/regurgitation Distension/bloating Dysphagia Diarrhea Constipation Fecal incontinence/soilage Nausea and vomiting Abdominal pain	Higher score = worse GI symptoms (1 wk)	Yes[95]	Yes[96]
QOLRAD (25 items)	QoL GERD/upper GI	Emotional distress sleep disturbance Vitality Food/drink problems Physical/social functioning	A low score indicates low quality of life, whereas a high score indicates better QoL (1 wk)	Yes[97]	Yes[98]
PAGI-QoL (30 items)	QoL Mood	Daily activities Clothing Diet/food habits Relationship Psychological well-being Distress	0 (lowest QoL) to 5 (highest QoL) (2 wk)	Yes[99]	No

Wexner Incontinence Score (5 item)	Lower GI Fecal incontinence	Stool frequency, consistency (gas, liquid, solid) Pad use/lifestyle alteration	Lower score = less incontinence (score 0–20) a score of ≥9 is considered clinically significant (4 wk)	Yes[100]	Yes, but not validated[101]
FISI (4 item)	Lower GI fecal incontinence	Stool frequency, consistency (gas, liquid, solid, mucus)	Lower score = less incontinence Maximum score 61 (1 mo)	Yes[74]	No

Abbreviations: GERD, gastroesophageal reflux disease; PAGI-QoL, Patient Assessment of Upper Gastrointestinal Disorders–Quality of Life; PROMIS-GI, Patient-Reported Outcomes Measurement Information System–Gastrointestinal Symptom Scales; QOLRAD, Quality of Life in Reflux and Dyspepsia; UCLA SCTC GIT, University of California Scleroderma Clinical Trial Consortium Gastrointestinal Tract.

there are fewer data to support the use of stimulant laxatives.[59] For patients with slow colonic transit (see later discussion), osmotic laxatives may be indicated initially, whereas patients with normal colonic transit may benefit from a trial of stimulant laxatives; however, not all guidelines support this practice.[57,60] Prosecretory agents, such as linaclotide and lubiprostone, are recommended in idiopathic constipation and have also been found to improve symptoms of constipation in SSc.[59,61,62]

Investigations for constipation. Blood tests are recommended to look for anemia, inflammation, hypothyroidism, hypercalcemia, and celiac disease.[54] Abdominal plain radiograph is an easy, accessible tool for excluding pseudo-obstruction and assessing complications of constipation, including "wide mouth" diverticula and colonic dilatation.[63] Its use in diagnosing constipation is limited, with no correlation to colonic transit studies and considerable interobserver variability in reporting of fecal loading.[64,65]

Colonic transit studies can help differentiate between normal transit and slow transit constipation, which has therapeutic implications. There exist 3 main methods for assessing colonic transit. The first involves the ingestion of a capsule of radiopaque markers, followed by abdominal radiograph on day 1 and day 6. The second, scintigraphy, involves the ingestion of a coated capsule or meal containing an isotope with images acquired through use of a gamma camera at specific time points up to 72 hours. The newest method uses a wireless motility capsule (which measures pH as it travels through the bowel), allowing assessment of whole gut transit times. Although this method has been shown to have 87% agreement relative to radiopaque marker methods in the general population, its utility in patients with SSc is yet to be assessed.[65,66]

Anorectal manometry (discussed later) can be used to evaluate pelvic floor dysfunction (or "outlet obstruction").[57] This condition is important to identify, as it often does not respond to laxative therapy. Treatment for pelvic floor dysfunction consists of physiotherapy and biofeedback training.[57]

Additional management of constipation. Pyridostigmine (an acetylcholinesterase inhibitor used in autoimmune gastric dysmotility) has been found to improve symptoms of constipation in SSc in 1 retrospective cohort study.[67] Prucalopride has also been shown to both increase bowel motions and improve symptoms of constipation in an open-label crossover study of 40 patients with SSc and may be indicated in patients with slow colonic transit.[68]

Insoluble fiber supplementation (such as psyllium husk) is recommended in chronic idiopathic constipation.[69] Although fiber supplementation may have some use in patients with SSc with difficulty emptying but a normal urge to void, it is not well tolerated in patients with SSc, causing bloating/distension and flatulence.[63,70] Fiber can also worsen gastroparesis and slow colonic transit time; therefore, caution should be taken to rule out slow colonic transit before commencement.[71]

Fecal incontinence

Fecal incontinence (FI) is estimated to be present in 27% to 38% of patients with SSc, although this may be an underestimation, as patients often feel uncomfortable discussing the associated symptoms (**Fig. 3**).[72] Symptoms may include loss of fecal contents (with or without prior urge to defecate) or leakage of stool without awareness, perianal pruritus, skin irritation, or infection.[73]

Assessment of fecal incontinence. For assessment of symptoms, the Wexner incontinence score is frequently used in the general population. The Faecal Incontinence

Table 3
Management

Medication	Common Doses	Uses	Serious Adverse Effects
Prokinetics	Prucalopride 2 mg daily	Constipation ↓ Gastroparesis symptoms	
	Octreotide (50 μg subcutaneously nightly)	SIBO (100% cure rate) CIPO	
SIBO antibiotic	Rifaximin 1200-1600mg/d for 10-14 d	SIBO	
	Neomycin 500 mg twice daily for 10 d	SIBO (with methane production on breath testing)	Nephrotoxicity, auditory ototoxicity, and vestibular ototoxicity (usually irreversible)
	Ciprofloxacin 500 mg twice daily for 7–10 d	SIBO	Prolonged QT interval Seizures Tendon rupture
	Metronidazole 500 mg twice daily OR 500 mg 3× daily OR 250 mg 3× daily for 7–10 d	SIBO	Confusion Encephalopathy
	Augmentin duo forte 875/125 mg twice daily OR amoxicillin 500 mg 3× daily for 1 wk	SIBO	C difficile Hypersensitivity reactions Hepatotoxicity
Acetylcholinesterase inhibitor	Pyridostigmine (30–60 mg 3× daily)	Constipation	
Colonic secretory agent	Linaclotide (high dose >145 μg daily, low dose <145 μg daily)	Constipation	

Abbreviation: CIPO, chronic intestinal pseudo-obstruction.

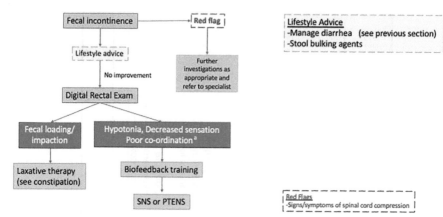

Fig. 3. Fecal incontinence. ARM, anorectal manometry. [a]ARM $\pm$ Balloon expulsion test if needed.

Severity Score (FISI) is another general questionnaire that has been used in SSc.[74] If there is associated urinary retention or other symptoms and signs suggestive of cauda equina syndrome or spinal cord compression, imaging with MRI should be considered.

Initial management. Although no guidelines exist for management of FI in SSc, the American College of Gastroenterology (ACG) recommends initial digital rectal examination to assess anal resting tone and squeeze pressures and to rule out local pathologic condition and fecal loading/impaction.[73,75] Following this, conservative management, including correction of predisposing factors like diarrhea, constipation, and SIBO, is recommended before further, more invasive, investigations.[72]

Investigations for fecal incontinence. Anorectal manometry can be used to measure both anorectal motor and sensory function and to direct treatment.[75] It involves insertion of a catheter into the anus and rectum, measuring the following: (a) pressures at rest; (b) pressures during squeezing and coughing; (c) rectoanal coordination during simulated defecation; as well as (d) rectal sensation thresholds.[76] Rectal sensation is measured through inflation of a balloon inserted in the rectum with balloon volumes recorded at points of first sensation, urge to void or desire to defecate volume, and maximum tolerated volume. The balloon expulsion test provides a measure of the patient's ability to expel a balloon from the rectum (measured in time taken) and, if abnormal, should be confirmed with abnormal coordination during push maneuver on anorectal manometry. In SSc, common findings include low resting anal pressure (hypotonia), decreased rectal sensation and compliance as well as impaired or absent rectoanal inhibitory reflex, which plays a role in maintaining continence.[55,77] Studies of consecutive patients with SSc have shown that manometric abnormalities are also present in asymptomatic patients, although given the cross-sectional study design, it is unknown whether this is predictive of future symptoms.[78,79]

For the assessment of anatomical abnormalities, both MRI and ultrasound can be used to complement anorectal manometry. Endoanal ultrasound is considered the gold standard for assessment of internal anal sphincter defects, whereas MRI is considered superior for investigating the external anal sphincter and is better able to assess atrophy.[80] Although these imaging modalities are recommended by the

ACG in patients during preoperative evaluations, their role in the management of patients with SSc is not well defined.[81–83]

Additional management of fecal incontinence in systemic sclerosis. Biofeedback training is a noninvasive management strategy for FI. It describes a program that encompasses education regarding defecation, anal squeeze exercises, and rectal sensory retraining. In a retrospective review of 301 female patients with FI, biofeedback training resulted in improvement in 67% wherein the only predictor of outcome was urge incontinence.[84,85] In SSc, a retrospective study of 13 women with SSc and FI showed an improvement in symptom scores, quality of life (QoL), and anal squeeze pressure following a 6-week biofeedback session, with sustained improvement over 6 months of follow-up.[86]

Neuromodulation of the sacral nerves through low-voltage stimulation has been shown to be an effective intervention in patients with FI who do not respond to initial management.[87] Sacral nerve stimulation (SNS) involves direct stimulation of the sacral nerve roots through an implanted device (inserted during surgery), whereas percutaneous tibial nerve stimulation (PTNS) stimulates the sacral nerves noninvasively and indirectly through the tibial nerve.[88] A recent meta-analysis found SNS to be more effective than PTNS; however, it is more costly and more invasive.[87,88] Although PTNS has been shown to improve FI in numerous studies, there have also been 2 double-blind, placebo-controlled trials showing no effect over placebo.[89,90] In SSc, results of SNS are mixed and based only on 2 small case series.[91,92] PTNS was investigated in a small, randomized single-blind trial of 13 patients with SSc with FI whereby a symptomatic improvement over placebo was seen.[93]

SUMMARY AND RECOMMENDATIONS

Lower GI symptoms are a frequently encountered problem for clinicians managing patients with SSc. The current management practices are focused on the treatment of symptoms with little information available on how to use GI investigations in daily practice. This review has demonstrated how to integrate the objective assessment of common lower GI symptoms into clinical care with the aim of guiding clinical decision making. Understanding the type of abnormal GI function that is affecting a patient and determining which parts of the gut are impacted can help clinicians to target therapy more precisely.

There are several limitations in the field that will be a focus of future research. First, although we are able to extrapolate from existing guidelines in the field of gastroenterology, guidelines to screen and/or objectively assess for SSc-related GI complications are needed to standardize care. Second, as the majority of published studies in the SSc GI literature are cross-sectional in design, there is a paucity of longitudinal studies identifying the risk factors that differentiate patients at high versus low risk of disease progression. Third, there is much uncertainty related to predicting the temporal trajectories and outcomes of patients with SSc-related GI disease. As a result, determining the efficacy of various drugs in the prevention or modification of disease progression is challenging. Future prospective longitudinal studies are warranted to address these gaps in knowledge and to lay the foundations for interventional studies of novel therapies.

CLINICS CARE POINTS

Diarrhea practice points

- Diarrhea can be due to a number of pathologic conditions, and careful history can help direct investigations.
- Acute diarrhea (<4 weeks) should prompt investigation of infectious causes.
- If red flags are present (including weight loss, blood, or mucous in bowel motions, unexplained anemia, or elevated calprotectin), gastroscopy and colonoscopy should be undertaken.
- Small intestinal bacterial overgrowth occurs in a third of patients with systemic sclerosis and can be diagnosed with either glucose or lactulose breath testing. However, as these tests have poor sensitivity for small intestinal bacterial overgrowth, empiric antibiotic treatment may be pursued when clinically appropriate.

Constipation practice points
- Constipation is common in systemic sclerosis, and a trial of lifestyle recommendations should be undertaken before investigation if no red flag symptoms are present.
- Caution should be taken when prescribing fiber in patients with systemic sclerosis, as it may worsen bloating and delayed gastric emptying, and slow colonic transit.
- Prucalopride, pyridostigmine, and linaclotide may improve constipation in patients with systemic sclerosis.

Fecal incontinence practice points
- Fecal incontinence prevalence is likely underestimated in systemic sclerosis studies owing to patient hesitancy to report symptoms.
- Correction of precipitating factors (such as diarrhea or loose stools) can improve symptoms.
- Biofeedback training and neurofeedback (such as sacral nerve stimulation and percutaneous tibial nerve stimulation) demonstrate benefit in patients with systemic sclerosis with fecal incontinence.

FUNDING STATEMENT

NIH/NIAMS K23 AR071473, Rheumatology Research Foundation, Scleroderma Research Foundation, and Jerome L. Greene Foundation to Z.H. McMahan.

REFERENCES

1. Gu YS, Kong J, Cheema GS, et al. The immunobiology of systemic sclerosis. Semin Arthritis Rheum 2008;38(2):132–60.
2. Ebert E. Gastric and enteric involvement in progressive systemic sclerosis. J Clin Gastroenterol 2008;42(1):5–12.
3. Faezi ST, Paragomi P, Shahali A, et al. Prevalence and severity of depression and anxiety in patients with systemic sclerosis: an epidemiologic survey and investigation of clinical correlates. J Clin Rheumatol 2017;23(2):80–6.
4. Bodukam V, Hays RD, Maranian P, et al. Association of gastrointestinal involvement and depressive symptoms in patients with systemic sclerosis. Research Support, N.I.H., Extramural. Rheumatology 2011;50(2):330–4.
5. Frantz C, Avouac J, Distler O, et al. Impaired quality of life in systemic sclerosis and patient perception of the disease: a large international survey. Semin Arthritis Rheum 2016;46(1):115–23.
6. Franck-Larsson K, Graf W, Rönnblom A. Lower gastrointestinal symptoms and quality of life in patients with systemic sclerosis: a population-based study. Eur J Gastroenterol Hepatol 2009;21(2):176–82.
7. Sharif R, Mayes MD, Nicassio PM, et al. Determinants of work disability in patients with systemic sclerosis: a longitudinal study of the GENISOS cohort. Semin Arthritis Rheum 2011;41(1):38–47.
8. Basta F, Afeltra A, Margiotta DPE. Fatigue in systemic sclerosis: a systematic review. Systematic Review. Clin Exp Rheumatol 2018;36 Suppl 113(4):150–60.

9. Horsley-Silva JL, Umar SB, Vela MF, et al. The impact of gastroesophageal reflux disease symptoms in scleroderma: effects on sleep quality. Dis Esophagus 2019;32(5):doy136.
10. Steen VD, Medsger TA Jr. Severe organ involvement in systemic sclerosis with diffuse scleroderma. Arthritis Rheum 2000;43(11):2437–44.
11. Hoffmann-Vold A-M, Volkmann ER. Gastrointestinal involvement in systemic sclerosis: effects on morbidity and mortality and new therapeutic approaches. Journal of Scleroderma and Related Disorders 2019;6(1):37–43.
12. Richard N, Hudson M, Wang M, et al. Severe gastrointestinal disease in very early systemic sclerosis is associated with early mortality. Rheumatology 2019;58(4):636–44.
13. Schmeiser T, Saar P, Jin D, et al. Profile of gastrointestinal involvement in patients with systemic sclerosis. Original Paper. Rheumatol Int: Clinical and Experimental Investigations 2012;32(8):2471.
14. Trezza M, Krogh K, Egekvist H, et al. Bowel problems in patients with systemic sclerosis. Scand J Gastroenterol 1999;34(4):409–13.
15. Shane AL, Mody RK, Crump JA, et al. 2017 Infectious Diseases Society of America clinical practice guidelines for the diagnosis and management of infectious diarrhea. Clin Infect Dis 2017;65(12):e45–80.
16. Feng X, Li XQ, Jiang Z. Prevalence and predictors of small intestinal bacterial overgrowth in systemic sclerosis: a systematic review and meta-analysis. Review. Clin Rheumatol 2021;11:11.
17. Polkowska-Pruszynska B, Gerkowicz A, Szczepanik-Kulak P, et al. Small intestinal bacterial overgrowth in systemic sclerosis: a review of the literature. Systematic Review. Arch Dermatol Res 2019;311(1):1–8.
18. Miller JB, Gandhi N, Clarke J, et al. Gastrointestinal involvement in systemic sclerosis: an update. J Clin Rheumatol 2018;24(6):328–37.
19. Adarsh MB, Sharma SK, Sinha SK, et al. Gastrointestinal dysmotility and infections in systemic sclerosis- an indian scenario. observational study. Curr Rheumatol Rev 2018;14(2):172–6.
20. Bae S, Allanore Y, Furst DE, et al. Associations between a scleroderma-specific gastrointestinal instrument and objective tests of upper gastrointestinal involvements in systemic sclerosis. Clin Exp Rheumatol 2013;31(2 Suppl 76):57–63.
21. Arasaradnam RP, Brown S, Forbes A, et al. Guidelines for the investigation of chronic diarrhoea in adults: British Society of Gastroenterology. Gut 2018;67(8):1380–99.
22. O'Brien L, Wall CL, Wilkinson TJ, et al. What are the pearls and pitfalls of the dietary management for chronic diarrhoea? Nutrients 2021;13(5):1393.
23. Cangemi DJ, Lacy BE. Management of irritable bowel syndrome with diarrhea: a review of nonpharmacological and pharmacological interventions. Therapeutic Advances in Gastroenterology 2019;12. 1756284819878950.
24. Iriondo-DeHond A, Uranga JA, Del Castillo MD, et al. Effects of coffee and its components on the gastrointestinal tract and the brain–gut axis. Nutrients 2020;13(1):88.
25. Marie I, Leroi AM, Gourcerol G, et al. Fructose malabsorption in systemic sclerosis. observational study. Medicine 2015;94(39):e1601.
26. Marie I, Leroi AM, Gourcerol G, et al. Lactose malabsorption in systemic sclerosis. Aliment Pharmacol Ther 2016;44(10):1123–33.
27. Doerfler B, Allen TS, Southwood C, et al. Medical Nutrition Therapy for Patients With Advanced Systemic Sclerosis (MNT PASS): A Pilot Intervention Study.

Research Support, N.I.H., Extramural Research Support, Non-U.S. Gov't. Journal of Parenteral & Enteral Nutrition 2017;41(4):678–84.

28. Lomer MC, Parkes G, Sanderson J. lactose intolerance in clinical practice-myths and realities. Aliment Pharmacol Ther 2008;27(2):93–103.

29. Shepherd SJ, Gibson PR. Fructose malabsorption and symptoms of irritable bowel syndrome: guidelines for effective dietary management. J Am Diet Assoc 2006;106(10):1631–9.

30. Lacy BE, Pimentel M, Brenner DM, et al. ACG clinical guideline: management of irritable bowel syndrome. Journal of the American College of Gastroenterology 2021;116(1).

31. Khoshini R, Dai S-C, Lezcano S, et al. A systematic review of diagnostic tests for small intestinal bacterial overgrowth. Dig Dis Sci 2008;53(6):1443–54.

32. Tillman R, King C, Toskes P. Continued experience with the xylose breath test-evidence that the small bowel culture as the gold standard for bacterial overgrowth may be tarnished. Gastroenterology 1981;80(5):1304.

33. Eckburg PB, Bik EM, Bernstein CN, et al. Diversity of the human intestinal microbial flora. Science 2005;308(5728):1635–8.

34. Grace E, Shaw C, Whelan K, et al. Small intestinal bacterial overgrowth-prevalence, clinical features, current and developing diagnostic tests, and treatment. Aliment Pharmacol Ther 2013;38(7):674–88.

35. Losurdo G, Leandro G, Ierardi E, et al. Breath tests for the non-invasive diagnosis of small intestinal bacterial overgrowth: a systematic review with meta-analysis. Journal of Neurogastroenterology and Motility 2020;26(1):16.

36. Kaye SA, Lim SG, Taylor M, et al. Small bowel bacterial overgrowth in systemic sclerosis: detection using direct and indirect methods and treatment outcome. Comparative Study Research Support, Non-U.S. Gov't. Br J Rheumatol 1995; 34(3):265–9.

37. Gasbarrini A, Corazza GR, Gasbarrini G, et al. Methodology and indications of H2-breath testing in gastrointestinal diseases: the Rome Consensus Conference. Aliment Pharmacol Ther 2009;29(Suppl 1):1–49.

38. Polkowska-Pruszynska B, Gerkowicz A, Rawicz-Pruszynski K, et al. The role of fecal calprotectin in patients with systemic sclerosis and small intestinal bacterial overgrowth (SIBO). Diagnostics 2020;10(8):13.

39. Marie I, Leroi AM, Menard JF, et al. Fecal calprotectin in systemic sclerosis and review of the literature. Review. Autoimmunity Reviews. 2015;14(6):547–54.

40. Kilcoyne A, Kaplan JL, Gee MS. Inflammatory bowel disease imaging: current practice and future directions. World J Gastroenterol 2016;22(3):917–32.

41. Maaser C, Sturm A, Vavricka SR, et al. ECCO-ESGAR Guideline for diagnostic assessment in ibd part 1: initial diagnosis, monitoring of known IBD, detection of complications. Journal of Crohn's and Colitis 2019;13(2):144–164K.

42. Maconi G, Nylund K, Ripolles T, et al. EFSUMB recommendations and clinical guidelines for intestinal ultrasound (GIUS) in inflammatory bowel diseases. Ultraschall in der Medizin-European Journal of Ultrasound 2018;39(03):304–17.

43. Novak KL, Nylund K, Maaser C, et al. Expert consensus on optimal acquisition and development of the international bowel ultrasound segmental activity score [IBUS-SAS]: a reliability and inter-rater variability study on intestinal ultrasonography in crohn's disease. Journal of Crohn's and Colitis. 2021;15(4):609–16.

44. Gemignani L, Savarino V, Ghio M, et al. Lactulose breath test to assess oro-cecal transit delay and estimate esophageal dysmotility in scleroderma patients. Clinical Trial. Seminars in Arthritis & Rheumatism 2013;42(5):522–9.

45. Parodi A, Sessarego M, Greco A, et al. Small intestinal bacterial overgrowth in patients suffering from scleroderma: clinical effectiveness of its eradication. Am J Gastroenterol 2008;103(5):1257–62.

46. Low K, Hwang L, Hua J, et al. A combination of rifaximin and neomycin is most effective in treating irritable bowel syndrome patients with methane on lactulose breath test. J Clin Gastroenterol 2010;44(8):547–50.

47. Zhong C, Qu C, Wang B, et al. Probiotics for preventing and treating small intestinal bacterial overgrowth. J Clin Gastroenterol 2017;51(4):300–11.

48. Garcia-Collinot G, Madrigal-Santillan EO, Martinez-Bencomo MA, et al. Effectiveness of Saccharomyces boulardii and Metronidazole for Small Intestinal Bacterial Overgrowth in Systemic Sclerosis. Clinical Trial Research Support, Non-U.S. Gov't. Dig Dis Sci 2020;65(4):1134–43.

49. Revaiah PC, Kochhar R, Rana SV, et al. Risk of small intestinal bacterial overgrowth in patients receiving proton pump inhibitors versus proton pump inhibitors plus prokinetics. JGH open 2018;2(2):47–53.

50. Soudah HC, Hasler WL, Owyang C. Effect of octreotide on intestinal motility and bacterial overgrowth in scleroderma. N Engl J Med 1991;325(21):1461–7.

51. Madrid AM, Hurtado C, Venegas M, et al. Long-term treatment with cisapride and antibiotics in liver cirrhosis: effect on small intestinal motility, bacterial overgrowth, and liver function. Am J Gastroenterol 2001;96(4):1251–5.

52. Roland BC, Ciarleglio MM, Clarke JO, et al. Small intestinal transit time is delayed in small intestinal bacterial overgrowth. J Clin Gastroenterol 2015;49(7): 571–6.

53. Aziz I, Whitehead WE, Palsson OS, et al. An approach to the diagnosis and management of Rome IV functional disorders of chronic constipation. Expert Rev Gastroenterol Hepatol 2020;14(1):39–46.

54. Lacy BE, Mearin F, Chang L, et al. Bowel disorders. Gastroenterology 2016; 150(6):1393–407. e5.

55. Sallam H, McNearney TA, Chen JD. Systematic review: pathophysiology and management of gastrointestinal dysmotility in systemic sclerosis (scleroderma). Research Support, Non-U.S. Gov't Review Systematic Review. Aliment Pharmacol Ther 2006;23(6):691–712.

56. McMahan ZH, Tucker AE, Perin J, et al. The relationship between gastrointestinal transit, Medsger GI severity, and UCLA GIT 2.0 symptoms in patients with systemic sclerosis. Arthritis Care Res 2020;16:16.

57. Locke GR, Pemberton JH, Phillips SF. American Gastroenterological Association medical position statement: Guidelines on constipation. Gastroenterology 2000; 119(6):1761–6.

58. Gao R, Tao Y, Zhou C, et al. Exercise therapy in patients with constipation: a systematic review and meta-analysis of randomized controlled trials. Scand J Gastroenterol 2019;54(2):169–77.

59. Ford AC, Suares NC. Effect of laxatives and pharmacological therapies in chronic idiopathic constipation: systematic review and meta-analysis. Gut 2011;60(2):209–18.

60. Hansi N, Thoua N, Carulli M, et al. Consensus best practice pathway of the UK scleroderma study group: gastrointestinal manifestations of systemic sclerosis. Clin Exp Rheumatol 2014;32(6 Suppl 86):214–21.

61. Ford AC, Moayyedi P, Lacy BE, et al. American College of Gastroenterology monograph on the management of irritable bowel syndrome and chronic idiopathic constipation. Journal of the American College of Gastroenterology 2014;109:S2–26.

62. Dein EJ, Wigley FM, McMahan ZH. Linaclotide for the treatment of refractory lower bowel manifestations of systemic sclerosis. BMC Gastroenterol 2021; 21(1):174.
63. Sattar B, Chokshi RV. Colonic and anorectal manifestations of systemic sclerosis. Review. Curr Gastroenterol Rep 2019;21(7):33.
64. Cowlam S, Vinayagam R, Khan U, et al. Blinded comparison of faecal loading on plain radiography versus radio-opaque marker transit studies in the assessment of constipation. Clin Radiol 2008;63(12):1326–31.
65. Rao SSC, Meduri K. What is necessary to diagnose constipation? Best Pract Res Clin Gastroenterol 2011;25(1):127–40.
66. Rao SS, Kuo B, McCallum RW, et al. Investigation of colonic and whole-gut transit with wireless motility capsule and radiopaque markers in constipation. Clin Gastroenterol Hepatol 2009;7(5):537–44.
67. Ahuja NK, Mische L, Clarke JO, et al. Pyridostigmine for the treatment of gastrointestinal symptoms in systemic sclerosis. Research Support, Non-U.S. Gov't. Semin Arthritis Rheum 2018;48(1):111–6.
68. Vigone B, Caronni M, Severino A, et al. Preliminary safety and efficacy profile of prucalopride in the treatment of systemic sclerosis (SSc)-related intestinal involvement: results from the open label cross-over PROGASS study. Randomized Controlled Trial Research Support, Non-U.S. Gov't. Arthritis Res Ther 2017; 19(1):145.
69. Suares N, Ford A. Systematic review: the effects of fibre in the management of chronic idiopathic constipation. Aliment Pharmacol Ther 2011;33(8):895–901.
70. McMahan ZH, Hummers LK. Systemic sclerosis—challenges for clinical practice. Nat Rev Rheumatol 2013;9(2):90–100.
71. Butt S, Emmanuel A. Systemic sclerosis and the gut. Expert Rev Gastroenterol Hepatol 2013;7(4):331–9.
72. Richard N, Hudson M, Baron M, et al. Clinical correlates of faecal incontinence in systemic sclerosis: Identifying therapeutic avenues. Rheumatology 2017; 56(4):581–8.
73. Sbeit W, Tawfik Khoury AM. Diagnostic approach to faecal incontinence: what test and when to perform? World J Gastroenterol 2021;27(15):1553.
74. Rockwood TH, Church JM, Fleshman JW, et al. Patient and surgeon ranking of the severity of symptoms associated with fecal incontinence. Dis Colon Rectum 1999;42(12):1525–31.
75. Wald A, Bharucha AE, Cosman BC, et al. ACG clinical guideline: management of benign anorectal disorders. Journal of the American College of Gastroenterology 2014;109(8):1141–57.
76. Carrington EV, Heinrich H, Knowles CH, et al. The International Anorectal Physiology Working Group (IAPWG) recommendations: Standardized testing protocol and the London classification for disorders of anorectal function. Neuro Gastroenterol Motil 2020;32(1):e13679.
77. Sallam HS, McNearney TA, Chen JZ. Anorectal motility and sensation abnormalities and its correlation with anorectal symptoms in patients with systemic sclerosis: a preliminary study. ISRN Gastroenterol 2011;2011:402583.
78. Fynne L, Worsøe J, Laurberg S, et al. Faecal incontinence in patients with systemic sclerosis: is an impaired internal anal sphincter the only cause? Scand J Rheumatol 2011;40(6):462–6.
79. Luciano L, Granel B, Bernit E, et al. Esophageal and anorectal involvement in systemic sclerosis: a systematic assessment with high resolution manometry. Clin Exp Rheumatol 2016;34 Suppl 100(5):63–9.

80. Albuquerque A. Endoanal ultrasonography in fecal incontinence: current and future perspectives. World J Gastrointest Endosc 2015;7(6):575–81.
81. Pinto RA, Correa Neto IJF, Nahas SC, et al. Functional and anatomical analysis of the anorectum of female scleroderma patients at a center for pelvic floor disorders. Arq Gastroenterol 2018;1(Suppl 1):47–51, 55 Suppl.
82. deSouza NM, Williams AD, Wilson HJ, et al. Fecal incontinence in scleroderma: assessment of the anal sphincter with thin-section endoanal MR imaging. Radiology 1998;208(2):529–35.
83. Delaney F, Fenlon H, Buckley B, et al. Multimodality imaging of the gastrointestinal manifestations of scleroderma. Clin Radiol 2021;76(9):640–9.
84. Mazur-Bialy AI, Kołomańska-Bogucka D, Opławski M, et al. Physiotherapy for prevention and treatment of fecal incontinence in women—systematic review of methods. J Clin Med 2020;9(10):3255.
85. Mazor Y, Prott G, Jones M, et al. Factors associated with response to anorectal biofeedback therapy in patients with fecal incontinence. Clin Gastroenterol Hepatol 2021;19(3):492–502. e5.
86. Collins J, Mazor Y, Jones M, et al. Efficacy of anorectal biofeedback in scleroderma patients with fecal incontinence: a case–control study. Scand J Gastroenterol 2016;51(12):1433–8.
87. Jarrett M, Mowatt G, Glazener CM, et al. Systematic review of sacral nerve stimulation for faecal incontinence and constipation. Journal of British Surgery 2004; 91(12):1559–69.
88. Simillis C, Lal N, Qiu S, et al. Sacral nerve stimulation versus percutaneous tibial nerve stimulation for faecal incontinence: a systematic review and meta-analysis. Int J Colorectal Dis 2018;33(5):645–8.
89. Leroi AM, Siproudhis L, Etienney I, et al. Transcutaneous electrical tibial nerve stimulation in the treatment of fecal incontinence: a randomized trial (CONSORT 1a). Am J Gastroenterol 2012;107(12):1888–96.
90. Knowles CH, Horrocks EJ, Bremner SA, et al. Percutaneous tibial nerve stimulation versus sham electrical stimulation for the treatment of faecal incontinence in adults (CONFIDeNT): a double-blind, multicentre, pragmatic, parallel-group, randomised controlled trial. Lancet 2015;386(10004):1640–8.
91. Butt S, Alam A, Cohen R, et al. Lack of effect of sacral nerve stimulation for incontinence in patients with systemic sclerosis. Colorectal Dis 2015;17(10): 903–7.
92. Kenefick N, Vaizey C, Nicholls R, et al. Sacral nerve stimulation for faecal incontinence due to systemic sclerosis. Gut 2002;51(6):881–3.
93. Butt S, Alam A, Raeburn A, et al. PWE-183 preliminary significant findings from a randomised control trial of posterior tibial nerve stimulation in systemic sclerosis associated faecal incontinence. Gut 2014;63(Suppl 1):A206.
94. Khanna D, Hays R, Maranian P, et al. Reliability, validity, and minimally important differences of the UCLA scleroderma clinical trial consortium gastrointestinal tract (UCLA SCTC 2.0) instrument. Arthritis Rheum 2009;10:603.
95. Spiegel BMR, Hays RD, Bolus R, et al. Development of the NIH Patient-Reported Outcomes Measurement Information System (PROMIS) gastrointestinal symptom scales. Am J Gastroenterol 2014;109(11):1804–14.
96. Nagaraja V, Hays RD, Khanna PP, et al. Construct validity of the patient-reported outcomes measurement information system gastrointestinal symptom scales in systemic sclerosis. Arthritis Care Res 2014;66(11):1725–30.

97. Wiklund IK, Junghard O, Grace E, et al. Quality of Life in Reflux and Dyspepsia patients. Psychometric documentation of a new disease-specific questionnaire (QOLRAD). Eur J Surg Suppl 1998;(583):41–9.

98. McMahan ZH, Frech T, Berrocal V, et al. Longitudinal assessment of patient-reported outcome measures in systemic sclerosis patients with gastroesophageal reflux disease - scleroderma clinical trials consortium. Research Support, Non-U.S. Gov't. J Rheumatol 2019;46(1):78–84.

99. de la Loge C, Trudeau E, Marquis P, et al. Cross-cultural development and validation of a patient self-administered questionnaire to assess quality of life in upper gastrointestinal disorders: the PAGI-QOL. Qual Life Res 2004;13(10): 1751–62.

100. Jorge JM, Wexner SD. Etiology and management of fecal incontinence. Dis Colon Rectum 1993;36(1):77–97.

101. Thoua NM, Schizas A, Forbes A, et al. Internal anal sphincter atrophy in patients with systemic sclerosis. Research Support, Non-U.S. Gov't. Rheumatology 2011;50(9):1596–602.

Treatment of Inflammatory Arthritis in Systemic Sclerosis

Cristiane Kayser, MD, PhD*,
Lucas Victória de Oliveira Martins, MD, MSc

KEYWORDS

- Systemic sclerosis • Scleroderma • Overlap conditions • Treatment • Arthritis
- Arthropathy

KEY POINTS

- The identification of inflammatory arthritis has important implications in the treatment of systemic sclerosis (SSc).
- Although joint involvement is common in SSc, overlap with rheumatoid arthritis (SSc-RA) should be considered.
- Low-dose corticosteroids, methotrexate, hydroxychloroquine, and non-tumor necrosis factor (TNF) biologics for more severe cases can be considered for the treatment of arthritis in SSc.

INTRODUCTION

Systemic sclerosis (SSc) is a heterogeneous autoimmune disease, with varying clinical manifestations and multisystemic involvement. SSc may be associated with the presence of other connective tissue diseases, including overlap with rheumatoid arthritis (SSc-RA).[1] Nonetheless, articular involvement is frequent in SSc, and it is often difficult to distinguish between SSc-RA overlap and primary articular involvement due to SSc.[2] However, the presence of SSc-RA or arthritis implies changes in the assessment of the disease symptoms and pharmacological management of patients. In this review, we describe the features of joint involvement in SSc, including SSc-RA, and how the pharmacological management of SSc is influenced by the coexistence of arthritis.

Arthritis in Systemic Sclerosis

Articular involvement is a common complication of SSc that can affect 46% to 95% of patients.[3] This complication can occur with different manifestations, such as polyarthralgia, inflammatory arthritis, friction rubs, joint contractures, and

Rheumatology Division, Escola Paulista de Medicina, Federal University of São Paulo (UNIFESP), Rua Botucatu 740, 3 andar, São Paulo, São Paulo 04023-062, Brazil
* Corresponding author.
E-mail address: cristiane.kayser@unifesp.br

Rheum Dis Clin N Am 49 (2023) 337–343
https://doi.org/10.1016/j.rdc.2023.01.008
0889-857X/23/

overlapping RA.[4] It has been shown to strongly contribute to disability, reducing the daily living activities, with a major impact on the quality of life in SSc.[5]

The SSc arthritis pattern varies from an oligoarticular to a polyarticular pattern, non-erosive to erosive, with acute or insidious onset, and with an intermittent or chronic course.[3,4] The most common symptoms are generalized arthralgia and joint stiffness, and they contribute to disability and poor quality of life. Arthralgia or arthritis may be the first presenting symptom of SSc preceding or coinciding with the diagnosis of the disease, highlighting the importance of this manifestation in SSc.[6] Inflammatory arthritis prevalence in SSc is estimated in 16% with hands (particularly the metacarpophalangeal and proximal interphalangeal joints) and wrists being the most commonly affected joints.[2,7] Data from the European Scleroderma Trials and Research (EUSTAR) cohort showed that the presence of synovitis was more frequent in patients with diffuse cutaneous subset, within the first 5 years of the disease, and was associated with elevated levels of acute phase reactants.[2]

A wide range of frequencies of overlapping SSc-RA have been described, varying from 1.7% to 17.5% depending on the study, with a mean prevalence estimated at 4.2%.[8,9] The presence of SSc-RA overlap is associated with a limited cutaneous subset, erosive arthritis, and higher titers of anticyclic citrullinated peptide (CCP) antibodies and rheumatoid factor (RF) in several studies.[1,8,10] However, RF positivity occurs in 30% to 50% of patients with SSc and is not specific and does not distinguish patients with joint involvement from those without.[11,12] Anti-CCP antibody positivity occurs in 1% to 15% of patients with SSc and is more specific and highly associated with RA overlap, particularly if high titers are found.[3,10,13,14] Indeed, different studies have confirmed the value of anti-CCP antibody for the identification of patients with SSc-RA overlap, with a sensitivity of 50% to 100% and a specificity of 95%.[12,13] In other studies, U1RNP, U3RNP, and RNA polymerase 3 antibodies have been associated with joint involvement.[15]

Radiographic abnormalities vary and include periarticular osteopenia, joint space narrowing, and erosive arthritis, which can be found in 18% of patients, especially in the wrist and metacarpophalangeal and proximal interphalangeal joints.[3,16] In those patients with SSc-RA overlap, erosions are similar to those found in RA. In addition, power Doppler ultrasonography is a useful method for detecting inflammation, synovial proliferation, synovitis, and erosions. One study showed that ultrasonography was superior to clinical examination alone in identifying synovitis and tenosynovitis.[17] MRI is also a promising tool, with higher sensitivity for the detection of synovitis and osseous erosion in inflammatory arthropathy due to SSc.[18]

Treatment of Arthritis in Systemic Sclerosis

The management of arthritis in SSc includes nonpharmacological (physical and occupational therapy) and pharmacological treatment (**Fig. 1**). Nonetheless, there is a lack of robust evidence for the treatment of SSc arthritis. Only small or open-label studies that address the treatment of SSc arthritis are available, and there have been no large randomized clinical trials that have evaluated arthritis in SSc.[4] Furthermore, outcome measures for SSc arthritis remain poorly defined. Most measurement tools available in SSc-arthritis that assess clinical examination, functional assessments, and assessments of quality of life, and radiographic imaging are not well validated.[19]

Therefore, the treatment of SSc arthritis is generally extrapolated from those used in RA and other rheumatic diseases.[4,20] Treatment choice should also consider the presence of other organ involvement, such as skin, lung, or gastrointestinal tract involvement. **Table 1** summarizes the different conventional synthetic disease-modifying antirheumatic drugs (csDMARDs), biologic DMARDs (bDMARDs), and other drugs

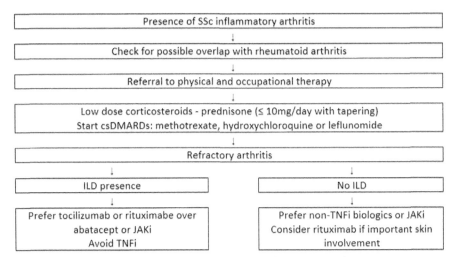

Fig. 1. Suggested algorithm for the treatment of SSc inflammatory arthritis. csDMARDs, conventional synthetic disease-modifying antirheumatic drugs; ILD, interstitial lung disease; JAKi, janus kinase inhibitors; SSc, systemic sclerosis; TNFi, TNF inhibitors.

commonly used to treat arthritis in SSc and the necessary precautions for safe use in those patients.

There is no adequate evidence for the use of nonsteroidal anti-inflammatory drugs in SSc arthritis but they can be used briefly for relief from pain and stiffness.[7] They should be used with caution in patients with gastroesophageal disease, gastric antral vascular ectasia, and renal and cardiac dysfunction.[7,20] Low-dose corticosteroids (prednisone ≤10 mg/d) or corticosteroids injections are relatively safe and might be used for the symptomatic treatment of inflammatory arthritis. Prednisone dose of 15 mg/d or greater should be avoided due to the risk of scleroderma renal crisis, especially in patients with early diffuse SSc and those with anti-RNA polymerase III antibodies.[4,20]

Although csDMARDs have not been properly studied in a controlled randomized trial in SSc arthritis, methotrexate, hydroxychloroquine, and leflunomide can be used based on consensus recommendations.[21,22] Commonly, methotrexate is the first choice for the treatment of SSc arthritis due to its extensive use in RA, modest benefit in the treatment of skin thickening and the possibility of subcutaneous use, especially in patients with SSc with significant gastrointestinal involvement. Hydroxychloroquine and leflunomide have limited literature available but they can be considered in patients who have failed to methotrexate.[20–22]

For patients with refractory arthritis, bDMARDs, with preference given to the use of non-TNF bDMARDs may be considered based on expert opinion.[20–22] Observational studies with tocilizumab, rituximab, and abatacept derived from the EUSTAR cohort showed a reduction in joint outcomes, such as tender and swollen joint count, DAS28 ESR and DAS28 CRP, in SSc.[23–25] In a recent phase II randomized clinical trial of SSc, abatacept showed no difference from placebo in secondary arthritis endpoints and also in the primary endpoint (modified Rodnan skin score) but due to the experience of its use in RA, it can be considered in SSc arthritis or SSc-RA overlap.[26] Most of the trials with tocilizumab or rituximab in SSc have focused on the treatment of skin thickening or interstitial lung disease (ILD) showing some benefits in those situations.[27,28] Moreover, in some of these studies, rituximab and tocilizumab also

Table 1
Pharmacological therapy for arthritis in systemic sclerosis

Drug	Other Indications in SSc	Precautions/Side Effects in SSc
NSAIDs	–	Esophageal involvement, gastric antral vascular ectasia, renal, or cardiac dysfunction
Corticosteroids	–	Scleroderma renal crisis (prednisone >15 mg/d)
csDMARDs		
Methotrexate	Skin	Hepatotoxicity If GI involvement, prefer subcutaneous administration
Hydroxychloroquine	–	Ophthalmologic screening
Leflunomide	–	Hepatotoxicity
bDMARDs		
Tocilizumab	ILD	Higher risk of infection
Abatacept	–	Higher risk of infection
Rituximab	ILD and skin	Higher risk of infection
TNF inhibitors	–	TNF inhibitor–induced pulmonary fibrosis Higher risk of infection
tsDMARDs		
JAK inhibitors	–	Higher risk of infection Cardiovascular events Malignancy

Abbreviations: bDMARDs, biologic disease-modifying antirheumatic drugs; csDMARDs, conventional synthetic disease-modifying antirheumatic drugs; GI, gastrointestinal; ILD, interstitial lung disease; NSAIDs, nonsteroidal anti-inflammatory drugs; SSc, systemic sclerosis; TNF, tumor necrosis factor; tsDMARDs, targeted synthetic disease-modifying antirheumatic drugs.

demonstrated improvement for SSc arthritis.[27,29] In this scenario, the use of rituximab or tocilizumab in csDMARD-refractory SSc arthritis may be considered especially in patients with concomitant SSc ILD or skin thickening.[20,21]

Regarding TNF inhibitors, they have not clearly demonstrated efficacy for the treatment of SSc, and only small observational studies showed some improvement in SSc arthritis with etanercept or infliximab.[30] However, there is concern about the possibility of pulmonary fibrosis induced by TNF inhibitors. There are several studies in RA showing a possible association of TNF inhibitors with new onset or worsening of ILD in patients with RA.[31,32] Thus, as ILD is a common and severe manifestation in SSc, it is recommended the avoidance of the use of TNF inhibitors in these patients, and other biologics agents may be preferred. Moreover, more data about their efficacy and safety in patients with SSc are needed.[4,31]

Other treatments have been evaluated, with mixed results. A small study with tofacitinib in SSc showed improvement of synovitis on ultrasound.[33] Mycophenolate mofetil and cyclophosphamide already have evidence for ILD and cutaneous involvement; however, it is unclear whether they are effective in treating SSc arthritis.[4] A small pilot study with 7 patients showed improvement of SSc arthritis with intravenous immunoglobulin.[34]

Nonpharmacological treatment should also be indicated, including education, rehabilitation, and occupational therapy.[20,21] Therapeutic education is crucial for the management of arthritis in SSc and should be indicated for all patients. Education and counselling contribute to improving the patient's quality of life, treatment adherence, and patient outcome.[35] Rehabilitation and occupational therapy can reduce disability and improves hand function, aerobic capacity, and/or muscle strength.[36] However, most of the studies are small and larger studies to determine the efficacy of rehabilitation techniques, and occupational therapy are needed.

SUMMARY

In summary, articular involvement is common in SSc; however, SSc-RA overlap is less frequent. Management includes nonpharmacological and pharmacological treatment, such as low-dose corticosteroids and csDMARDs, as well as tocilizumab or rituximab for refractory arthritis. Finally, pharmacological management of SSc-RA arthritis should consider the presence of other organic involvements of SSc and the safety profile of drugs in SSc.

CLINICS CARE POINTS

- In systemic sclerosis, the presence of inflammatory arthritis is common and may be due to disease involvement or an overlap with RA.
- Few studies have evaluated the management of articular involvement in SSc and treatment is mainly derived from RA.
- Treatment choice should take into account the presence of other systemic involvement, such as skin or lung.
- Low-dose corticosteroids and conventional DMARDs such as methotrexate and hydroxychloroquine can be used for inflammatory disease.
- For arthritis refractory to conventional DMARDs, treatment with bDMARDs or tsDMARDs may be considered, avoiding the use of TNFi.
- Validated outcome measures and large randomized controlled clinical trials are needed to assess the efficacy of existing and new medications for this disabling complication in SSc.
- Limited cutaneous subset, erosive arthritis, and high titers of rheumatoid factor or anti-CCP are associated with overlap with RA.

DISCLOSURE

The authors have nothing to disclose.

REFERENCES

1. Iaccarino L, Gatto M, Bettio S, et al. Overlap connective tissue disease syndromes. Autoimmun Rev 2013;12(3):363–73.
2. Avouac J, Walker U, Tyndall A, et al. Characteristics of joint involvement and relationships with systemic inflammation in systemic sclerosis: Results from the EULAR Scleroderma Trial and Research Group (EUSTAR) database. J Rheumatol 2010;37(7):1488–501.
3. Avouac J, Clements PJ, Khanna D, et al. Articular involvement in systemic sclerosis. Rheumatology 2012;51(8):1347–56.
4. Blank RB, Nwawka OK, Yusov AA, et al. Inflammatory arthritis in systemic sclerosis: what to do? J Scleroderma Relat Disord 2019;4(1):3–16.
5. Sandqvist G, Eklund M, Åkesson A, et al. Daily activities and hand function in women with scleroderma. Scand J Rheumatol 2004;33(2):102–7.

6. Baron M, Lee P, Keystone EC. The articular manifestations of progressive systemic sclerosis (scleroderma). Ann Rheum Dis 1982;41(2):147–52.
7. Morrisroe KB, Nikpour M, Proudman SM. Musculoskeletal manifestations of systemic sclerosis. Rheum Dis Clin North Am 2015;41(3):507–18.
8. Elhai M, Avouac JÔ, Kahan A, et al. Systemic sclerosis at the crossroad of poly-autoimmunity. Autoimmun Rev 2013;12(11):1052–7.
9. Avouac J, Guerini H, Wipff J, et al. Radiological hand involvement in systemic sclerosis. Ann Rheum Dis 2006;65(8):1088–92.
10. Morita Y, Muro Y, Sugiura K, et al. Anti-cyclic citrullinated peptide antibody in systemic sclerosis. Clin Exp Rheumatol 2008;26(4):542–7.
11. Pakozdi A, Nihtyanova S, Moinzadeh P, et al. Clinical and serological hallmarks of systemic sclerosis overlap syndromes. J Rheumatol 2011;38(11):2406–9.
12. Polimeni M, Feniman D, Skare TS, et al. Anti-cyclic citrullinated peptide anti-bodies in scleroderma patients. Clin Rheumatol 2012;31(5):877–80.
13. Ueda-Hayakawa I, Hasegawa M, Kumada S, et al. Usefulness of anti-cyclic citrul-linated peptide antibody and rheumatoid factor to detect rheumatoid arthritis in patients with systemic sclerosis. Rheumatology 2010;49(11):2135–9.
14. Riccardi A, Martinroche G, Contin-Bordes C, et al. Erosive arthritis autoantibodies in systemic sclerosis. Semin Arthritis Rheum 2022;52:151947.
15. Steen VD. Autoantibodies in systemic sclerosis. Semin Arthritis Rheum 2005; 35(1):35–42.
16. Chapin R, Hant FN. Imaging of Scleroderma. Rheum Dis Clin North Am 2013; 39(3):515–46.
17. Elhai M, Guerini H, Bazeli R, et al. Ultrasonographic hand features in systemic sclerosis and correlates with clinical, biologic, and radiographic findings. Arthritis Care Res 2012;64(8):1244–9.
18. Abdel-Magied RA, Lotfi A, Abdelgawad EA. Magnetic resonance imaging versus musculoskeletal ultrasonography in detecting inflammatory arthropathy in sys-temic sclerosis patients with hand arthralgia. Rheumatol Int 2013;33(8):1961–6.
19. Lóránd V, Bálint Z, Komjáti D, et al. Validation of disease activity indices using the 28 joint counts in systemic sclerosis. Rheumatology 2016;55(10):1849–58.
20. Roofeh D, Khanna D. Management of systemic sclerosis: the first five years. Curr Opin Rheumatol 2020;32(3):228–37.
21. Hachulla E, Agard C, Allanore Y, et al. French recommendations for the manage-ment of systemic sclerosis. Orphanet J Rare Dis 2021;16.
22. Fernández-Codina A, Walker KM, Pope JE. Treatment algorithms for systemic sclerosis according to experts. Arthritis Rheumatol 2018;70(11):1820–8.
23. Elhai M, Meunier M, Matucci-Cerinic M, et al. Outcomes of patients with systemic sclerosis-associated polyarthritis and myopathy treated with tocilizumab or aba-tacept: a EUSTAR observational study. Ann Rheum Dis 2013;72(7):1217–20.
24. Elhai M, Boubaya M, Distler O, et al. Outcomes of patients with systemic sclerosis treated with rituximab in contemporary practice: a prospective cohort study. Ann Rheum Dis 2019;78(7):979–87.
25. Castellví I, Elhai M, Bruni C, et al. Safety and effectiveness of abatacept in sys-temic sclerosis: The EUSTAR experience. Semin Arthritis Rheum 2020;50(6): 1489–93.
26. Khanna D, Spino C, Johnson S, et al. Abatacept in early diffuse cutaneous sys-temic sclerosis: results of a phase ii investigator-initiated, multicenter, double-blind, randomized, placebo-controlled trial. Arthritis Rheumatol 2020;72(1): 125–36.

27. Khanna D, Lin CJF, Furst DE, et al. Tocilizumab in systemic sclerosis: a randomised, double-blind, placebo-controlled, phase 3 trial. Lancet Respir Med 2020;8(10):963–74.

28. Ebata S, Yoshizaki A, Oba K, et al. Safety and efficacy of rituximab in systemic sclerosis (DESIRES): a double-blind, investigator-initiated, randomised, placebo-controlled trial. Lancet Rheumatol 2021;3(7):e489–97.

29. Yarkan Tuğsal H, Zengin B, Kenar G, et al. Rituximab on lung, skin, and joint involvement in patients with systemic sclerosis: a case series study and review of the literature. Int J Rheum Dis 2022;25(7):755–68.

30. Phumethum V, Jamal S, Johnson SR. Biologic therapy for systemic sclerosis: a systematic review. J Rheumatol 2011;38(2):289–96.

31. Perez-Alvarez R, Perez-de-Lis M, Diaz-Lagares C, et al. Interstitial lung disease induced or exacerbated by TNF-targeted therapies: analysis of 122 cases. Semin Arthritis Rheum 2011;41(2):256–64.

32. Huang Y, Lin W, Chen Z, et al. Effect of tumor necrosis factor inhibitors on interstitial lung disease in rheumatoid arthritis: angel or demon? Drug Des Devel Ther 2019;13:2111–25.

33. Karalilova RV, Batalov ZA, Sapundzhieva TL, et al. Tofacitinib in the treatment of skin and musculoskeletal involvement in patients with systemic sclerosis, evaluated by ultrasound. Rheumatol Int 2021;41(10):1743–53.

34. Nacci F, Righi A, Conforti ML, et al. Intravenous immunoglobulins improve the function and ameliorate joint involvement in systemic sclerosis: A pilot study. Ann Rheum Dis 2007;66(7):977–9.

35. Saketkoo LA, Frech T, Varjú C, et al. A comprehensive framework for navigating patient care in systemic sclerosis: a global response to the need for improving the practice of diagnostic and preventive strategies in SSc. Best Pract Res Clin Rheumatol 2021;35(3).

36. Liem SIE, Vlieland TPMV, Schoones JW, et al. The effect and safety of exercise therapy in patients with systemic sclerosis: a systematic review. Rheumatol Adv Pract 2019;3(2):rkz044.

Pulmonary Hypertension
How to Best Treat the Different Scleroderma Phenotypes?

Benjamin D. Korman, MD[a,*], Daniel J. Lachant, DO[b],
Flavia V. Castelino, MD[c]

KEYWORDS

- Scleroderma • Systemic sclerosis • Pulmonary hypertension • Screening
- Treatment

KEY POINTS

- Systemic sclerosis associated pulmonary hypertension (SSc-PH) is highly heterogeneous due to the various clinical phenotypes and varying mechanisms of PH in each patient with SSc.
- Accurate and early diagnosis of SSc-PH is essential to allow for optimal targeted treatment.
- Careful phenotyping of PH in SSc is important because the therapy required for each of these forms of PH is different.

INTRODUCTION

Systemic sclerosis (SSc) is a complex and heterogenous disease characterized by skin fibrosis and variable degrees of internal organ involvement including the heart and lungs.[1] Pulmonary hypertension (PH) is a leading cause of morbidity and mortality among patients with SSc, with estimates of about 30% of SSc deaths attributable to PH.[2]

PH in SSc patients is heterogenous due to the various clinical phenotypes of SSc and a variety of physiologic processes, which can potentially contribute to this pathologic condition, most commonly pulmonary arterial hypertension (PAH). As symptoms are often underreported in SSc, early screening and accurate diagnosis of lung disease is of particular importance, and early treatment is associated with

[a] Division of Allergy, Immunology, and Rheumatology, University of Rochester Medical Center, 601 Elmwood Avenue, Box 695, Rochester, NY 14642, USA; [b] Division of Pulmonary and Critical Care Medicine, University of Rochester Medical Center, 601 Elmwood Avenue, Box 692, Rochester, NY 14642, USA; [c] Division of Rheumatology, Massachusetts General Hospital, 55 Fruit Street, Yawkey 4B, Boston, MA 02114, USA
* Corresponding author.
E-mail address: benjamin_korman@urmc.rochester.edu

Rheum Dis Clin N Am 49 (2023) 345–357
https://doi.org/10.1016/j.rdc.2023.01.015
0889-857X/23/© 2023 Elsevier Inc. All rights reserved.

better clinical outcomes. Assessment of risk factors and screening tests, including pulmonary function testing (PFT), high-resolution computerized tomography (CT) of the chest, and echocardiography are important tools in the initial evaluation of patients with SSc. Historically, systemic sclerosis associated pulmonary arterial hypertension (SSc-PAH) patients have been less responsive to treatments compared with idiopathic PAH.[3] Extensive research has led to an improved understanding of the mediators involved in the pathogenesis of PAH, development of novel targeted therapeutics for SSc-PAH and advanced treatment approaches, which we will outline in this review.

Classification and Definitions

PH encompasses a heterogenous group of conditions defined by an elevated mean pulmonary arterial pressure (PAP) and the clinical phenotype of PH in SSc can be quite variable. PAH is characterized by progressive pulmonary arterial vasculopathy with increased pulmonary vascular resistance (PVR) and PAP leading to increased right ventricular (RV) load, RV dysfunction, and premature death.[4]

The World Health Organization (WHO) classifies patients with PH into 5 categories based on the cause (**Table 1**).[5] Although patients with SSc are susceptible to all forms of PH, WHO Group 1, PAH, is the most common type affecting patients with SSc. Pulmonary veno-occlusive disease (PVOD) can also complicate SSc and explain some SSc patients in Group 1.[6] Other types of PH, including Group 2, pulmonary hypertension due to left heart disease, and Group 3, pulmonary hypertension due to chronic lung disease, are seen given the prevalence of heart disease and interstitial

Table 1		
World Health Organization clinical classification of pulmonary hypertension		
Group	**Potential Causes**	
Group 1	Pulmonary Arterial Hypertension • Idiopathic • Heritable • Drug and toxin • Associated with: CTD, HIV, portal hypertension, congenital heart disease, schistosomiasis • PVOD	
Group 2	PH due to left heart disease	
Group 3	PH due to lung disease and/or hypoxia • Obstructive lung disease • Restrictive lung disease • Mixed restrictive/obstructive pattern	
Group 4	Chronic thromboembolic PH (CTEPH)	
Group 5	PH with unclear multifactorial mechanisms • Hematologic disorders: chronic hemolytic anemia, myeloproliferative disorders, splenectomy • Systemic disorders: sarcoidosis, pulmonary histiocytosis, lymphangioleiomyomatosis • Metabolic disorders: glycogen storage disease, Gaucher disease, thyroid disorders • Other	

Causes that are classified under each of the WHO pulmonary hypertension subsets. Patients with SSc often have physiology which makes them qualify for multiple WHO classes.

Abbreviations: CTD, connective tissue disease; HIV, human immunodeficiency virus; PH, pulmonary hypertension; WHO, World Health Organization.

lung disease (ILD) in patients with SSc. Patients may also rarely present with Group 4 disease, chronic thromboembolic pulmonary hypertension because patients with SSc have an increased risk of venous thromboembolism, possibly due to an increased incidence of antiphospholipid antibodies.[7,8]

Given the multiple and often potentially overlapping causes for SSc-PH, the precise classification of PH can be challenging. Careful phenotyping of PH is thus very important and can affect treatment strategies and decisions. A right heart catherization (RHC) is imperative in the diagnosis of PH and can help differentiate the various types of PH, particularly the distinction between precapillary and postcapillary pulmonary hypertension. Traditional definitions of PAH have used a mean PAP greater than 25 mm Hg, with a pulmonary capillary wedge pressure 15 mm Hg or lesser, and a PVR 3 woods units or greater.[9] Revised evidence-based classification criteria now define a mean PAP greater than 20 mm Hg as abnormal for the purpose of early diagnosis.[10] Multiple studies in SSc-PAH have shown that patients with mPAP between 21 and 24 mm Hg have symptoms comparable to those who meet the old definition, and these patients have an increased risk to progress to 25 mm Hg or greater, with a higher mortality than patients with mPAP 20 mm Hg or lesser.[11,12] Therefore, by lowering the threshold for diagnosis, the new classification should allow for earlier treatment of these high-risk patients.

Pathophysiology

The primary pathophysiology in SSc-PH is thought to be due to loss and obstructive remodeling of the pulmonary vascular bed, which increases PVR and results in right heart failure.[13] At a cellular level, pathologic lesions demonstrate an accumulation of pulmonary artery smooth muscle cells, fibroblasts, myofibroblasts, and pericytes in the pulmonary arterial wall, which lead to the occlusion of the vascular lumen and intimal fibrosis, coupled with loss of precapillary arteries and infiltration of a perivascular inflammatory cell population.

Endothelial dysfunction in PAH is characterized by the impairment of vasodilatation as well as procoagulant properties, and inflammatory changes including an increased expression of adhesion molecules. This results in impaired angiogenesis and vascular repair as well as high shear stress and low oxygen tension, which maintain the vascular dysfunction.[13]

Three key molecular pathways that are significantly dysregulated in PAH endothelial cells are the nitric oxide (NO), endothelin, and prostaglandin pathways, which mediate vasodilation and/or limit vasoconstriction, and each is impaired in SSc endothelial cells. Treatments targeting these 3 pathways are the primary mechanism of action of PAH therapy[14] and are described further in the treatment section.

Epidemiology and Risk Factors

The prevalence of SSc-PH is estimated to be 10% to 15% based on prior studies.[15,16] Risk factors for an increased risk for PAH in SSc include longer disease duration, limited cutaneous SSc (lcSSc), age greater than 60 years, elevated NT-proBNP, anti-centromere antibodies, and nucleolar pattern antinuclear antibody.[17] The PHAROS cohort and REVEAL registry are longitudinal studies that have provided valuable information regarding risk factors and clinical outcomes of patients with SSc-PAH.[18,19]

Historically, lcSSc has been associated with an increased risk for PAH; however, further studies have revealed that PAH is present in both diffuse and limited disease, with some studies showing a similar prevalence in both SSc subsets.[20-22] Patients with lcSSc frequently have prominent vascular manifestations of Raynaud and telangiectasias, the latter of which has correlated with the development of PAH.[23]

Interestingly, digital ulcers, a severe manifestation of Raynaud's, which often responds to vasodilatory medication used in PAH, has not been shown to be associated with PAH.[24]

Screening

Patients who are diagnosed and treated early for PAH have significantly improved outcomes, including long-term survival, compared with those who are diagnosed later in the disease course. The use of a detection strategy using systematic screening in the REVEAL registry led to a 4-fold improvement in mortality compared with routine clinical practice, with an increase in 5-year survival from 17% to 64%[25] while an Australian group found that 3-year survival in a screened cohort was 94.7% compared with 42.7% in an unscreened/prevalent PAH group.[26]

Most patients with SSc should undergo routine screening through a combination of testing including echocardiography, PFT, and biomarker assessment with these noninvasive tests being used to identify patients at high risk for PAH that should undergo invasive hemodynamic testing.[27] Noninvasive measures found to correlate with PAH include an echocardiogram demonstrating an elevated PA pressure (right ventricular systolic pressure [RVSP] >40 mm Hg) and/or any degree of RV dysfunction, PFT findings with diffusion capacity for carbon monoxide (DLCO) less than 60% predicted or an FVC/DLCO ratio greater than 1.6, and an elevated serum NT-proBNP.[28] Although each of these tests is individually useful, most have poor predictive value for PAH in individual patients and therefore screening requires a combination of these approaches to achieve optimal specificity and specificity. Additional methodologies including cardiopulmonary exercise testing and right heart catheterization during exercise have been suggested as an additional means of detection of SSc-PA,[29–31] although additional high-quality studies need to be done to better understand their role in screening and diagnosis.

A variety of screening approaches have been developed to allow for an early detection of SSc-PAH, with the DETECT[32] (using multiple parameters and a scoring system) and Australian Scleroderma Interest Group (ASIG)[33] (primarily utilizing BNP and PFT parameters), The ESC/ERS[34] (echocardiographic parameters) screening protocols to determine whether patients are at high risk and warrant RHC. The Sixth World Symposium of Pulmonary Hypertension recommends that in patients with SSc with DLCO less than 80% of predicted, annual PAH screening should be performed, which includes identification of increased risk by (1) DETECT, (2) the ESC/ERS recommendations, (3) FVC/DLCO ratio >1.6, and (4) NT-proBNP (N terminal pro-B natriuretic peptide) greater than 2-fold upper limit of normal and that if any of these are positive, patients should be referred for RHC[34]; the detailed list of variables used to make these assessments is outlined in **Table 2**.

Treatment

General principles, treatment, and screening for comorbid conditions

The WHO has developed a functional classification system to categorize PH according to clinical symptoms and severity.[35] In general, targeted therapy is recommended for patients with functional class (FC) II or higher, and the goal of treatment is to improve FC. In addition to various targeted therapies discussed in later discussion, the following general strategy can be applied to all types of SSc-PH. Volume optimization should be achieved with the use of diuretics, usually a loop diuretic in combination with aldosterone blockade. Resting, exertional, and nocturnal hypoxemia should be treated with supplemental oxygen to relieve hypoxic vasoconstriction.[36] Evaluating and treating sleep disorder breathing is important[37] because sleep disorder breathing

Table 2
Screening algorithms recommended for determination of need for invasive hemodynamic monitoring in SSc-PAH

Assessment	1. DETECT	2. ESC/ERS Risk Stratification	3. FVC/DLCO Ratio	4. NT-proBNP
	Step 1: Clinical Variables FVC % predicted/DLCO % predicted Current/past telangiectasias Serum anticentromere antibodies	Assess each of the following: Signs of right heart failure Progression of symptoms and clinical manifestations Syncope		
Variables considered	Serum NT-proBNP Serum urate Right-axis deviation on electrocardiogram Step 2: Echocardiographic Right atrium area TR velocity	WHO-FC 6MWD BNP or NT-proBNP Echocardiography cMRI Hemodynamics		
Should lead to RHC if	Scoring at steps 1 > 300 and step 2 > 35	Scoring indicates intermediate or high risk	>1.6	>2× upper limit of normal

Abbreviations: 6MWD, 6 min walk distance; cMRI, cardiac magnetic resonance imaging; DLCO, diffusion capacity for carbon monoxide, FVC; forced vital capacity, NT-proBNP; N terminal B natriuretic peptide, TR; tricuspid regurgitation, WHO-FC; world health organization functional class.

is common in SSc-PH and can contribute to worsening PH. Iron deficiency is also frequently seen in SSc-PH and is associated with worse outcomes.[38] There is limited data about intravenous iron supplementation in SSc-PH.[39] Based on our experience using the iron deficiency criteria from FAIR-HF[40] and CONFIRM-HF,[41] intravenous iron helps improve symptoms of dyspnea and quality of life. SSc patients are at high risk of gastrointestinal hemorrhage.[42] When the iron deficiency is present, expert gastroenterology evaluation is important to minimize blood loss. Other causes of anemia, including vitamin B12 and folate deficiencies should be considered.[43] We will discuss targeted therapies for the treatment of the various SS-PH phenotypes in later discussion (**Table 3**).

Management of SSc-PAH (World Health Organization Class I)

There are limited randomized clinical trials in SSc-PAH, and most data and treatment algorithms are adapted from idiopathic PAH and smaller series of patients with SSc.[44,45] In general, treatment decisions are based on severity of PAH and RV function with the ultimate goal of achieving low risk status.[44] There are multiple different assessments available that use a combination of factors including FC, 6-minute walk test distance, and NT-pro BNP/BNP when calculating risk.[46–48] Early initiation of vasodilator therapy is important to help preserve the pulmonary vasculature by preventing progressive remodeling that increases PVR.[49] To ensure adequate treatment response, follow-up is typically recommended every 3 to 6 months when initiating therapy.[44] Patients with SSc-PAH are complex and can be difficult to manage therefore comanagement with a Pulmonary Hypertension Association Comprehensive Care Center or a specialized center is important and improves outcomes.[45]

Table 3
Management of pulmonary hypertension

Class	Therapies	WHO Group	Comment
Phosphodiesterase type 5 inhibitors (NO)	Sildenafil Tadalafil	1	Typically given in combination with an ERA. Cannot combine with guanylate cyclase stimulator
Guanylate cyclase stimulators (NO)	Riociguat	1,4	Cannot combine with phosphodiesterase type 5 inhibitor. Typically given in combination with ERA
Endothelin Receptor Antagonists (ERA)	Bosentan Macitentan Ambrisentan	1,4	Typically given in combination with an NO pathway drug. Bosentan is not commonly used because of hepatotoxicity risk
Prostacyclin analogs	Epoprostenol	1	Continuous intravenous delivery. Typically added on background therapy
	Treprostinil	1,3	Parenteral (subcutaneous, intravenous), oral, and inhalational delivery Inhalational can be used for Group 3 PH.
	Iloprost	1	Inhalational delivery. Typically added on background therapy
Prostacyclin IP receptor agonist	Selexipag	1	Typically added on background therapy
Calcium channel blocker	Amlodipine	1	Idiopathic PAH if vasoreactive testing is positive
Balloon pulmonary angioplasty		4	Expert CTEPH Center
Pulmonary thromboendarterectomy		4	Expert CTEPH Center
Diuretics (loop + aldosterone antagonist)		1,2,3,4,5	Clinically indicated based on fluid retention.
Intravenous iron		1,2,3,4,5	Clinically indicated
Supplemental oxygen		1,2,3,4,5	Clinically indicated for resting, exertional, nocturnal hypoxemia
Anticoagulation		4	Not recommended to treat group 1 PAH
Immunosuppression			Not recommended to treat group 1 PAH

Treatment modalities used in different forms of SSc-PH are separated by class and then by WHO groups for which they are indicated.

Abbreviations: CTEPH, Chronic Thromboembolic Pulmonary Hypertension; ERA, endothelin receptor antagonist; NO, nitric oxide; PAH, pulmonary arterial hypertension; PH, pulmonary hypertension.

In PAH, endothelial function is impaired, which results in reduced NO synthase,[50] increased production of endothelin-1,[51] and reduced prostacyclin synthase.[52] By targeting these 3 different pathways, vasodilation and inhibition of smooth muscle proliferation is achieved.[53] The NO pathway is targeted with either a phosphodiesterase type-5 inhibitor (sildenafil and tadalafil) or through direct stimulation by soluble guanylate cyclase stimulator (riociguat). Both therapies work to increase cyclic guanosine monophosphate (cGMP). Phosphodiesterase inhibitors should not be used in combination with soluble guanylate cyclase stimulators due to risk of hypotension. The endothelin-1 pathway is targeted by endothelin receptor antagonists. Endothelin-1 binds to ET_A receptor and results in vasoconstriction and cellular proliferation. ET_A receptors can be blocked by selective ET_A receptor antagonist (ambrisentan) or nonselective ET_A-ET_B receptor antagonist (bosentan and macitentan). The theoretic benefit of selective ET_A blockade is ET_B receptors help with vasodilation and antiproliferation. Bosentan[54] is less commonly used because of the risk of hepatotoxicity. Prostacyclin analogs bind to the IP receptor and increase cyclic adenosine monophosphate (cAMP). The current approved agents are epoprostenol (intravenous), treprostinil (parenteral, oral, and inhaled), iloprost (inhaled), and selexipag (IP receptor agonist, oral).

SSc-PAH patients are rarely vasodilator responsive during RHC and, therefore, are not treated with high-dose calcium channel blockers.[55,56] WHO FC I patients can be monitored closely off therapy with frequent reassessment. Less commonly, monotherapy can be used in low-risk patients.[44] Sildenafil monotherapy[57] and riociguat[58] are effective in SSc-PAH. There has not been any subgroup analysis reported with tadalafil in SSc-PAH, and there is less data supporting monotherapy with endothelin receptor antagonists.

Most commonly, SSc-PAH patients are treated with initial upfront combination therapy, such as tadalafil and ambrisentan. The AMBITION trial, in which 24% of patients had SSc found that the combination therapy for PAH was associated with lower clinical failure than monotherapy.[59] In a post hoc analysis, the combination treatment strategy had reduced risk for clinical failure in SSc-PAH.[60] A smaller multicenter study showed combination therapy resulted in improvement in hemodynamics, RV size and function assessed by cardiac magnetic resonance imaging, and improvement in functional status after 36 weeks of treatment in 24 treatment naïve scleroderma PAH patients.[61] In intermediate risk PAH patients, switching the phosphodiesterase inhibitors for riociguat is a reasonable strategy based on the REPLACE study.[62] Since SSc-PAH patients are at high risk for progression, prostacyclin therapy is often added on background vasodilator therapy. In FC II/III patients, selexipag (an oral selective nonprostanoid prostacyclin receptor agonist) reduced hospitalization and disease progression.[63] Subcutaneous treprostinil was shown to improve symptoms, exercise capacity, and hemodynamics in PAH-associated with connective tissue disease.[64] In a very small study of 5 patients with scleroderma PAH, aerosolized iloprost improved 6-min walk test distance and reduced pulmonary pressures.[65] Intravenous epoprostenol was shown to improve 6MWT distance, hemodynamics, and FC in scleroderma PAH.[66] Familiarity with prostacyclin therapy is important when treating these patients. In severe refractory cases, lung transplantation should be pursued.

Management of Patients with World Health Organization Class II Pulmonary Hypertension (Secondary to Lung Disease)

Until recently, there were no specific treatment considerations for PH secondary to ILD. Riociguat previously showed an increased risk of harm,[67] and bosentan showed no benefit.[68] Inhaled treprostinil showed a 31m improvement in 6-minute walk test distance (6MWD) compared with placebo.[69] In the connective tissue disease-ILD subgroup, there was a 43.5 m increase in 6MWD with treprostinil. It is not clear if the benefit is prostacyclin specific, the mode of delivery, or both, and inhaled treprostinil should be considered in this group. Beyond therapy for PH in the setting of ILD, treatment of SSc-ILD has also advanced significantly with the recent approvals of tocilizumab, a monoclonal antibody against IL-6 receptor, and nintedanib, an antifibrotic agent. As both these agents are relatively new and will be used in large numbers of patients with SSc-ILD, ongoing and future studies with these agents in SSc-ILD should be able to assess for the development and protection of PH in these patients.

Management of World Health Organization Class III (Secondary to Left Heart) and IV (Thromboembolic) Pulmonary Hypertension in Systemic Sclerosis

SSc is associated with pulmonary venous hypertension resulting in PH in the setting of often subtle cardiac involvement. Imaging studies using cardiac MRI have shown that one-third of patients with SSc have diastolic dysfunction and around 1 in 5 have myocardial delayed-contrast enhancement suggestive of myocardial fibrosis.[70] Moreover, a hemodynamic study showed that more than 50% of patients diagnosed with SSc-PH had postcapillary PH, and that one-third of the precapillary patients with PAH were reclassified as displaying occult postcapillary PH when subjected to a fluid challenge.[71] This suggests that left-heart disease and heart failure with preserved ejection fraction are likely underdiagnosed and undertreated in SSc and may reflect part of why PAH treatment in SSc is less successful than PAH due to other more uniform causes.

In heart failure with a preserved ejection fraction, aldosterone blockade with spironolactone[72] and sodium-glucose cotransporter 2 inhibitors were shown to reduce the risk of hospitalization.[73] There are currently no specific FDA-approved therapies for mixed precapillary and postcapillary pulmonary hypertension. Involvement of a cardiologist specializing in heart failure is valuable in managing these complicated patients because they often have poor survival relative to other SSc-PH subtypes.

Patients with SSc, particularly those with antiphospholipid antibodies, are at risk for developing deep venous thrombosis, pulmonary emboli, and chronic thromboembolic pulmonary hypertension. In these instances, CT angiography and ventilation perfusion (VQ) scans are diagnostically useful and evaluation at a chronic thromboembolic pulmonary hypertension center is needed to evaluate for interventions such as pulmonary thromboendarterectomy, balloon pulmonary angioplasty, or medical vasodilator therapy. Empiric anticoagulation is not recommended in SSc-PH[74] in contrast to other forms of PH where it has some purported benefit.[75]

Role of Immunomodulation in SSc-PH

Patients with SSc are frequently treated with immunomodulatory therapy for indications including skin disease, ILD, arthritis, and muscle disease. However, unlike other forms of connective-tissue disease PAH such as systemic lupus erythematosus and mixed connective tissue disease where immunomodulation has shown to lead to improved PAH outcomes,[76,77] patients with SSc-PAH have been generally considered to be refractory to immunomodulatory therapy. This is based largely on earlier studies that have shown that cyclophosphamide and glucocorticoid therapy has not been shown to be beneficial in SSc-PAH.[78] A recent multicenter study showed rituximab in SSc-PAH was safe and well tolerated. Despite being on background vasodilator therapy, there was suggestion that rituximab improved 6MWD but was not statistically significant.[79] Prospective studies are needed to determine whether early initiation of tocilizumab or mycophenolate is beneficial in SSc-PH.

SUMMARY

Pulmonary hypertension in SSc is a multifactorial illness, which can have features of any of the WHO PH classes and often results from more than one pathophysiology. Advances in diagnosis and screening have allowed for earlier detection and treatment of less severe disease, which should improve outcomes. Treatment modalities are evolving and most patients will require a combination of therapies and care from an interdisciplinary team of specialists in rheumatology, pulmonology, and cardiology. A better understanding of disease mechanisms has led to novel diagnostic and treatment strategies to specifically address each patient's PH phenotype and improve outcomes in this challenging disease.

CLINICS CARE POINTS

- SSc patients are at risk for multiple different types of PH and management should be tailored to the specific subtype of PH
- Patients with SSc at should be assessed for risk of PH and undergo screening to improve early detection
- Most patients with SSc-PAH should be treated with combination therapy including a phosphodiesterase inhibitor and an endothelin receptor blocker

DISCLOSURES

D.J. Lachant reports consulting and speaking fees from United Therapeutics and Bayer. The University of Rochester receives research funds from United Therapeutics, United States. F.V. Castelino reports consulting fees from Boehringer Ingelheim.

REFERENCES

1. Denton CP, Khanna D. Systemic sclerosis. Lancet 2017;390(10103):1685-99.
2. Steen VD, Medsger TA. Changes in causes of death in systemic sclerosis, 1972-2002. Ann Rheum Dis 2007;66(7):940-4.
3. Ramjug S, Hussain N, Hurdman J, et al. Idiopathic and Systemic Sclerosis-Associated Pulmonary Arterial Hypertension: A Comparison of Demographic, Hemodynamic, and MRI Characteristics and Outcomes. Chest 2017;152(1): 92-102.
4. Lai YC, Potoka KC, Champion HC, et al. Pulmonary arterial hypertension: the clinical syndrome. Circ Res 20 2014;115(1):115-30.
5. Nef HM, Mollmann H, Hamm C, et al. Pulmonary hypertension: updated classification and management of pulmonary hypertension. Heart 2010;96(7):552-9.
6. Gunther S, Jais X, Maitre S, et al. Computed tomography findings of pulmonary venoocclusive disease in scleroderma patients presenting with precapillary pulmonary hypertension. Arthritis Rheum 2012;64(9):2995-3005
7. Schoenfeld SR, Choi HK, Sayre EC, et al. Risk of Pulmonary Embolism and Deep Venous Thrombosis in Systemic Sclerosis: A General Population-Based Study. Arthritis Care Res 2016;68(2):246-53.
8. Balanescu P, Ladaru A, Balanescu E, et al. Association of anti phosphatidyl ethanolamine antibodies and low complement levels in systemic sclerosis patients-results of a cross-sectional study. Scand J Clin Lab Invest 2015;75(6):476-81.

9. Badesch DB, Champion HC, Gomez Sanchez MA, et al. Diagnosis and assessment of pulmonary arterial hypertension. J Am Coll Cardiol 2009;54(1 Suppl): S55–66.

10. Simonneau G, Montani D, Celermajer DS, et al. Haemodynamic definitions and updated clinical classification of pulmonary hypertension. Eur Respir J 2019; 53(1):1801913.

11. Valerio CJ, Schreiber BE, Handler CE, et al. Borderline mean pulmonary artery pressure in patients with systemic sclerosis: transpulmonary gradient predicts risk of developing pulmonary hypertension. Arthritis Rheum 2013;65(4):1074–84.

12. Bae S, Saggar R, Bolster MB, et al. Baseline characteristics and follow-up in patients with normal haemodynamics versus borderline mean pulmonary arterial pressure in systemic sclerosis: results from the PHAROS registry. Ann Rheum Dis 2012;71(8):1335–42.

13. Humbert M, Guignabert C, Bonnet S, et al. Pathology and pathobiology of pulmonary hypertension: state of the art and research perspectives. Eur Respir J 2019;53(1).

14. Zanin-Silva DC, Santana-Goncalves M, Kawashima-Vasconcelos MY, et al. Management of Endothelial Dysfunction in Systemic Sclerosis: Current and Developing Strategies. Front Med 2021;8:788250.

15. Phung S, Strange G, Chung LP, et al. Prevalence of pulmonary arterial hypertension in an Australian scleroderma population: screening allows for earlier diagnosis. Intern Med J 2009;39(10):682–91.

16. Avouac J, Airo P, Meune C, et al. Prevalence of pulmonary hypertension in systemic sclerosis in European Caucasians and metaanalysis of 5 studies. J Rheumatol 2010;37(11):2290–8.

17. Jiang Y, Turk MA, Pope JE. Factors associated with pulmonary arterial hypertension (PAH) in systemic sclerosis (SSc). Autoimmun Rev 2020;19(9):102602.

18. Chung L, Farber HW, Benza R, et al. Unique predictors of mortality in patients with pulmonary arterial hypertension associated with systemic sclerosis in the REVEAL registry. Chest 2014;146(6):1494–504.

19. Kolstad KD, Li S, Steen V, et al. Long-Term Outcomes in Systemic Sclerosis-Associated Pulmonary Arterial Hypertension From the Pulmonary Hypertension Assessment and Recognition of Outcomes in Scleroderma Registry (PHAROS). Chest 2018;154(4):862–71.

20. Hinchcliff M, Fischer A, Schiopu E, et al. Pulmonary Hypertension Assessment and Recognition of Outcomes in Scleroderma (PHAROS): baseline characteristics and description of study population. J Rheumatol 2011;38(10):2172–9.

21. Hunzelmann N, Genth E, Krieg T, et al. The registry of the German Network for Systemic Scleroderma: frequency of disease subsets and patterns of organ involvement. Rheumatology 2008;47(8):1185–92.

22. Steen V, Medsger TA Jr. Predictors of isolated pulmonary hypertension in patients with systemic sclerosis and limited cutaneous Involvement. Arthritis Rheum 2003; 48(2):516–22.

23. Shah AA, Wigley FM, Hummers LK. Telangiectases in scleroderma: a potential clinical marker of pulmonary arterial hypertension. J Rheumatol 2010;37(1): 98–104.

24. Khimdas S, Harding S, Bonner A, et al. Associations with digital ulcers in a large cohort of systemic sclerosis: results from the Canadian Scleroderma Research Group registry. Arthritis Care Res 2011;63(1):142–9.

25. Humbert M, Yaici A, de Groote P, et al. Screening for pulmonary arterial hypertension in patients with systemic sclerosis: clinical characteristics at diagnosis and long-term survival. Arthritis Rheum 2011;63(11):3522–30.
26. Morrisroe K, Stevens W, Sahhar J, et al. Epidemiology and disease characteristics of systemic sclerosis-related pulmonary arterial hypertension: results from a real-life screening programme. Arthritis Res Ther 2017;19(1):42.
27. Vachiery JL, Coghlan G. Screening for pulmonary arterial hypertension in systemic sclerosis. Eur Respir Rev 2009;18(113):162–9.
28. Young A, Nagaraja V, Basilious M, et al. Update of screening and diagnostic modalities for connective tissue disease-associated pulmonary arterial hypertension. Semin Arthritis Rheum 2019;48(6):1059–67.
29. Santaniello A, Casella R, Vicenzi M, et al. Cardiopulmonary exercise testing in a combined screening approach to individuate pulmonary arterial hypertension in systemic sclerosis. Rheumatology 2020;59(7):1581–6.
30. Walkey AJ, Ieong M, Alikhan M, et al. Cardiopulmonary exercise testing with right-heart catheterization in patients with systemic sclerosis. J Rheumatol 2010;37(9):1871–7.
31. Kovacs G, Olschewski H. Potential role of exercise echocardiography and right heart catheterization in the detection of early pulmonary vascular disease in patients with systemic sclerosis. J Scleroderma Relat Disord 2019;4(3):219–24.
32. Coghlan JG, Denton CP, Grunig E, et al. Evidence-based detection of pulmonary arterial hypertension in systemic sclerosis: the DETECT study. Ann Rheum Dis 2014;73(7):1340–9.
33. Thakkar V, Stevens WM, Prior D, et al. N-terminal pro-brain natriuretic peptide in a novel screening algorithm for pulmonary arterial hypertension in systemic sclerosis: a case-control study. Arthritis Res Ther 2012;14(3):R143.
34. Frost A, Badesch D, Gibbs JSR, et al. Diagnosis of pulmonary hypertension. Eur Respir J 2019;53(1).
35. Galie N, Humbert M, Vachiery JL, et al. 2015 ESC/ERS Guidelines for the Diagnosis and Treatment of Pulmonary Hypertension. Rev Esp Cardiol 2016; 69(2):177.
36. Dunham-Snary KJ, Wu D, Sykes EA, et al. Hypoxic Pulmonary Vasoconstriction: From Molecular Mechanisms to Medicine. Chest 2017;151(1):181–92.
37. Nokes BT, Raza HA, Cartin-Ceba R, et al. Individuals With Scleroderma May Have Increased Risk of Sleep-Disordered Breathing. J Clin Sleep Med 2019; 15(11):1665–9.
38. Ruiter G, Lanser IJ, de Man FS, et al. Iron deficiency in systemic sclerosis patients with and without pulmonary hypertension. Rheumatology 2014;53(2): 285–92.
39. Neumann M, Wong KA, Lazo K, et al. Iron therapy as a novel treatment of scleroderma-related pulmonary hypertension: A case report and literature review. Respirology Case Reports 2022;10(2):e0904.
40. Anker SD, Comin Colet J, Filippatos G, et al. Ferric Carboxymaltose in Patients with Heart Failure and Iron Deficiency. N Engl J Med 2009;361(25):2436–48.
41. Ponikowski P, van Veldhuisen DJ, Comin-Colet J, et al. Beneficial effects of long-term intravenous iron therapy with ferric carboxymaltose in patients with symptomatic heart failure and iron deficiency. Eur Heart J 2015;36(11):657–68.
42. Shreiner AB, Murray C, Denton C, et al. Gastrointestinal Manifestations of Systemic Sclerosis. J Scleroderma Relat Disord 2016;1(3):247–56.
43. Wielosz E, Majdan M. Haematological abnormalities in systemic sclerosis. Reumatologia 2020;58(3):162–6.

44. Galiè N, Channick RN, Frantz RP, et al. Risk stratification and medical therapy of pulmonary arterial hypertension. Eur Respir J 2019;53(1):1801889.

45. Klinger JR, Elliott CG, Levine DJ, et al. Therapy for Pulmonary Arterial Hypertension in Adults: Update of the CHEST Guideline and Expert Panel Report. Chest 2019;155(3):565–86.

46. Kylhammar D, Kjellström B, Hjalmarsson C, et al. A comprehensive risk stratification at early follow-up determines prognosis in pulmonary arterial hypertension. Eur Heart J 2018;39(47):4175–81.

47. Boucly A, Weatherald J, Savale L, et al. Risk assessment, prognosis and guideline implementation in pulmonary arterial hypertension. Eur Respir J 2017;50(2): 1700889.

48. Benza RL, Kanwar MK, Raina A, et al. Development and Validation of an Abridged Version of the REVEAL 2.0 Risk Score Calculator, REVEAL Lite 2, for Use in Patients With Pulmonary Arterial Hypertension. Chest 2021;159(1):337–46.

49. Vachiéry J-L, Gaine S. Challenges in the diagnosis and treatment of pulmonary arterial hypertension. Eur Respir Rev 2012;21(126):313.

50. Giaid A, Saleh D. Reduced expression of endothelial nitric oxide synthase in the lungs of patients with pulmonary hypertension. N Engl J Med 1995;333(4):214–21.

51. Giaid A, Yanagisawa M, Langleben D, et al. Expression of endothelin-1 in the lungs of patients with pulmonary hypertension. N Engl J Med 1993;328(24): 1732–9.

52. Tuder RM, Cool CD, Geraci MW, et al. Prostacyclin synthase expression is decreased in lungs from patients with severe pulmonary hypertension. Am J Respir Crit Care Med 1999;159(6):1925–32.

53. Hassoun PM. Pulmonary Arterial Hypertension. N Engl J Med 2021;385(25): 2361–76.

54. Humbert M, Segal ES, Kiely DG, et al. Results of European post-marketing surveillance of bosentan in pulmonary hypertension. Eur Respir J 2007;30(2):338.

55. Hassoun PM. Therapies for scleroderma-related pulmonary arterial hypertension. Expert Rev Respir Med 2009;3(2):187–96.

56. Humbert M, Sitbon O, Chaouat A, et al. Pulmonary arterial hypertension in France: results from a national registry. Am J Respir Crit Care Med 2006; 173(9):1023–30.

57. Badesch DB, Hill NS, Burgess G, et al. Sildenafil for pulmonary arterial hypertension associated with connective tissue disease. J Rheumatol 2007;34(12): 2417–22.

58. Humbert M, Coghlan JG, Ghofrani HA, et al. Riociguat for the treatment of pulmonary arterial hypertension associated with connective tissue disease: results from PATENT-1 and PATENT-2. Ann Rheum Dis 2017;76(2):422–6.

59. Galiè N, Barberà JA, Frost AE, et al. Initial Use of Ambrisentan plus Tadalafil in Pulmonary Arterial Hypertension. N Engl J Med 2015;373(9):834–44.

60. Coghlan JG, Galiè N, Barberà JA, et al. Initial combination therapy with ambrisentan and tadalafil in connective tissue disease-associated pulmonary arterial hypertension (CTD-PAH): subgroup analysis from the AMBITION trial. Ann Rheum Dis 2017;76(7):1219–27.

61. Hassoun PM, Zamanian RT, Damico R, et al. Ambrisentan and Tadalafil Up-front Combination Therapy in Scleroderma-associated Pulmonary Arterial Hypertension. Am J Respir Crit Care Med 2015;192(9):1102–10.

62. Hoeper MM, Al-Hiti H, Benza RL, et al. Switching to riociguat versus maintenance therapy with phosphodiesterase-5 inhibitors in patients with pulmonary arterial

hypertension (REPLACE): a multicentre, open-label, randomised controlled trial. Lancet Respir Med 2021;9(6):573–84.

63. Gaine S, Chin K, Coghlan G, et al. Selexipag for the treatment of connective tissue disease-associated pulmonary arterial hypertension. Eur Respir J 2017; 50(2):1602493.

64. Oudiz RJ, Schilz RJ, Barst RJ, et al. Treprostinil, a Prostacyclin Analogue, in Pulmonary Arterial Hypertension Associated With Connective Tissue Disease. Chest 2004;126(2):420–7.

65. Launay D, Hachulla E, Hatron PY, et al. Aerosolized iloprost in CREST syndrome related pulmonary hypertension. J Rheumatol 2001;28(10):2252–6.

66. Badesch DB, Tapson VF, McGoon MD, et al. Continuous intravenous epoprostenol for pulmonary hypertension due to the scleroderma spectrum of disease. A randomized, controlled trial. Ann Intern Med 2000;132(6):425–34.

67. Nathan SD, Behr J, Collard HR, et al. Riociguat for idiopathic interstitial pneumonia-associated pulmonary hypertension (RISE-IIP): a randomised, placebo-controlled phase 2b study. Lancet Respir Med 2019;7(9):780–90.

68. Corte TJ, Keir GJ, Dimopoulos K, et al. Bosentan in pulmonary hypertension associated with fibrotic idiopathic interstitial pneumonia. Am J Respir Crit Care Med 2014;190(2):208–17.

69. Waxman A, Restrepo-Jaramillo R, Thenappan T, et al. Inhaled Treprostinil in Pulmonary Hypertension Due to Interstitial Lung Disease. N Engl J Med 2021;384(4): 325–34.

70. Hachulla AL, Launay D, Gaxotte V, et al. Cardiac magnetic resonance imaging in systemic sclerosis: a cross-sectional observational study of 52 patients. Ann Rheum Dis 2009;68(12):1878–84.

71. Fox BD, Shimony A, Langleben D, et al. High prevalence of occult left heart disease in scleroderma-pulmonary hypertension. Eur Respir J 2013;42(4):1083–91.

72. Pitt B, Pfeffer MA, Assmann SF, et al. Spironolactone for Heart Failure with Preserved Ejection Fraction. N Engl J Med 2014;370(15):1383–92.

73. Anker SD, Butler J, Filippatos G, et al. Empagliflozin in Heart Failure with a Preserved Ejection Fraction. N Engl J Med 2021;385(16):1451–61.

74. Khan MS, Usman MS, Siddiqi TJ, et al. Is Anticoagulation Beneficial in Pulmonary Arterial Hypertension? Circulation: Cardiovascular Quality and Outcomes 2018; 11(9):e004757.

75. Roldan T, Villamanan E, Rios JJ, et al. Assessment of the quality of anticoagulation management in patients with pulmonary arterial hypertension. Thromb Res 2017;160:83–90.

76. Jais X, Launay D, Yaici A, et al. Immunosuppressive therapy in lupus- and mixed connective tissue disease-associated pulmonary arterial hypertension: a retrospective analysis of twenty-three cases. Arthritis Rheum 2008;58(2):521–31.

77. Kommireddy S, Bhyravavajhala S, Kurimeti K, et al. Pulmonary arterial hypertension in systemic lupus erythematosus may benefit by addition of immunosuppression to vasodilator therapy: an observational study. Rheumatology 2015;54(9): 1673–9.

78. Sanchez O, Sitbon O, Jaïs X, et al. Immunosuppressive Therapy in Connective Tissue Diseases-Associated Pulmonary Arterial Hypertension. Chest 2006; 130(1):182–9.

79. Zamanian RT, Badesch D, Chung L, et al. Safety and Efficacy of B-Cell Depletion with Rituximab for the Treatment of Systemic Sclerosis-associated Pulmonary Arterial Hypertension: A Multicenter, Double-Blind, Randomized, Placebo-controlled Trial. Am J Respir Crit Care Med 2021;204(2):209–21.

Health Care Utilization
What Is the Cost of Caring for Scleroderma?

Kathleen Morrisroe, MBBS, FRACP, PhD[a,b,]*, Nora Sandorfi, MD[c],
Murray Barron, MD[d]

KEYWORDS

- Systemic sclerosis • Scleroderma • Economic burden • Health care utilization
- Health care cost • Indirect cost • Unemployment • Productivity

KEY POINTS

- Systemic sclerosis (SSc) is associated with significant economic burden with the average annual per patient total cost ranging between USD$26,000 and USD$30,000 across several countries.
- SSc is associated with significant health care utilization and associated cost, with an average annual direct cost per patient with SSc of USD$9106 to USD$28,257.
- SSc is associated with significant unemployment and lost productivity equating to an annual indirect cost per patient of USD$5524 to USD$19,842.
- To allow greater generalizability and transferability of monetary results, we propose that future cost of illness studies provide their cost as a percentage relative to their country's respective national gross domestic product.

INTRODUCTION

Systemic sclerosis (SSc), also known as scleroderma, is a chronic multisystem auto-immune connective tissue disease characterized by progressive fibrosis of the skin and internal organs.[1] SSc can be distinguished into two clinical subtypes based on the extent of skin involvement, with limited SSc (lcSSc) having skin involvement restricted to the fingers (sclerodactyly), distal extremities (distal to the elbows and knees) and face, whilst in diffuse SSc (dcSSc), the proximal extremities and trunk are also affected.[1] The epidemiology of SSc varies worldwide, with lower estimates of prevalence (<150 per million) and incidence (<10 per million per year) reported in Northern Europe and Japan, and higher estimates of prevalence (276 to 443 per

[a] Department of Medicine, The University of Melbourne at St Vincent's Hospital (Melbourne), 41 Victoria Parade, Fitzroy 3065, Victoria, Australia; [b] Department of Rheumatology, St Vincent's Hospital (Melbourne), 41 Victoria Parade, Fitzroy 3065, Victoria, Australia; [c] University of Pennsylvania, White Building, 5th Floor, 3400 Spruce Street, Philadelphia, PA 19104, USA; [d] Division of Rheumatology, Suite A710, 3755 Cote Street Catherine Road, Montreal, Quebec H3T 1E2, Canada
* Corresponding author.
E-mail address: kathleen.morrisroe@svha.org.au

Rheum Dis Clin N Am 49 (2023) 359–375
https://doi.org/10.1016/j.rdc.2023.01.016
0889-857X/23/© 2023 Elsevier Inc. All rights reserved.

million) and incidence (14 to 21 per million per year) in Southern Europe, North America and Australia.[1] Owing to its' progressive disease phenotype and the potential for multi-organ irreversible vascular and fibrotic damage, individuals with SSc require a multimodal team approach to care and lifelong follow-up necessitating significant health care utilization. As such, despite its rarity, SSc is one of the costliest of the rheumatic diseases, with the health care cost of patients with SSc, in terms of dollars per annum, exceeding that of age and sex-matched counterparts with inflammatory arthritis and/or inflammatory myopathies.[2,3]

Furthermore, SSc occurs during peak working age and given the near universal involvement of the hands with manifestations including sclerodactyly, synovitis, joint contractures, Raynaud's phenomenon and digital ulceration, it is not uncommon for patients with SSc to report impairment of hand function resulting in difficulties with employment and work productivity in addition to self-care and household chores.[4,5] As such, SSc also has the potential to have a significant economic burden as a consequence of unemployment and lost productivity.

From a health economic perspective, cost of illness studies are vital in recognizing and understanding the true burden of a disease and the potential impact that new interventions can have in reducing this burden. Economic studies can quantify both the direct costs of the disease, which reflect the costs of health care service utilization, and the indirect costs of the disease which include the costs resulting from lost employment and work productivity attributable to the morbidity and premature mortality of that disease. Because of their significant impact on physical function, indirect costs for the rheumatic diseases can far exceed their direct health care associated costs.[6] Unfortunately certain costs such as the out of pocket expenses for transport to and from the health service appointments, over the counter medical supplies such as dressings and skin care products for digital ulcers, and the significant costs of off-label use of medications and/or experimental treatment are difficult to capture for inclusion in these cost-of-illness studies reviewed here.

This review article highlights the economic burden associated with SSc as a consequence of the direct costs, predominantly comprising health care utilization costs, and the indirect costs attributable to SSc from unemployment and lost productivity. We adopted a pragmatic approach to our review, thereby conducting a broad scoping literature review. We searched the PubMed database for articles written in the English language using the following keywords: "Systemic sclerosis," "Scleroderma," "health care utilization," "economic burden," "cost," "unemployment," and "work productivity." We identified 40 articles, 25 of which are included herein. We excluded 15 as they were not directly related to this review on the economic burden of SSc.

The Cost of Systemic Sclerosis Worldwide

The worldwide literature quantifying the cost attributable to SSc and its disease manifestations are summarized in **Tables 1** and **2**, respectively, and displayed graphically in **Fig. 1**. Given the significant cost variability between studies, we have outlined each of the study's methodology, cost ascertainment and inclusions in **Table 3** to enable a greater understanding of cost variations between studies and countries. In addition, given the inability to compare currencies and time periods, we have converted all costs to the 2022 equivalent US dollars (USD$) to allow for cost comparison. Cost conversion was performed on the May 8th, 2022.

United States

There were six studies which estimated the cost of SSc in the United States between 1994 and 2015. Four studies estimated only the direct cost of SSc[7-10] and the

Table 1
Total cost of systemic sclerosis

Country Year Published	Year Currency	Annual Mean/Median per Patient Cost in Author's Currency			2022 Cost in USD$		
		Direct	Indirect	Total	Direct	Indirect	Total
France							
Lopez-Bastida et al,[16] 2016	2012 EUR€	11,933	9624	21,557	14,799	11,934	26,733
Chevreul et al,[17] 2015	2013 EUR€	8452	10,526	22,459	10,315	12,847	27,412
Germany							
Lopez-Bastida et al,[16] 2016	2012 EUR€	18,896	11,901	30,797	23,431	14,757	38,190
Sweden							
Lopez-Bastida et al,[16] 2016	2012 EUR€	10,171	2557	12,728	12,612	3170	15,783
UK							
Gayle et al,[23] 2020	2016 GBP£	1496			2035		
Lopez-Bastida et al,[16] 2016	2012 EUR€	12,098	14,444	26,542	15,004	17,913	32,917
Italy							
Lopez-Bastida et al,[16] 2016	2012 EUR€	10,899	1701	12,560	13,515	2108	15,575
Belotti Masserini et al,[33] 2003	2001 EUR€	11,073			17,301		
Hungary							
Lopez-Bastida et al,[16] 2016	2012 EUR€	2346	2261	4607	2909	2803	5712

(continued on next page)

Table 1
(continued)

Country Year Published	Year Currency	Annual Mean/Median per Patient Cost in Author's Currency			2022 Cost in USD$		
		Direct	Indirect	Total	Direct	Indirect	Total
Minier et al,[19] 2010	2006 EUR€	4,229	5,390	9,619	5,928	7,556	13,485
Spain							
Lopez-Bastida et al,[6] 2016	2012 EUR€	14,162	7,478	21,640	17,562	9,273	26,839
Lopez-Bastida et al,[18] 2014	2011 EUR€	13,738	7,303	21,042	17,417	9,258	26,670
Canada							
McCormick et al,[13] 2013	2010 CAD$	10,673			10,619		
Bernatsky et al,[2] 2009	2007 CAD$	5,038	13,415	18,453	5,215	13,888	19,103
United States							
Zhou et al,[12] 2019	2015 USD$	18,069	4,554	22,623	21,917	5,524	27,441
RamPoudel et al,[7] 2018	2013 USD$	8,885			10,965		
Fischer et al,[25] 2018	2014 USD$	18,513 to 23,268			22,483 to 28,257		
Furst et al,[10] 2012	2009 USD$	17,365			23,271		
Nietert[9] 2001	1995 USD$	14,948 median 8,441			28,199 median 15,924		
Wilson et al,[11] 1997	1994 USD$	4,694	10,228	14,959	9,106	19,842	29,020

	Year	Currency		
Singapore				
Xiang[15] 2022	2020	SPD$	66,289	47,640
Australia				
Morrisroe et al,[5] 2018	2015	AUD$	67,595	52,468
Morrisroe et al,[14] 2017	2015	AUD$	11,607	9,009

References for conversions (done May 8th, 2022) https://www.inflationtool.com/euro; https://www.xe.com/currencyconverter/; https://www.bankofcanada.ca/rates/related/inflation-calculator/; https://www.bankofengland.co.uk/monetary-policy/inflation/inflation-calculator; https://www.in2013dollars.com/brazil/inflation; https://www.usinflationcalculator.com/https://www.rba.gov.au/calculator/.

Abbreviations: D, direct cost; I, indirect cost; SSc, systemic sclerosis; T, total cost.

Table 2
Cost of systemic sclerosis disease manifestations

Country Year Published	Year Currency	Annual Mean/Median per Patient Cost in Author's Currency			2022 Cost in USD$		
		Direct	Indirect	Total	Direct	Indirect	Total
SSc-ILD							
Belgium							
Davidsen et al,[20] 2021	2019 EUR€	9,293			10,788		
Finland							
Davidsen et al,[20] 2021	2019 EUR€	13,857			16,087		
Greece							
Davidsen et al,[20] 2021	2019 EUR€	6,191			7,186		
Netherlands							
Davidsen et al,[20] 2021	2019 EUR€	10,751			12,480		
Norway							
Davidsen et al,[20] 2021	2019 EUR€	16,333			18,960		
Portugal							
Davidsen et al,[20] 2021	2019 EUR€	8,696			10,095		
Sweden							
Davidsen et al,[20] 2021	2019 EUR€	25,354			29,433		
Denmark							
Knarborg et al,[21] 2022	2020 EUR€	20,275	14,097	29,725	21,022	15,556	33,851

Reference	Year, currency						
Davidsen et al,[20] 2021	2019 EUR€	17,480					20,292
France							
Cottin et al,[22] 2021	2017 EUR€	25,753					27,692
UK							
Gayle et al,[23] 2020	2016 GBP,£	6,375					8,672
United States							
Zhou et al,[24] 2019	2015 USD$	25,977	5,640	33,195	31,510	6,841	40,265
Fischer et al,[25] 2018	2014 USD $	31,285 to 55,446			37,994 to 67,336		
Australia							
Morrisroe et al,[26] 2020	2015 AUD$	8,375			6,504		
SSc-PAH							
United States							
Fischer et al,[25] 2018	2014 USD $	44,454 to 63,320			53,987 to 76,898		
Australia							
Morrisroe et al,[27] 2019	2015 AUD$	9,612			8,878		
Digital ulceration							
Australia							
Morrisroe et al,[28] 2019	2015 AUD$	46,364			32,497		
Italy							
Cozzi et al,[29] 2010	2009 EUR€	23,730			30,301		

References for conversions (done May 8th, 2022) https://www.inflationtool.com/euro; https://www.xe.com/currencyconverter/; https://www.bankofcanada.ca/rates/related/inflation-calculator/; https://www.bankofengland.co.uk/monetary-policy/inflation/inflation-calculator; https://www.in2013dollars.com/brazil/inflation; https://www.usinflationcalculator.com/ https://www.rba.gov.au/calculator/.

Abbreviations: D, direct cost; DU, digital ulceration; I, indirect cost; ILD, interstitial lung disease; PAH, pulmonary arterial hypertension; SSc, systemic sclerosis; T, total cost.

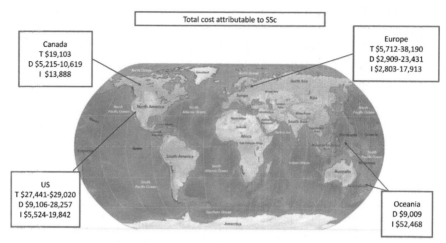

Fig. 1. Total cost attributable to SSc by continent in 2022 equivalent US dollars.

remaining two studies estimated both the direct and indirect costs attribuF to SSc.[11,12] Taken together the average annual total cost per patient with SSc ranged between USD$27,441 and USD$29,020, with the direct cost ranging between USD$9106-USD$28,257 and indirect cost ranging between USD$5524 and USD$19,842 (see **Table 1**). The wide range of direct costs reported in these studies is largely related to which health care costs were included in the study's cost calculation (summarized in **Table 3**). The study's, which reported the lower cost estimate (USD$10,965-USD$15,924) did not include the cost of medications and/or outpatient services.[7,9] The indirect cost attributable to SSc, including both the cost of lost productivity and unemployment, was substantial (USD$5524 to USD$19,842).[11,12] In the two study's which estimated indirect cost, the cost was predominantly driven by lost productivity accounting for 70% and 82% of the indirect cost, respectively.[11,12]

Unlike Wilson and colleagues[11] who found that the indirect cost attributable to SSc was higher than the direct cost accounting for 68% of the total cost (USD$19,842 and USD$9106, respectively), Zhou and colleagues[12] found that the direct cost attributable to SSc was larger than the indirect cost accounting for 79% of the total cost (USD$21,917 vs USD$5524, respectively). Interestingly, in both studies, the direct cost was sourced from large government-based claims databases and included the cost of hospitalization, outpatient/ambulatory care services and medication cost. Zhou and colleagues,[12] with costs calculated in 2015, found that their health care cost was predominantly driven by outpatient services (~37%), followed by hospitalization and medication costs (~33% and ~26%, respectively). Wilson and colleagues,[11] with costs calculated in 1994, found that their health care cost was predominantly driven by hospitalization (~45%), followed by medications (22%) and outpatient services (19%). The latter study's medication cost is not comparable to present day cost given the lack of availability at that time of the more costly pulmonary arterial hypertension vasodilatory therapy and antifibrotic agent and may account for the lower direct cost attributable to SSc.[11]

Canada

There were two Canadian cost of illness studies calculating cost between 2007 and 2010; one calculated the annual direct cost per patient with SSc as USD$10,619[13]

Table 3
Study methodology and inclusion criteria

Country Year Published	Cost Ascertainment		Cost Inclusion							
	Private Database	Government Database	Direct Cost						Indirect Cost	
			Hospitalization	ED Visits	Outpatient	Laboratory Tests	Drugs	Home Care	Lost Productivity	Early Retirement
France										
Cottin et al,[22]2021		X	X				X			
Lopez-Bastida et al,[16] 2016	X	X	X	X	X	X	X	X	X	X
Chevreul et al,[17] 2015	X		X	X	X	X	X		X	X
Germany										
Lopez-Bastida et al,[16] 2016	X	X	X	X	X	X	X	X	X	X
Sweden										
Lopez-Bastida et al,[16] 2016	X	X	X	X	X	X	X	X	X	X
Italy										
Lopez-Bastida et al,[16] 2016	X	X	X	X	X	X	X	X	X	X
Cozzi et al,[29] 2010, Italy		X	X				X			
Belotti Masserini et al,[33] 2003		X	X				X			
Spain										
Lopez-Bastida et al,[16] 2016	X	X	X	X	X	X	X	X	X	X

(continued on next page)

Table 3
(continued)

Country Year Published	Cost Ascertainment		Cost Inclusion							
			Direct Cost						Indirect Cost	
	Private Database	Government Database	Hospitalization	ED Visits	Outpatient	Laboratory Tests	Drugs	Home Care	Lost Productivity	Early Retirement
Lopez-Bastida et al,[18] 2014		X	X	X	X	X	X		X	X
Hungary										
Lopez-Bastida et al,[16] 2016	X	X	X	X	X	X	X	X	X	X
Minier et al,[19] 2010		X	X		X	X	X	X	X	X
Denmark										
Knarborg et al,[21] 2022, *Denmark*		X	X		X		X	X		
Davidsen et al,[20] 2021	X		X		X	X	X	X		
Belgium										
Davidsen et al,[20] 2021	X		X		X	X	X			
Finland										
Davidsen et al,[20] 2021	X		X		X	X	X			
Norway										
Davidsen et al,[20] 2021	X		X		X	X	X			
Portugal										
Davidsen et al,[20] 2021	X		X		X	X	X			
Netherlands										
Davidsen et al,[20] 2021	X		X		X	X	X			
Greece										
Davidsen et al,[20] 2021	X		X		X	X	X			

Study								
UK								
Gayle et al,[23] 2020		X	X			X	X	X
Lopez-Bastida et al,[16] 2016	X	X	X		X	X	X	X
Canada								
McCormick et al,[13] 2013		X	X		X	X		
Bernatsky et al,[2] 2009	X	X	X		X	X	X	X
United States								
Zhou et al,[12] 2019		X	X		X	X	X	X
Zhou et al,[24] 2019		X	X		X	X	X	X
RamPoudel et al,[7] 2018		X	X		X			
Fischer et al,[25] 2018		X	X		X	X		
Furst et al,[10] 2012		X	X		X	X		
Nietert,[9] 2001		X	X		X			
Wilson et al,[11] 1997		X	X		X	X	X	X
Singapore								
Xiang,[15] 2022	X						X	X
Australia								
Morrisroe et al,[26] 2020		X	X		X	X	X	
Morrisroe et al,[28] 2019		X	X		X	X	X	
Morrisroe et al,[5] 2018	X	X	X		X		X	X
Morrisroe et al,[27] 2019		X	X		X	X	X	
Morrisroe et al,[14] 2017		X	X		X	X	X	

Abbreviation: ED, emergency department.

and the other as USD$19,103 (consisting of a direct cost of USD$5215 and indirect cost of USD$13,888).[2] Similar to the Wilson and colleagues study,[11] Bernatsky and colleagues[2] found that the indirect cost (predominantly from lost productivity) was the main driver of the total cost. In addition, Bernatsky and colleagues[2] also noted that the more severe disease subtype, diffuse SSc, was more costly in terms of annual health care dollars and lost productivity, than the limited disease subtype.

Oceania

Three studies, two in Australia and one in Singapore, calculated the annual cost of SSc in Oceania between 2015 and 2020, estimating a direct cost of USD$9009[14] and indirect cost of USD$47,640 to 52,468 resulting from lost employment and reduced productivity.[5,15] Direct costs in this study were driven by hospitalization and emergency department presentations, followed by medication cost and the cost of outpatient services (accounting for 44%, 31.2% and 24.4% of the direct cost, respectively). The direct cost of SSc in this study is lower than that reported in the US studies mentioned above, which may be a reflection of the different health care systems but also a reflection of cost ascertainment, with the Australian study calculating cost of the public health care, whereas the US study estimated cost based on claims in private insurance databases.

Europe

There are six European cost of illness studies published between 2003 and 2020, four of which calculated the total annual cost per patient with SSc and two calculated only the direct cost (see **Tables 1** and **3**). Two studies estimated the total annual cost per patient with SSc in France[16,17] and in Spain[16,18] to be between USD$26,670 and USD$27,412, inclusive of a direct cost of USD$10,315 to USD$17,562 and an indirect cost of USD$9258 to USD$12,847.[16,17] These are comprehensive cost-of-illness studies, with cost ascertainment and inclusion similar to the US studies above, including the cost of hospitalization, ED presentation, outpatient services, and medication cost in addition to the cost of lost unemployment and productivity, which may explain their cost equivalence (US total cost USD$27,441 to USD$29,020). A slightly higher total annual cost for SSc was reported in a German and UK cost of illness study[16] showing an annual cost per patient with SSc of USD$32,917 to USD$38,190, inclusive of a direct cost of USD$15,004 to USD$23,431 and indirect cost of USD$14,757 to USD$17,913 (see **Table 1**). In contrast, the total annual cost per patient with SSc in Italy, Sweden and Hungary seem to be lower despite the cost ascertainment and inclusion being similar (see **Table 3**), with a total annual cost per patient with SSc of USD$15,575 to USD$15,783 in Sweden and Italy (inclusive of a direct cost between USD$12,612 and USD$13,515 and indirect cost between USD$2108- USD$3170),[16] and a total annual cost per patient with SSc in Hungary of USD$5712 to USD$13,485 (inclusive of a direct cost between USD$2909 and USD$5928 and indirect cost between USD$2803 and USD$7556).[16,19] It must be noted however that the cost of professional and informal care reported across these countries, despite similar methodology, was significantly lower in the UK, Sweden and Hungary,[16] and in some cases not recorded, likely contributing to the lower total cost calculated in these respective countries.

The significantly lower total cost among patients with SSc in Hungary, compared with other European countries in addition to US and Canada, highlights the need for a better method of cost comparison between countries, which integrates the countries respective socioeconomic status. This point is further discussed below.

The Cost of Systemic Sclerosis-Associated Cardiopulmonary Manifestations and Digital Ulceration

There are seven studies estimating the cost of SSc associated interstitial lung disease (SSc-ILD) between 2014 and 2019, including four European studies,[20–23] two US studies[24,25] and one Australian study[26] (see **Table 2**). These studies highlight the significant cost associated with SSc-ILD with the two studies estimating the total annual cost per SSc-ILD patient of USD$33,851 to USD$40,265 (inclusive of a direct cost of USD$21,022 to USD$31,510 and indirect cost of USD$6841 to USD$15,556). The driver of health care costs in these studies was inpatient hospitalization, followed by outpatient services and medication costs (accounting 39% to 58.9%, 37% to 28.3% and 2.6% to 7.3% of the direct cost, respectively).[21,24]

Two studies estimated the direct cost of SSc associated pulmonary arterial hypertension (SSc-PAH) between 2014 and 2015, with a direct annual cost per SSc-PAH patient to be USD$9612 with an annual society cost of USD$53,987-USD$76,898[25,27] (see **Table 2**). These studies differ in their inclusion of medication cost, specifically the cost of PAH specific vasodilator therapy. In the US study, PAH vasodilator therapy was included in the direct health care cost and was found to be the main driver of cost, accounting for 51% of the total cost, followed by hospitalization and outpatient services (16% and 4.2%, respectively).[25] In the Australian study,[27] medication was not included in the total cost, and the main driver of health care cost was hospitalization followed by outpatient services.

Two studies estimated the direct health care cost of SSc related digital ulceration (DU), including the inpatient cost of intravenous iloprost, with a reported annual direct health care cost of USD$30,301 to USD$32,497.[28,29] The average direct costs per DU patient was USD$9743 driven predominantly by hospitalization, outpatient services and medication cost (51%, 36% and 2.7%, respectively).

Indirect Cost in Systemic Sclerosis

Compared with the general US population, patients with SSc reported more days of work loss (21.3 vs 6.8; adjusted incidence risk ratio (IRR) 2.6, 95% CI 2.1 to 3.2), including more medically related absenteeism (11.0 vs 4.8; adjusted IRR 2.3, 95% CI 2.0 to 2.6) and days of disability (10.2 vs 2.0; adjusted IRR 2.1, 95% CI 1.7 to 2.7; $P < .0001$).[12] Factors associated with reduced work productivity in an Australian SSc cohort included presence of synovitis and sicca symptoms, whereas tertiary education was protective.[5] In addition, 20% of those working age in an Australian SSc cohort were unemployed. Unemployment was associated with the presence of DU (OR 3.9, 95%CI 1.7 to 9.1, $P = .002$), dcSSc (OR 2.2, 95%CI 1.3 to 3.5, $P = .002$), sicca symptoms (OR 2.7, 95%CI 1.6 to 4.4, $P < .001$), PAH (OR 2.2, 95%CI 1.1 to 4.5, $P = .02$) and the presence of a physical job (OR 1.8, 95%CI 1.1 to 3.1, $P = .03$) and PAH (OR 2.2, 95%CI 1.1 to 4.5, $P = .02$).[30]

The Average Total Cost of Systemic Sclerosis

Taking in account the differences in each study's costing methodologies and excluding certain non-calculable, such as OTC medications, the average annual per patient total cost of SSc is between USD$26,000 and USD$30,000 across several countries.

Determinants of Health Care Service Utilization and Associated Cost

Studies have consistently shown that patients with SSc use health care resources at a higher rate than the background general population and therefore have a higher associated health care cost.[10,12] Patients with SSc are more frequently hospitalized than age- and sex-matched population peers with a higher average length of stay (LOS) whilst in hospital. This was nicely illustrated in a recent US retrospective population-based cohort study showing a relative risk for hospitalization of 1.78 (95%CI 1.52 to 2.08) among patients with SSc compared with general population controls equating to a hospitalization rate of 31.9 vs 17.9 per 100 person years, respectively.[31] In addition, they found that hospitalization rate was increased with increasing age and was highest in the first 5 years following SSc diagnosis (RR 2.16, 95%CI 1.70 to 2.74). After the first 5 years, the hospitalization rate deceased steadily, with no difference in hospitalization rate found after 15 years from SSc diagnosis.[31]

The most common reason for hospitalizations across SSc cohorts include disorders of the circulatory, respiratory, digestive, and musculoskeletal/connective tissue system.[7,14,31] SSc itself is the primary reason for hospitalization in over one-third of hospitalizations, with infection accounting for nearly a quarter of admissions.[7,31] The annual median [interquartile range (IQR)] hospitalization rate per patient with SSc among SSc cohorts ranges between 5 (IQR 2 to 11) with a median LOS of 1 to 8 days.[7,9,13,14,32] Of concern is the in-hospital mortality rate of 5% reported in one large US study,[7] with mortality being independently associated with acute kidney injury, ILD, PAH, cachexia, infection (aspiration/respiratory infection), in addition to the co-morbidities of hypertension, diabetes mellitus, coronary artery disease and cerebrovascular disease.[7] Noteworthy, several these comorbidities have been shown to also be independently associated with a higher risk of hospitalization in other SSc cohorts including the presence of coronary artery disease (HR 1.64, 95%CI 1.01 to 2.64), diabetes mellitus (HR 2.99, 95%CI 1.71 to 5.22), hypertension (HR 1.83, 95%CI 1.33 to 2.52) and PAH (HR 2.08, 95%CI 1.26 to 3.43).[14,31] Additional determinants of health care use and associated cost in SSc include older age (>65 year old), male gender, greater disease severity including the presence of dcSSc, PAH, ILD, DU, renal and gastrointestinal involvement.[2,10,14,27]

Challenges with Quantifying the Cost of Systemic Sclerosis

As can be seen from the tables, there is large variability in the results of the different studies. Some of this is due to different methodologies and some undoubtedly due to very different socioeconomic factors across countries. Higher-income countries have a higher capacity to spend on their health care systems and thus it may be expected that their costs seem higher. One possible way for future studies to adjust for these inter-country economic disparities may be to present these direct and indirect costs as a percentage relative to each country's respective national gross domestic product (GDP). This cost relative to GDP/capita may allow for better generalizability of study results. Unfortunately, the necessary conversions of costs relative to GDP/capita was beyond the scope of this review.

Furthermore, the direct health care cost of SSc is undoubtedly underestimated in the studies included in this review for several reasons. As seen in the most of the studies estimating direct cost In SSc, medication cost is a significant contributor to overall direct cost, often being the second or third highest contributor to direct health care cost, so it is understandable that if medications were not included in the study the total direct costs would seem lower. In addition, there are several medications, such as Rituximab or Tocilizumab. currently used off label in SSc as regulatory agencies have not yet approved such drugs for a SSc indication, thus these medications would be funded as an out-of-pocket cost or compassionate access. Furthermore, over the last 5 years, there has been increasing confidence in the use of transplantation in the treatment of SSc, including stem cell transplantation, lung and heart transplantation. The substantial cost of these transplantations would not have been captured in the included economic studies which included costing performed between 1994 and 2016. In addition, preventative care and out of pocket cost to the patient and their caregivers are often not included in economic studies as they are very difficult to reliably estimate. A limitation of this review in using inflation rates to calculate the cost of SSc in 2022 USD$ lies in the assumption that the health care costs align with changes in inflation rather than changes within each specific countries health care system. Nevertheless, it allows us to make direct comparisons between studies done at different times in different countries.

SUMMARY

The economic burden of SSc, including both the health care utilization cost and cost resulting from unemployment and lost productivity, is substantial and is likely underestimated in many studies. To allow greater generalizability and transferability of monetary results, we propose that future cost of illness studies provide their cost as a percentage relative to their country's respective national GDP.

CLINICS CARE POINTS

- The economic burden of SSc is substantial and is likely underestimated in many studies.
- Recognising the impact of disease on the individuals work life is important, such as impact on employment and productivity.

AUTHORS' CONTRIBUTIONS

K. Morrisroe: literature review, design and preparation of article. N. Sandorfi: literature review, design and preparation of article. M. Barron: literature review, design and preparation of article.

DISCLOSURE

All authors have read and approved the final article. No author declares a conflict of interest.

AVAILABILITY OF DATA AND MATERIALS

Not applicable.

FUNDING

K. Morrisroe holds a National Health and Medical Research Council of Australia Investigator Grant (APP1197169).

REFERENCES

1. Allanore Y, Simms R, Distler O, et al. Systemic sclerosis. Nat Rev Dis Prim 2015; 1(1):15002.
2. Bernatsky S, Hudson M, Panopalis P, et al. The cost of systemic sclerosis. Arthritis Rheum 2009;61(1):119–23.

3. Bernatsky S, Panopalis P, Pineau CA, et al. Healthcare costs of inflammatory my-opathies. J Rheumatol 2011;38(5):885–8.
4. Sandqvist G, Eklund M. Daily occupations–performance, satisfaction and time use, and relations with well-being in women with limited systemic sclerosis. Disabil Rehabil 2008;30(1):27–35.
5. Morrisroe K, Sudararajan V, Stevens W, et al. Work productivity in systemic scle-rosis, its economic burden and association with health-related quality of life. Rheumatology 2018;57(1):73–83.
6. Batko B, Rolska-Wójcik P, Władysiuk M. Indirect Costs of Rheumatoid Arthritis Depending on Type of Treatment-A Systematic Literature Review. Int J Environ Res Public Health 2019;16(16):2966.
7. Ram Poudel D, George M, Dhital R, et al. Mortality, length of stay and cost of hos-pitalization among patients with systemic sclerosis: results from the National Inpatient Sample. Rheumatology 2018;57(9):1611–22.
8. Fischer A, Zimovetz E, Ling C, et al. Humanistic and cost burden of systemic sclerosis: A review of the literature. Autoimmun Rev 2017;16(11):1147–54.
9. Nietert PJ, Silverstein MD, Silver RM. Hospital admissions, length of stay, charges, and in-hospital death among patients with systemic sclerosis. J Rheumatol 2001;28(9):2031–7.
10. Furst DE, Fernandes AW, Iorga SR, et al. Annual medical costs and healthcare resource use in patients with systemic sclerosis in an insured population. J Rheumatol 2012;39(12):2303–9.
11. Wilson L. Cost-of-illness of scleroderma: the case for rare diseases. Semin Arthritis Rheum 1997;27(2):73–84.
12. Zhou Z, Fan Y, Tang W, et al. Economic Burden among Commercially Insured Pa-tients with Systemic Sclerosis in the United States. J Rheumatol 2019;46(8):920–7.
13. McCormick N, Marra C, Sayre EC, et al. Longitudinal analysis of direct medical costs for systemic sclerosis patients: a population- based study 2013.
14. Morrisroe K, Stevens W, Sahhar J, et al. Quantifying the direct public health care cost of systemic sclerosis: A comprehensive data linkage study. Medicine (Baltim) 2017;96(48):e8503.
15. Xiang L, Kua SMY, Low AHL. Work Productivity and Economic Burden of Sys-temic Sclerosis in a Multiethnic Asian Population. Arthritis Care Res 2022;74(5):818–27.
16. López-Bastida J, Linertová R, Oliva-Moreno J, et al. Social/economic costs and health-related quality of life in patients with scleroderma in Europe. Eur J Health Econ 2016;17(Suppl 1):109–17.
17. Chevreul K, Brigham KB, Gandré C, et al. The economic burden and health-related quality of life associated with systemic sclerosis in France. Scand J Rheu-matol 2015;44(3):238–46.
18. López-Bastida J, Linertová R, Oliva-Moreno J, et al. Social economic costs and health-related quality of life in patients with systemic sclerosis in Spain. Arthritis Care Res 2014;66(3):473–80.
19. Minier T, Péntek M, Brodszky V, et al. Cost-of-illness of patients with systemic sclerosis in a tertiary care centre. Rheumatology 2010;49(10):1920–8.
20. Davidsen JR, Miedema J, Wuyts W, et al. Economic Burden and Management of Systemic Sclerosis-Associated Interstitial Lung Disease in 8 European Countries: The BUILDup Delphi Consensus Study. Adv Ther 2021;38(1):521–40.

21. Knarborg M, Løkke A, Hilberg O, et al. Direct and indirect costs of systemic sclerosis and associated interstitial lung disease: A nationwide population-based
cohort study. Respirology 2022;27(5):341–9.
22. Cottin V, Larrieu S, Boussel L, et al. Epidemiology, Mortality and Healthcare
Resource Utilization Associated With Systemic Sclerosis-Associated Interstitial
Lung Disease in France. Front Med 2021;8:699532.
23. Gayle A, Schoof N, Alves M, et al. Healthcare Resource Utilization Among Patients in England with Systemic Sclerosis-Associated Interstitial Lung Disease:
A Retrospective Database Analysis. Adv Ther 2020;37(5):2460–76.
24. Zhou Z, Fan Y, Thomason D, et al. Economic Burden of Illness Among Commercially Insured Patients with Systemic Sclerosis with Interstitial Lung Disease in the
USA: A Claims Data Analysis. Adv Ther 2019;36(5):1100–13.
25. Fischer A, Kong AM, Swigris JJ, et al. All-cause Healthcare Costs and Mortality in
Patients with Systemic Sclerosis with Lung Involvement. J Rheumatol 2018;45(2):
235–41.
26. Morrisroe K, Stevens W, Sahhar J, et al. The clinical and economic burden of systemic sclerosis related interstitial lung disease. Rheumatology 2020;59(8):
1878–88.
27. Morrisroe K, Stevens W, Sahhar J, et al. The economic burden of systemic sclerosis related pulmonary arterial hypertension in Australia. BMC Pulm Med 2019;
19(1):226.
28. Morrisroe K, Stevens W, Sahhar J, et al. Digital ulcers in systemic sclerosis: their
epidemiology, clinical characteristics, and associated clinical and economic
burden. Arthritis Res Ther 2019;21(1):299.
29. Cozzi F, Tiso F, Lopatriello S, et al. The social costs of digital ulcer management in
sclerodema patients: an observational Italian pilot study. Joint Bone Spine 2010;
77(1):83–4.
30. Morrisroe K, Huq M, Stevens W, et al. Determinants of unemployment amongst
Australian systemic sclerosis patients: results from a multicentre cohort study.
Clin Exp Rheumatol 2016;34(Suppl 100):79–84.
31. Coffey CM, Sandhu AS, Crowson CS, et al. Hospitalization Rates Are Highest in
the First 5 Years of Systemic Sclerosis: Results From a Population-based Cohort
(1980-2016). J Rheumatol 2021;48(6):877–82.
32. Sanna S, Casula L, Perra D, et al. AB0788 Epidemiology of systemic sclerosis in
sardinia. analysis of hospitalization data in the decade 2001-2010. Ann Rheum
Dis 2013;72(Suppl 3):A1031–.
33. Belotti Masserini A, Zeni S, Cossutta R, et al. [Cost-of-illness in systemic sclerosis: a retrospective study of an Italian cohort of 106 patients]. Reumatismo
2003;55(4):245–55.

Expanding the Treatment Team

What Is the Role for Occupational Therapy, Physical Therapy, Wound Care, and Nutritional Support in Systemic Sclerosis?

Tracy M. Frech, MD, MS[a],*, Janet L. Poole, PhD, OTR/L[b],
Maureen Murtaugh, PhD, RDN[c], Marco Matucci-Cerinic, MD, PhD[d]

KEYWORDS

- Occupational therapy • Physical therapy • Wound care • Nutrition
- Systemic sclerosis

KEY POINTS

- Coordination of ancillary services is a critical aspect of SSc treatment.
- Implementation of an occupational therapist, physical therapist, wound care expert, and nutritional support specialist into the care plan is a critical component of management.
- Longitudinal use of instruments and questionnaires can detect changes in limitations for patients with SSc and demonstrate improvement with therapy interventions.
- Telemedicine options for ancillary services must address payment and regulatory barriers as well as potential challenges to the treatment process.

INTRODUCTION

Multiorgan system inflammation, vascular dysfunction, and fibrosis characterize systemic sclerosis (SSc). Comanagement of patients with SSc by rheumatologists, pulmonologists, and gastroenterologists requires diagnostics to help determine a treatment plan for joints, muscles, lungs, and the gastrointestinal tract.[1] Coordination of ancillary services is a critical aspect of SSc treatment, and implementation of an

 ᵃ Department of Internal Medicine, Vanderbilt University Medical Center, Nashville, TN, USA; ᵇ Occupational Therapy Graduate Program, Department of Pediatrics, University of New Mexico, Albuquerque, NM, USA; ᶜ Department of Internal Medicine, Division of Epidemiology, University of Utah, Salt Lake City, UT, USA; ᵈ Division of Rheumatology and Scleroderma Unit, AOU Careggi, Florence and Department of Experimental and Clinical Medicine, University of Florence, Italy
* Corresponding author. 1161 Medical Center North, T-3113b, Nashville, TN 37323.
E-mail address: tracy.frech@vumc.org

Rheum Dis Clin N Am 49 (2023) 377–387
https://doi.org/10.1016/j.rdc.2023.01.009
0889-857X/23/© 2023 Elsevier Inc. All rights reserved.

occupational therapist, physical therapist, wound care expert, and nutrition support specialist into the care plan is a critical component of management. An interdisciplinary approach to SSc can address limitations in quality of life through directed assessments and personalized treatment plans.[2]

OCCUPATIONAL AND PHYSICAL THERAPY

Occupational therapy (OT) and physical therapy (PT) are key members of the treatment team to preserve mobility and participation in meaningful life activities for people with SSc. Although an occupational therapist can help address the structural and functional changes of the hands and face, a physical therapist can assist in large joint mobility and strength training and endurance, and both assist in improving functionality. The prevalence of functional and work disability is high and people with SSc can become work disabled within 5 years after diagnosis.[3] Pain, fatigue, stress, anxiety, and depression are symptoms that affect participation in meaningful life activities including work. Self-management is a key component of management of chronic conditions such as SSc, and OT and PT can help people set goals around physical activity, hand and face exercises, and use of strategies to manage fatigue and pain. These can lead to increased self-efficacy and empowerment that can increase functional and work ability and reduce anxiety and depression. Fatigue is one of the top most bothersome symptoms reported by people with SSc.[4] OT plays a key role in teaching people energy management strategies that can be used at work and in daily life activities. Tools to combat fatigue include the use of assistive devices and ergonomic adaptations, pacing, prioritizing, and planning for task completion, sleep, and test breaks.[5] Physical activity and exercise have been shown to reduce fatigue in patients with SSc and improve cardiopulmonary functioning.[6] Physical therapists are the ideal team members to prescribe graded aerobic and strengthening programs and to monitor cardiac and pulmonary function during and after exercise programs. Patients are advised to be more active and exercise but are often not sure what exercises to do or how to get started.[7]

HAND AND FACE ASSESSMENT AND INTERVENTION IN SYSTEMIC SCLEROSIS

SSc can cause range of motion (ROM) limitations both in the edematous and sclerotic phase of the disease.[8] All planes of wrist motion, metacarpophalangeal and proximal interphalangeal flexion/extension, and thumb abduction, opposition and flexion are affected. The prevention of small joint contractures and their management are best achieved by the principles of occupational hand therapy.[9] Strategies to maintain or improve hand function are necessary at the time of SSc diagnosis and throughout the course of the disease.[10,11] Specific exercises for the hand are described in the literature and on the National Scleroderma Foundation website (http://www.scleroderma.org/site/DocServer/Form16c_low_res.pdf?docID=19809&AddInterest=1281): and Taking Charge of Systemic Sclerosis (https://www.selfmanagescleroderma.com/). The use of manual lymphatic drainage, compression[12] and/or heat (paraffin wax, hot packs, warm water)[11,13] can heat up the tissues before patient performs the exercises.

There are instruments that are specific to assessment of SSc hand dysfunction, which are helpful for establishing a baseline measurement. These include measurement of finger-to-palm distance and handgrip strength, as well as formal instruments such as the Cochin Hand Function Scale (CHFS; also called the Duruöz Hand Index) and Hand Mobility in Scleroderma (HAMIS) test.[14,15]

The CHFS consists of 18 self-administered items that assess the ability to perform daily hand-related activities in patients with hand arthritis.[16] Due to redundancies in some items, a short-form CHFS of 6 items (CHFS-6) was developed using optimal test assembly and equivalency methods to measure hand disability in SSc.[17] The CHFS and CHFS-6 are valid and easy-to-use tools for hand involvement in SSc, which can be used in clinical or research setting.[15] There is a culturally adapted Swedish as well as Indian version of Cochin Hand Function Scale (I-CHFS), which are valid and reliable.[18,19]

The HAMIS consists of 9 items that assess all movements in an ordinary ROM-measured hand test and takes approximately 10 minutes to perform.[20,21] The HAMIS is demonstrated to be valid and reliable in English and Italian.[22] This instrument is sensitive to change and a useful outcome measure in hand rehabilitation but was subsequently modified (mHAMIS) to 4 items with less equipment needed in order to provide a more feasible test for use in clinical trials.[23]

If a patient has a digital ulcer (DU), the Hand Disability in Systemic Sclerosis-Digital Ulcers (HDISS-DU) can be used to determine the impact on hand function.[24] Additionally, a patient reported outcome, the Hand scleroDerma lived Experience (HAnDE) scale that assesses functional, esthetic, relational, existential, and emotional dimensions of the lived experience due to hand involvement in SSc, is being tested for use in future trials and clinical practice.[25]

Specific recommendations for the treatment of microstomia in patients with SSc are limited but include therapy evaluation and cessation of tobacco.[26,27] Mouth augmentation and oral stretching exercises are recommended for patients with reduced oral aperture.[28] Specific exercises for the face and mouth opening are described on the National Scleroderma Foundation website (http://www.scleroderma.org/site/Doc Server/Form_16c_low_res.pdf?docID=19809&AddInterest=1281) and Taking Charge of Systemic Sclerosis (https://www.selfmanagescleroderma.com/). A ruler can be used to measure mouth opening can be used by patient to monitor mouth opening. In addition, along with oral opening, the Mouth Handicap in Systemic Sclerosis (MHISS) scale, which has excellent reliability and good construct validity, can be used to assess the effectiveness of oral interventions.[29] Patient-tailored rehabilitation may improve limitations in mouth opening, and help with patient education about mouth and dental hygiene, periodontal maintenance, and treatment of sicca syndrome.[27]

Physical Activity and Exercise in Systemic Sclerosis

Physical activity and aerobic exercise programs, designed and supervised by physical therapists, are effective to improve aerobic capacity and strength. People with SSc can safely participate in a combination of aerobic, resistive, and stretching exercises.[6] Patients with cardiopulmonary involvement can engage in moderate aerobic intensive and moderate resistance but should be started and monitored by the treating physical therapist. Patients should be instructed to monitor blood pressure, heart rate and oximetry, preferably forehead, during exercise. Specific exercises, precautions and safety parameters for patients with muscle involvement should be monitored during graded resistive exercises.[6] Qualitative studies report the positive effects of these exercises on fatigue, well-being and function in daily life.[6] The Global Fellowship on Rehabilitation and Exercise (G-FoRSS) in Systemic Sclerosis reviews the scientific basis of and advocates for education and research of exercise as a systemic and targeted SSc disease-modifying treatment.[6]

In summary, rehabilitation professionals help people with SSc tailor activity options to their capacity while providing care and advice to preserve hand function, and promote self-management of symptoms and physical activity.[30] G-FoRSS advocates for education and research of exercise as a SSc disease-modifying treatment.[6] It is suggested that therapy comanagement care, in particular, for hand and oral dysfunction is underutilized in SSc and that initiatives to improve the quality and accessibility of OT and PT care for patients with SSc is needed.[31,32] The key for effective exercise therapy is consistency; starting gently and escalating with improvement to ensure compliance.[6] When used longitudinally, instruments can monitor and detect changes in patients with SSc who are doing exercise programs prescribed by OT and PT (**Box 1**).[10,12,33] Furthermore, regular review of progress and/or check up by OT and PT are recommended every 3 to 6 months to monitor changes to maintain better hand and overall function.[34]

WOUND CARE ASSESSMENT IN SYSTEMIC SCLEROSIS

Skin ulcers in SSc may be located on digits or extremities and may be related to ischemia, calcinosis, or trauma.[35] Ulcer management requires a dedicated multidisciplinary team that provides patient education and which is vigilant for detecting the development of infective complications and gangrene.[36] Successful treatment requires a combination of oral pharmaceutical therapies as well as appropriate locoregional wound therapies.[37,38] Calcinosis debulking of the hands and upper extremity can decrease pain scores and improve ROM.[39] Compression therapy if concurrent edema, and hyperbaric oxygen if concomitant osteomyelitis may be indicated.[40] Wound assessment in SSc may require hospitalization with comanagement by surgeons and wound care experts.[41–43] Debridement is difficult in immune-mediated wounds and it helps significantly to remove devitalized tissue, which usually delays healing.[37]

Critical aspects of wound assessment by interdisciplinary care teams include healing time, determination of the type/frequency of dressing change, and evaluation of infective complications (**Box 2**).[44] Health-care professionals managing patients with complex wounds require a particular level of expertise and education to ensure optimal wound care.[45] Although wound cleansing aims to remove debris, including dressing remnants and superficial slough from the wound, there is no standard protocol for SSc.[46] Wound dressings should match the level of drainage and depth of a wound.[47] Chronic wounds have additional dressing considerations, including moisture-retentive dressings, which allows for epithelial migration, angiogenesis, supports the presence and function growth factors, autolytic debridement, and preservation of electrical gradients.[48] Wound dressings include films, foams, hydrogels, hydrocolloids, and alginates that provide a moist environment but aim to have an

---

Box 1
Important instruments for SSc care team

Hand function
- Cochin Hand Function Scale (CHFS)[a] also known as the Duruöz Hand Index (DHI)
- Hand Mobility in Scleroderma (HAMIS)[a]
- Hand Disability in Systemic Sclerosis-Digital Ulcers (HDISS-DU)
- Hand scleroDerma lived Experience (HAnDE)

Mouth and nutrition
- Mouth Handicap in Systemic Sclerosis (MHISS)
- Malnutrition Universal Screening Tool (MUST)
- Subjective Global Assessment (SGA)
- European Prospective Investigation into Cancer and Nutrition Norfolk Food Frequency Questionnaire (EPIC-Norfolk FFQ)

[a]Modified shorter item scales exist.

Box 2
Aspects of wound care assessment
• Healing time
• Determination of the type of dressing
• Evaluation of infective complications
• Cleansing and debridement
• Determining frequency of repeat evaluation

optimal water vapor transmission rate and absorptive capacity.[49] For refractory wounds that need growth stimulation, tissue-engineered dressings are an option.[47,50]

Telemedicine holds promise for potential improvement in enhancing availability and reducing costs in SSc wound care assessment; however, the majority of severe ulcerations in SSc require in person care provided by nursing staff.[51,52] Computer-assisted planimetry methods of SSc-related DU area on photographs is reliable but further work is needed to move toward applying these methods as outcome measures in the clinical setting.[53] Nonetheless, the best approach to ulcer assessment in SSc likely includes prompt assessment by a telemedicine ulcer image upload to facilitate both a prompt assessment and comanagement with wound care services for optimized dressing selection and complication monitoring.

NUTRITIONAL ASSESSMENT IN SYSTEMIC SCLEROSIS

Nutritional risk and gastrointestinal involvement are frequent and closely correlated in patients with SSc.[54] Although serum albumin is not useful as a marker for malnutrition in SSc, assessment of body mass index (BMI) and unplanned weight loss (WL), and overall disease severity can be helpful.[55] Systematic screening for malnutrition in both the inpatient and outpatient settings is indicated due to its negative prognostic role.[56,57] Personalized nutritional counseling in an interdisciplinary setting may help address the unmet need of management of nutritional impairment in SSc.[58]

The most common tool used in SSc is the Malnutrition Universal Screening Tool (MUST) for adults, which was developed by the British Association of Enteral and Parenteral Nutrition and is recommended by the European Society of Clinical Nutrition and Metabolism due to its high degree of reliability and association with outcome.[59] The MUST is based on 3 clinical parameters associated with poor outcome: BMI, unintentional WL in the previous 3 to 6 months and absent nutritional intake for more than 5 days. In a study of 586 patients with SSc, univariate logistic regression analysis indicated that predictors of nutritional risk by MUST were diffuse disease, the number of GI symptoms, shorter disease duration, disease severity (physician global assessment), oral aperture, hemoglobin, abdominal distension on examination, and the physician's assessment of possible malabsorption.[60] In another study of 129 patients with SSc showed while it is effective, it may be a relatively poor tool for chronic and gradually progressive disorders.[61,62] Nonetheless, the study identified that severe malnutrition in patients with SSc is associated with reduced quality of life.

The Subjective Global Assessment (SGA) is a reliable method to assess nutritional status based on features of the history and physical examination.[63] This measurement tool includes 6 medical history and 5 physical examination variables to determine the risk of malnutrition without the need for precise body composition analysis. When 24 patients with SSc were assessed by both SGA and MUST, a third of the individuals classified as suspected or moderately malnourished by SGA were assessed at low risk by MUST.[64] The discrepancy in classification of impaired nutrition is possibly due to the inherent difference in the tools, since MUST is a screening tool for malnutrition and SGA is a more comprehensive nutritional assessment tool.

Dietary questionnaires can also be used to assess nutrition. The European Prospective Investigation into Cancer and Nutrition Norfolk Food Frequency Questionnaire (EPIC-Norfolk FFQ) assessed a detailed dietary intake in 42 patients with SSc and identified that dietary factors were connected to body composition and digestive symptoms.[58] The questionnaire contains 130 items (pertaining to the rate of consumption of certain foods, and alcoholic and nonalcoholic beverages). Additionally, the EPIC-Norfolk FFQ has a section regarding the patients' choice of breakfast cereal, the type and amount of milk consumed, food preparation, the fat used in cooking the meals, consumption of visible fat on meat, and intake of dietary supplements. In the SSc cohort, high sodium intake and frequent suboptimal energy consumption was identified.[58] The number of daily meals was not significantly correlated with MUST scores or the amount of weight lost in this study group.[58] These findings support the role for education provided by a dietitian.

Dietitians can help identify appropriate dietary recommendations, such as medical nutrition therapy and implementation of a low-fermentable oligosaccharides, disaccharides, monosaccharides, and polyol (low-FODMAP) diet.[65] A systematic review of open-label nonrandomized studies examining the role of probiotics, low FODMAP described data reported improvements in patient-reported outcome assessment of gastrointestinal symptoms after intervention with probiotic therapy and low-FODMAP diet but not following tailored dietary and nutritional counseling.[66] It should be noted, however, there was a high risk-of-bias for confounding variables and blinding of assessors in each of the 3 studies evaluated.[66] Iron deficiency anemia and vitamin D deficiency can improve with supplementation in SSc, supporting the role of a nutritional support protocol in optimizing care.[67]

CHALLENGES FOR CREATING A MULTIDISCIPLINARY TEAM

Coordination of SSc care between multiple providers is important for compliance to care recommendations but challenges exist in proper implementation (**Box 3**).[1] Telehealth options for OT/PT must address payment and regulatory barriers as well as challenges to the treatment process, particularly in establishing rapport with patients and other members of the health-care team.[68] Regular monitoring of blood pressure, heart rate, and, preferably, forehead oximetry with formal exercise programs may be required depending on SSc disease severity, which further challenges implantation on telehealth therapy options.[6] Medical nutrition therapy provided by registered dietitian nutritionists is largely uncompensated; thus, health centers are less likely to offer these evidence-based services and strengthen team-based care.[69] Costs constraints similarly limit the practices of wound care experts as economic constraints and the

---

Box 3
Challenges a multidisciplinary SSc care team

- Same day coordination of services
- Proper implementation of telehealth options for assessment and treatment
- Reimbursement for services
- Preventative treatment plans

movement toward value-based care demand outcome justification before adopting more costly products.[70] A focus on prevention rather than the management of damage is needed.[71]

SUMMARY

SSc-related impairments impede routine activities of daily living, which are not adequately addressed by the therapeutics prescribed by rheumatologists, pulmonologists, and gastroenterologists. A personalized approach to SSc requires a comprehensive assessment and care team. Questionnaires are helpful to identify restrictions in movement and risk of malnutrition; however, experts are needed to ensure a plan is put into place to address limitations. Telehealth may assist in wound triage and certain OT/PT interventions but further research is needed to understand proper implementation and effectiveness of remote care. Cost coverage and coordination of services is imperative for ensuring ancillary services are provided in a timely and effective basis to improve SSc outcomes.

FUNDING

TF's work is supported by VA Merit Award I01 CX002111.

DISCLOSURE

The authors have nothing to disclose.

CLINICS CARE POINTS

- A comprehensive care plan for SSc requires ancillary services to help a patient maintain function.
- Questionnaires can help identify SSc patients that benefit from specific ancillary services, monitor response to interventionl.

ACKNOWLEDGMENTS

Madeleine E. Frech assembled the articles and assisted in the creation of the article as a research assistant.

REFERENCES

1. Allred D, Frech T, McComber C, et al. Chronic multiorgan rare disease: the role of the nurse practitioner as a leader of the healthcare team. J Med Pract ManageJ Med Pract Manage 2017;32:413–6.
2. Almeida C, Almeida I, Vasconcelos C. Quality of life in systemic sclerosis. Autoimmun Rev 2015;14:1087–96.
3. Hudson M, Steele R, Lu Y, et al. Work disability in systemic sclerosis. J Rheumatol 2009;36:2481–6.
4. Maddali Bongi S, Del Rosso A, Mikhaylova S, et al. District disability, fatigue and mood disorders as determinants of health-related quality of life in patients with systemic sclerosis. Joint Bone Spine 2015;82(1):67–8.
5. Carandang K, Poole J, Connolly D. Fatigue and activity management education for individuals with systemic sclerosis: adaptation and feasibility study of an

intervention for a rare disease. Musculoskeletal Care 2022. https://doi.org/10.1002/msc.1617.

6. Pettersson H, Alexanderson H, Poole JL, et al. Exercise as a multi-modal disease-modifying medicine in systemic sclerosis: an introduction by The Global Fellowship on Rehabilitation and Exercise in Systemic Sclerosis (G-FoRSS). Best Pract Res Clin Rheumatol 2021;35:101695.

7. Harb S, Pelaez S, Carrier ME, et al. Barriers and facilitators to physical activity for people with scleroderma: a Scleroderma Patient-Centered Intervention Network (SPIN) Cohort study. Arthritis Care Res 2021. https://doi.org/10.1002/acr.24567.

8. Palmer DG, Hale GM, Grennan DM, et al. Bowed fingers. A helpful sign in the early diagnosis of systemic sclerosis. J Rheumatol 1981;8:266–72.

9. Young A, Namas R, Dodge C, et al. Hand impairment in systemic sclerosis: various manifestations and currently available treatment. Curr Treatm Opt Rheumatol 2016;2:252–69.

10. Landim SF, Bertolo MB, Marcatto de Abreu MF, et al. The evaluation of a home-based program for hands in patients with systemic sclerosis. J Hand Ther 2019;32:313–21.

11. Poole JL, Dodge C. Rehabilitation of the Hand and Upper Extremity, Seventh Edition, . Scleroderma: therapy. 7th editionVol.. Philadelphia, PA: Elsevier Inc; 2020. p. 1308–22.

12. Muller M, Klingberg K, Wertli MM, et al. Manual lymphatic drainage and quality of life in patients with lymphoedema and mixed oedema: a systematic review of randomised controlled trials. Qual Life Res 2018;27:1403–14.

13. Murphy SL, Poole JL, Chen YT, et al. Rehabilitation interventions in systemic sclerosis: a systematic review and future directions. Arthritis Care Res 2022;74:59–69.

14. Brower LM, Poole JL. Reliability and validity of the Duruoz Hand Index in persons with systemic sclerosis (scleroderma). Arthritis Rheum 2004;51:805–9.

15. Gheorghiu AM, Gyorfi H, Capotă R, et al. Reliability, validity, and sensitivity to change of the cochin hand functional disability scale and testing the new 6-item cochin hand functional disability scale in systemic sclerosis. J Clin Rheumatol 2021;27:102–6.

16. Duruoz MT, Poiraudeau S, Fermanian J, et al. Development and validation of a rheumatoid hand functional disability scale that assesses functional handicap. J Rheumatol 1996;23:1167–72.

17. Levis AW, Harel D, Kwakkenbos L, et al. Using optimal test assembly methods for shortening patient-reported outcome measures: development and validation of the cochin hand function scale-6: a Scleroderma Patient-Centered Intervention Network Cohort Study. Arthritis Care Res 2016;68:1704–13.

18. Bairwa D, Kavadichanda CG, Adarsh MB, et al. Cultural adaptation, translation and validation of Cochin Hand Function Scale and evaluation of hand dysfunction in systemic sclerosis. Clin Rheumatol 2021;40:1913–22.

19. Hesselstrand R, Nilsson JA, Sandqvist G. Psychometric properties of the Swedish version of the Scleroderma Health Assessment Questionnaire and the Cochin Hand Function Scale in patients with systemic sclerosis. Scand J Rheumatol 2013;42:317–24.

20. Sandqvist G, Eklund M. Hand Mobility in Scleroderma (HAMIS) test: the reliability of a novel hand function test. Arthritis Care Res 2000;13:369–74.

21. Sandqvist G, Eklund M. Validity of HAMIS: a test of hand mobility in scleroderma. Arthritis Care Res 2000;13:382–7.

22. Del Rosso A, Maddali-Bongi S, Sigismondi F, et al. The Italian version of the Hand Mobility in Scleroderma (HAMIS) test: evidence for its validity and reliability. Clin Exp Rheumatol 2010;28:S42–7.

23. Sandqvist G, Nilsson JA, Wuttge DM, et al. Development of a modified hand mobility in scleroderma (HAMIS) test and its potential as an outcome measure in systemic sclerosis. J Rheumatol 2014;41:2186–92.

24. Mouthon L, Poiraudeau S, Vernon M, et al. Psychometric validation of the Hand Disability in Systemic Sclerosis-Digital Ulcers (HDISS-DU(R)) patient-reported outcome instrument. Arthritis Res Ther 2020;22:3.

25. Sibeoni J, Dunogué B, Dupont A, et al. Development and validation of a patient-reported outcome in systemic sclerosis: the Hand scleroDerma lived Experience (HAnDE) scale. Br J Dermatol 2022;186:96–105.

26. Gonzalez CD, Pamatmat JJ, Hutto JC, et al. Review of the current medical and surgical treatment options for microstomia in patients with scleroderma. Dermatol Surg 2021;47:780–4.

27. Alantar A, Cabane J, Hachulla E, et al. Recommendations for the care of oral involvement in patients with systemic sclerosis. Arthritis Care Res 2011;63: 1126–33.

28. Maddali Bongi S, Passalacqua M, Landi G, et al. Rehabilitation of the face and temporomandibular joint in systemic sclerosis. Ther Adv Musculoskelet Dis 2021;13. 1759720X211020171.

29. Mouthon L, Rannou F, Bérezné A, et al. Development and validation of a scale for mouth handicap in systemic sclerosis: the Mouth Handicap in Systemic Sclerosis scale. Ann Rheum Dis 2007;66:1651–5.

30. Harb S, Cumin J, Rice DB, et al. Identifying barriers and facilitators to physical activity for people with scleroderma: a nominal group technique study. Disabil Rehabil 2021;43:3339–46.

31. Liem S, van Leeuwen NM, Vliet Vlieland T, et al. Physical therapy in patients with systemic sclerosis: physical therapists' perspectives on current delivery and educational needs. Scand J Rheumatol 2021;1–8. https://doi.org/10.1080/ 03009742.2021.1937306.

32. Liem SIE, van Leeuwen NM, Vliet Vlieland TPM, et al. Physical therapy in systemic sclerosis: the patient perspective. Arthritis Care Res 2021. https://doi.org/10. 1002/acr.24741.

33. Nguyen C, Bérezné A, Mestre-Stanislas C, et al. Changes over time and responsiveness of the Cochin hand function scale and mouth handicap in systemic sclerosis scale in patients with systemic sclerosis: a prospective observational study. Am J Phys Med Rehabil 2016;95:e189–97.

34. Waszczykowski M, Dziankowska-Bartkowiak B, Podgorski M, et al. Role and effectiveness of complex and supervised rehabilitation on overall and hand function in systemic sclerosis patients-one-year follow-up study. Sci Rep 2021;11: 15174.

35. Amanzi L, Braschi F, Fiori G, et al. Digital ulcers in scleroderma: staging, characteristics and sub-setting through observation of 1614 digital lesions. Rheumatology 2010;49(7):1374–82.

36. Hughes M, Bruni C, Ruaro B, et al. Digital ulcers in systemic sclerosis. Presse Med 2021;50:104064.

37. Lebedoff N, Frech TM, Shanmugam VK, et al. Review of local wound management for scleroderma-associated digital ulcers, J Scleroderma Relat Disord, 3, 2018, 66–70.

38. Hughes M, Allanore Y, El Aoufy K, et al. A practical approach to the management of digital ulcers in patients with systemic sclerosis: a narrative review. JAMA Dermatol 2021;157(7):851–8.

39. Klifto KM, Cho BH, Lifchez SD. Surgical debulking for symptomatic management of calcinosis cutis of the hand and upper extremity in systemic sclerosis. J Hand Surg Eur Vol 2021;46:928.e1–9.

40. Ubbink DT, Santema TB, Stoekenbroek RM. Systemic wound care: a meta-review of cochrane systematic reviews. Surg Technol Int 2014;24:99–111.

41. Beldner S, Rabinovich RV, Polatsch DB. Scleroderma of the hand: evaluation and treatment. J Am Acad Orthop Surg 2020;28:e686–95.

42. Ayello EA, Sibbald RG. Scleroderma and person/patient-centered concerns. Adv Skin Wound Care 2018;31:437.

43. Caetano J, Batista F, Amaral MC, et al. Acute hospitalization in a cohort of patients with systemic sclerosis: a 10-year retrospective cohort study. Rheumatol Int 2021. https://doi.org/10.1007/s00296-021-04983-4.

44. Lindholm C, Searle R. Wound management for the 21st century: combining effectiveness and efficiency. Int Wound J 2016;13(Suppl 2):5–15.

45. Eskes AM, Maaskant JM, Holloway S, et al. Competencies of specialised wound care nurses: a European Delphi study. Int Wound J 2014;11:665–74.

46. Pilcher M. Wound cleansing: a key player in the implementation of the TIME paradigm. J Wound Care 2016;25:S7–9.

47. Broussard KC, Powers JG. Wound dressings: selecting the most appropriate type. Am J Clin Dermatol 2013;14:449–59.

48. Powers JG, Morton LM, Phillips TJ. Dressings for chronic wounds. Dermatol Ther 2013;26:197–206.

49. Nuutila K, Eriksson E. Moist wound healing with commonly available dressings. Adv Wound Care 2021;10:685–98.

50. Frech TM, McNeill C, Lebiedz-Odrobina D, et al. Amniotic membrane dressings: an effective therapy for SSc-related wounds. Rheumatology 2019;58:734–6.

51. Jones SM, Banwell PE, Shakespeare PG. Telemedicine in wound healing. Int Wound J 2004;1:225–30.

52. Spinella A, Magnani L, De Pinto M. Management of systemic sclerosis patients in the COVID-19 era: the experience of an expert specialist reference center. Clin Med Insights Circ Respir Pulm Med 2021;15. 11795484211001349.

53. Simpson V, Hughes M, Wilkinson J, et al. Quantifying digital ulcers in systemic sclerosis: reliability of computer-assisted planimetry in measuring lesion size. Arthritis Care Res 2018;70:486–90.

54. Hvas CL, Harrison E, Eriksen MK, et al. Nutritional status and predictors of weight loss in patients with systemic sclerosis. Clin Nutr ESPEN 2020;40:164–70.

55. Baron M, Hudson M, Steele R, et al. Is serum albumin a marker of malnutrition in chronic disease? The scleroderma paradigm. J Am Coll Nutr 2010;29:144–51.

56. Codullo V, Cereda E, Crepaldi G, et al. Disease-related malnutrition in systemic sclerosis: evidences and implications. Clin Exp Rheumatol 2015;33:S190–4.

57. Cereda E, Codullo V, Klersy C, et al. Disease-related nutritional risk and mortality in systemic sclerosis. Clin Nutr 2014;33:558–61.

58. Burlui AM, Cardoneanu A, Macovei LA, et al. Diet in scleroderma: is there a need for intervention? Diagnostics 2021;11. https://doi.org/10.3390/diagnostics 11112118.

59. Stratton RJ, Hackston A, Longmore D, et al. Malnutrition in hospital outpatients and inpatients: prevalence, concurrent validity and ease of use of the 'malnutrition universal screening tool' ('MUST') for adults. Br J Nutr 2004;92:799–808.

60. Baron M, Hudson M, Steele R, et al. Malnutrition is common in systemic sclerosis: results from the Canadian scleroderma research group database. J Rheumatol 2009;36:2737–43.
61. Harrison E, Herrick AL, McLaughlin JT, et al. Malnutrition in systemic sclerosis. Rheumatology 2012;51:1747–56.
62. Preis E, Franz K, Siegert E, et al. The impact of malnutrition on quality of life in patients with systemic sclerosis. Eur J Clin Nutr 2018;72:504–10.
63. Baker JP, Detsky AS, Wesson DE, et al. Nutritional assessment: a comparison of clinical judgement and objective measurements. N Engl J Med 1982;306:969–72.
64. Murtaugh MA, Frech TM. Nutritional status and gastrointestinal symptoms in systemic sclerosis patients. Clinical nutrition 2013;32:130–5.
65. McMahan ZH, Hummers LK. Gastrointestinal involvement in systemic sclerosis: diagnosis and management. Curr Opin Rheumatol 2018;30:533–40.
66. Smith E, Pauling JD. The efficacy of dietary intervention on gastrointestinal involvement in systemic sclerosis: a systematic literature review. Semin Arthritis Rheum 2019;49:112–8.
67. Ortiz-Santamaria V, Puig C, Soldevillla C, et al. Nutritional support in patients with systemic sclerosis. Reumatol Clin 2014;10:283–7.
68. Lee AC, Davenport TE, Randall K. Telehealth physical therapy in musculoskeletal practice. J Orthop Sports Phys Ther 2018;48:736–9.
69. Braunstein N, Guerrero M, Liles S, et al. Medical nutrition therapy for adults in health resources & services administration-funded health centers: a call to action. J Acad Nutr Diet 2021;121:2101–7.
70. Sheckter CC, Meyerkord NL, Sinskey YL, et al. The optimal treatment for partial thickness burns: a cost-utility analysis of skin allograft vs. topical silver dressings. J Burn Care Res 2020;41:450–6.
71. Saketkoo LA, Frech T, Varjú C, et al. A comprehensive framework for navigating patient care in systemic sclerosis: a global response to the need for improving the practice of diagnostic and preventive strategies in SSc. Best Pract Res Clin Rheumatol 2021;35:101707.

Mental Health Considerations in Chronic Disease
What Is the Best Approach for Supporting a Scleroderma Patient?

Nancy Lazar, MSW, LCSW[a],*, Virginia D. Steen, MD[b]

KEYWORDS

- Scleroderma • Mental health • Anxiety • Depression • Social determinants of health
- SDOH • Psychosocial stressors • Self-management

KEY POINTS

- Individuals with scleroderma face intermittent, general, and scleroderma symptom–related psychosocial stressors, which are often associated with social determinants of health issues.
- All of these stressors directly affect their ability to care for themselves, their ability to engage in their life activities on a daily basis, and their overall quality of life.
- There is a prevalence of mental health issues, primarily depression and anxiety, within the scleroderma patient population.
- Considering the voice and main concerns of the scleroderma patient is an important focal point of patient-centered care.
- Directly asking patients about their scleroderma concerns, including their physical health, mental health, and social determinants of health stressors, as well as discussing ways for individuals to address these issues can have a positive impact on their disease self-management and, ultimately, their quality of life.

INTRODUCTION

Systemic sclerosis (SSc and scleroderma) is a complex and incurable connective tissue disease, affecting multiple organs, with significant morbidity and mortality.[1–4] Because this disease is chronic, severe, and systemic, quality of life is significantly affected in this patient population. Research has demonstrated that this disease has a substantial effect on health-related quality of life (HRoQL) when compared not

[a] Culver City, CA, USA; [b] Georgetown University - School of Medicine, Washington, DC 20007, USA
* Corresponding author.
E-mail address: intentionalitybh@gmail.com

Rheum Dis Clin N Am 49 (2023) 389–399
https://doi.org/10.1016/j.rdc.2023.01.010
0889-857X/23/© 2023 Elsevier Inc. All rights reserved.

only with individuals with other chronic illnesses but also with the general population.[3] HRQoL is defined as ". . . the influence of the disease and treatment on functioning and overall sense of life satisfaction perceived by the patient".[5] It is a construct, measured through patient self-report assessments, that identifies the impact health-related issues have on an individual's life, including their physical, mental, emotional and social functioning. Scleroderma-specific HRQoL-validated assessments are available to use in this patient population.[3] Individuals with scleroderma not only face general life worries but are also forced to endure specific stressors, caused by symptoms related to scleroderma, that directly affect their ability to care for themselves and their ability to engage in their life activities on a daily basis, which, ultimately, significantly affect their overall quality of life.[6] Some of the quality-of-life issues patients with SSc face include fatigue, limitations of daily functioning, and psychological distress, which can individually and collectively lead to ineffective disease management. Because there is no known cure for scleroderma, symptom management and disease modification are the primary focus of care in order to ensure the highest quality of life for this patient population as possible throughout the disease course.[5]

With psychological distress being an aspect of HRQoL, assessing and addressing any issues related to the mental health of individuals with scleroderma is important. There has been some but not adequate focus on the intersectionality between mental health and scleroderma in research. What has been examined to date has shown a prevalence of mental health issues for individuals with scleroderma. A study by Mozetta and colleagues[7] found that greater than 80% of their participants demonstrated a psychiatric disorder. In a more recent study, Seravina and colleagues[8] showed similar results, with 83% of their scleroderma participants having mental health disorders. The most prevalent mental health issues for individuals with scleroderma have been found to be anxiety and depression.[7–13]

The social and economic conditions of where individuals age, live, work, learn, and play, also known as social determinants of health (SDOH), are not only significant contributing factors for an individual's, a community's, and a population's health but are also more substantial influencers to health outcomes than the direct clinical care provided.[14] There has been significantly increasing evidence over more than the past 25 years of the strong impact SDOH have on health and health outcomes.[15] These health determinants can, in fact, be as large as a 90% contributing component of health outcomes.[16]

A common focus, within health care and with health care providers, is on access to care; however, the other areas of an individual's life, the SDOH, much similar to mental health, are not necessarily visible and, thus, are most often ignored despite the strong impact they have on a person's health status.[17] There is a bidirectionality to the relationship between SDOH and chronic diseases. Because of this bidirectional relationship, people who are afflicted by stressors related to SDOH have markedly higher health care costs. High health care expenditures not only put a strain on the individual and families but also put pressure on an already fragile health care system and available support resources at local, state, and federal levels.[18] For example, with the 2008 recession, food insecurity rates dramatically increased in the United States. These rates did begin to improve in 2010 and a decline in the prevalence of food insecurity in America began to be realized in 2011; however, these rates did not return to prerecession levels in spite of this recovery.[19,20] Leonard and colleagues[21] (2018) found, in their study, higher rates of both poor health and food insecurity in the southern region of the United States, particularly communities of Black, non-Hispanic members. The consequentiality of this exemplifies the increased need for support of likely shared social determinants as well as the fiscal and resource strain these occurrences place on the safety nets, including health care providers, not only in these specific communities but also on the county, state, and federal levels. With the co-occurrence of the high prevalence of mental health symptoms among individuals with scleroderma and general as well as scleroderma-specific SDOH issues, it is vital that these psychosocial stressors and mental health issues are identified, discussed, and incorporated into the care that is given to patients with scleroderma in order to assist with maintaining an optimal level of HRQoL for these patients.

DISCUSSION

Health care entities may not have the means available for any and/or all aspects of SDOH and mental health screenings and support services for scleroderma patients. These types of screenings take staff, time, patient agreement/willingness, and physical space to complete the screenings. Many health care settings do not have these resources available.[22] In addition, if these resources are available for the screenings to take place, the provider/facility/entity are then responsible for supporting and assisting with connecting an individual who has a positive screen with resources.[23] There is often little guidance, particularly in the outpatient clinic setting, on how to approach topics related to mental health and SDOH needs, and what assessment tool to use, for these nonpharmaceutical issues. In addition, many medical staff members/providers are not fully aware of the support resources that are available for the members of their patient populations in need and/or of where to look for and find these resources.[24] Because of this, supporting patient self-management for these nonpharmaceutical mental health and SDOH needs may be the only option providers have.

With improving HRQoL being a holistic goal of scleroderma treatment and status of HRQoL being from the patient's perspective, knowing individual patients' concerns and perceptions of their disease and treatment course necessitates consideration. HRQoL gives the provider a view into how each scleroderma patient believes they are functioning—physically, mentally, and within their day-to-day lives. By paying attention to the patients' voice, as the medical treatment plan is being developed and followed, scleroderma providers may improve on addressing the areas that are of concern for each patient as well as the areas that each patient is receptive to address in treatment; this can then assist with the relationship between the provider and patient as well as patient treatment compliance, which will have a positive impact on each patient's level of functioning and quality of life.[5,25]

The unknown cause of scleroderma, the unpredictability of this disease, and the variability of this disease course from patient to patient has been shown to have a significant impact on patients' perceptions of their disease and of themselves as they navigate their lives with this added burden.[1,5,25] Sumpton and colleagues[1] found that scleroderma participants in their study often perceived their care and treatment in a nihilistic manner, which, in turn, negatively affected their motivation to adhere to their treatment plan. In another study that uncovered the voice of patients with scleroderma, making sense of SSc, which included a strong desire to develop a cognitive understanding of the disease itself as well as to formulate a picture of what they have been experiencing, was identified as a priority for this patient population. Because mystery and uncertainty coincide with scleroderma, patients often develop their own ideas about why they have it. Self-deprecating thoughts, including thoughts of "Why me?" or "What did I do wrong?", are often some of the first thoughts people have after being diagnosed with scleroderma. These thoughts can reemerge and even persist as patients go through their disease course. A patient may think that they are being punished in some way or they did or did not do something to cause this. These types of thoughts are not helpful, can be quite painful emotionally, and can lead to ineffective coping strategies.[25] Arat and colleagues concluded that the patients' depictions of scleroderma and their particular illness presentation ". . . contribute more than classical disease characteristics to physical and mental health."[26] Therefore, these perceptions and how these perceptions affect each scleroderma patient's life, including the coping mechanisms that they are using, are important for providers to ask about and discuss with their patients as they provide care.

Another consequence of the incurability and heterogeneous nature of this disease is the negative impact it has on these patients' mental health statuses. As identified earlier, mental health issues are prevalent with this patient population. The impact mental health has on HRQoL of patients with SSc is also an important aspect of this care approach. Sierakowska and colleagues[5] demonstrated a significant correlation between anxiety and quality of life. Similar to what earlier cited studies showed, 80% of this study's participants were afflicted with anxiety and had a direct relationship with depression. With the current unprecedented times related to the COVID-19 Pandemic, Henry and colleagues[27] completed a longitudinal study where they tracked and analyzed the mental health symptoms, particularly related to anxiety and depression, of participants in their Scleroderma Patient-centered Intervention Network (SPIN) cohort and their SPIN-COVID-19 Cohort before and during the COVID-19 pandemic. Their findings showed a significant increase in symptoms related to anxiety initially, with return to prepandemic levels as the pandemic continued, and no significant change in frequency and/or severity of symptoms related to depression. The researchers, and patient members of their advisory and research teams, cited the higher susceptibility and poor outcomes if infected with the COVID-19 virus, the barriers to access to health care during the early stages of the pandemic, and the familiarity with social isolation individuals with scleroderma had before the quarantining restrictions were in place as probable reasons for these results.[27]

Understanding and focusing supportive care around the chronic and acute-on-chronic mental health symptoms, particularly related to anxiety and depression, that individuals who have scleroderma have to face in their daily lives, whether in the midst of a pandemic or not, can positively contribute to the impact this disease has on each person and, in turn, improve quality of life for these patients. In addition to anxiety and depression symptoms, it is very common for individuals who have a chronic illness to go through a grieving process when they are initially diagnosed and when they lose different levels of functioning as their disease progresses. Any type of loss can trigger a grief reaction. Encouraging patients to work through these emotions when they develop will assist each patient in going through the grief process fully. Each person grieves in his/her own way—there is no right or wrong way to grieve; however, it is important to allow oneself to feel the feelings that they have. Not only will these feelings dissipate over time, but the patient will also grow in self-awareness and emotional strength if they work through this process each time it arises.[28] If a patient has persistent feelings of sadness, hopelessness, and/or helplessness, if they feel stuck in their grief process or with any of the other issues listed earlier, and/or they would like more support, discussing and referring them for individual outpatient therapy is an important part of this supportive, patient-focused care approach. Cognitive behavioral therapy (CBT) is the primary, evidence-based therapeutic approach for addressing these mental health issues, especially symptoms related to depression and anxiety.[29,30] If a therapist/social worker is a part of the clinic, an internal referral can be completed. Otherwise, a referral to a community provider will be necessary. Individual therapy can be conducted in person; however, another consideration is telehealth therapy, which has been shown to be as effective as in-person and is often a convenient and helpful mode of care for individuals who have scleroderma, as their symptoms may preclude them from leaving their home and, thus, a barrier to care.[31,32] In addition, providing all patients with the local and/or national 24-hour crisis line contact information as well as instructing patients to call 911 or go directly to a hospital emergency room if they ever have thoughts of harming themselves and/or others is also an important conversation to have (**Fig. 1**).

Studies have also exposed the need for improved scleroderma-specific information for this patient population. The participants in the study by Mouthon and colleagues[25] highlighted a lack of understanding related to the mechanisms, cause, evolution, and symptoms of the disease. These individuals also identified the point of diagnosis as a critical point in their lives that differentiated between how their life was before and after receiving a formal scleroderma diagnosis. This study demonstrated that the manner in which the diagnosis was delivered to the patient, which included the words that the providers used during this conversation, was noteworthy, including the impact it had on the patients' emotional reactions. This moment often drove patients to turn to the Internet to research scleroderma and look for answers.[25] Appropriate, effective online information about patients with SSc tends to be scarce, which can contribute to and even exacerbate mental health symptoms, particularly anxiety.[1,25]

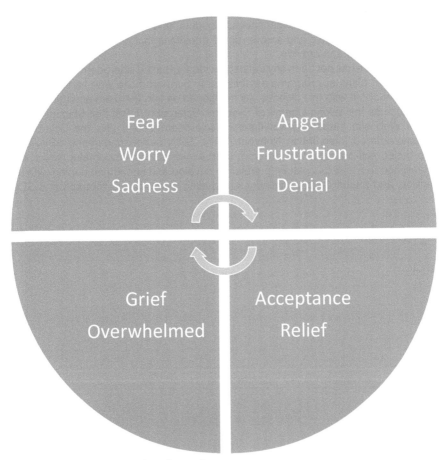

Fig. 1. Common emotions after diagnosis.

Because of the rare occurrence of SSc, patients may not know anyone else who has scleroderma, let alone anyone who has ever heard of scleroderma. Adding this to lack of effective and reliable informational resources, individuals with scleroderma can experience increased feelings related to isolation, disconnection, and being alone.[33] These feelings can be diminished just by knowing there are support groups and foundations and organizations available to them.[34] These groups/organizations can help patients locate others who have scleroderma and gain access to more information and education about this disease.[35] Taking initiative in this manner will, in turn, give patients knowledge and power. When an individual feels empowered, feelings of being alone slowly reduce. A piece of this supportive, patient-centered approach is connecting patients with others who have scleroderma, which includes referring patients to known online resources that are trustworthy in regard to the information that is given and the tone/manner in which it is presented, such as the SPIN Web site (http://www.spinsclero.com/en) and the TOSS Self-Manage Scleroderma Web site (https://www.selfmanagescleroderma.com); encouraging patients to join a scleroderma support group (**Fig. 2**); and clinics developing a sponsor program that connects newly diagnosed patients with those who have coped with living with this disease for a while. This allows patients, especially those who have been newly diagnosed with scleroderma, to gain a personal perceptive from someone who has been there. Although everyone's journey with scleroderma is unique to her/himself, gaining general information about someone else's experiences, thoughts, and feelings may allow others to gain a unique perceptive and answer some questions that only another person who has this diagnosis can provide.

To date, there has not been any defined, evidence-based scleroderma-specific self-management plans or programs established to support those who endure the challenges that come with this disease. As mentioned earlier, there are emerging internet sites, such as the Taking Charge of Systemic Sclerosis (TOSS) Self-Manage Scleroderma Web site (https://www.selfmanagescleroderma.com) and the Scleroderma Patient-centered Intervention Network (SPIN, SPIN self-management, SPIN-SELF) web-based self-management program (http://www.spinsclero.com/en), which were established to assist this patient population develop and strengthen coping with their physical and mental health challenges, including psychiatric symptoms and SDOH

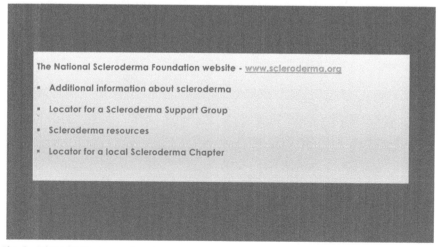

The National Scleroderma Foundation website - www.scleroderma.org

- Additional information about scleroderma
- Locator for a Scleroderma Support Group
- Scleroderma resources
- Locator for a local Scleroderma Chapter

Fig. 2. Scleroderma support groups.

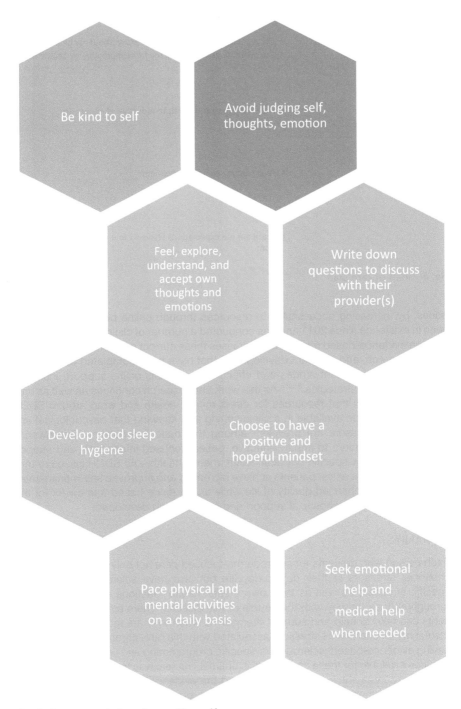

Fig. 3. Recommendations for positive self-care.

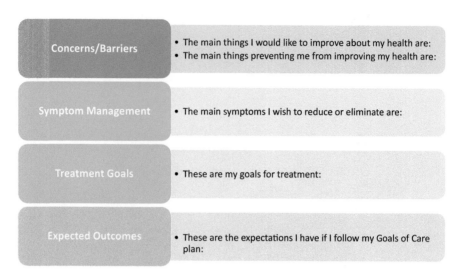

Fig. 4. Goals of care plan.

issues, by increasing accessibility to resources through online platforms. SPIN has been in existence since 2011 and has conducted a number of clinical trials to work toward an evidence-based model that addresses these current gaps in care. The efforts, clinical research, and program development that have been completed to date have demonstrated significant strides and effectiveness of this online support, including self-management strategies.[36,37] As this work and research continues as well as having the awareness that resources for direct mental health and wrap-around SDOH support may not be available in a clinic setting and knowing that psychological and psychosocial stressors are prevalent among this patient population, empowering scleroderma providers to impart effective, patient-focused information and support about scleroderma-specific physical health, mental health, and SDOH issues to their patients can further assist patients achieve increased and improved self-management and, ultimately, enhanced quality of life while an evidence-based framework for this patient-centered, psychosocial support and care is being developed.

SUMMARY

Each person who presents for scleroderma-focused care not only has their own psychosocial stressors in their day-to-day life but also have scleroderma symptom–specific stressors as well as their own mental health reactions at the start of and throughout their journey with the course of this disease. There are many actions patients can take to help and support themselves when they are faced with any of the mental health and SDOH stressors associated with this rare, chronic illness. Although having evidence-based, scleroderma-specific programming and wraparound support services available for these care needs is optimal, the reality is that there are generally limited resources within a clinic setting and the evidence-based approaches are in development; therefore, using the scleroderma providers to inform, discuss, and address these areas with their patients, using a patient-centered rather than provider-centered approach, can assist with more effective symptom and disease self-management, which will lead to the ultimate goal of scleroderma treatment— improve the quality of life for each patient.

CLINICS CARE POINTS

- Ask the questions about mental health status and SDOH issues at each patient encounter.
  - If validated assessments are used at a clinic visit, review them with the patient and ask related questions.
- Make recommendations for positive self-care (**Fig. 3**).
- Provide patients with information that is approachable and easy to read.
  - Create a new patient packet that includes comprehensive information related to the physical, mental, and psychosocial aspect of scleroderma.
  - Include material on what to expect for the disease course as well as for support services, such as in-person and/or on-line support groups, which can
    - Help a patient realize that there are other people who have been/are experiencing similar issues.
    - Bring relief and assist with feeling more empowered, thus decreasing feelings of being alone.
    - Aid with developing new skills, gaining more information and knowledge about scleroderma, learning additional coping skills, and receiving on-going support and encouragement.
    - Reduce any distress, depression, anxiety, or fatigue a patient might be feeling.
    - Provide an opportunity to develop a clearer understanding of what to expect with scleroderma, obtain practical advice, and compare information about resources.
- Have advance care planning discussions with each patient.
  - Encourage consideration and completion of a goals of care plan (**Fig. 4**) as well as an advance directive.
  - Offer guidance, as the following questions can do, to assist with this work.

Values
- How do your values/things that are important to you relate to your health care?
- Do you have specific beliefs that may influence your health care goals and wishes?
- Have you had experiences with family or friends where health care decisions had to be made?
- Reflect on these experiences and consider how they might affect your health care wishes.

Goals
- What is your understanding of what scleroderma is and how it affects you?
- What are your worries about your future?
- What is important to you in regard to your health care?

Wishes
- Are there conditions that you would or would not want certain treatment?
- Where would you want to be cared for in situations where advance care would be needed?
- Have you considered organ and tissue donation?

DISCLOSURE

The authors have nothing to disclose.

REFERENCES

1. Sumpton D, Thakkar V, O'Neill S, et al. It's Not Me, "It's Not Really Me." insights from patients on living with systemic sclerosis: an interview study. Arthritis Care Res 2017;69(11):1733–42.
2. Murphy SL, Kratz AL, Whibley D, et al. Fatigue and its association with social participation, functioning, and quality of life in systemic sclerosis. Arthritis Care Res 2021;73(3):415–22.

3. van Leeuwen NM, Ciaffi J, Liem SIE, et al. Health-related quality of life in patients with systemic sclerosis: evolution over time and main determinants. Rheumatology (Oxford, England) 2021;60(8):3646–55.
4. Denton CP, Khanna D. Systemic sclerosis. Lancet 2017;390(10103):1685–99.
5. Sierakowska M, Doroszkiewicz H, Sierakowska J, et al. Factors associated with quality of life in systemic sclerosis: a cross-sectional study. Qual Life Res 2019; 28(12):3347–54.
6. Bretterklieber A, Painsi C, Avian A, et al. Impaired quality of life in patients with systemic sclerosis compared to the general population and chronic dermatoses. BMC Res Notes 2014;7(1):594.
7. Mozzetta A, Antinone V, Alfani S, et al. Mental health in patients with systemic sclerosis: a controlled investigation. J Eur Acad Dermatol Venereol 2008;22(3): 336–40.
8. Seravina OF, Lisitsyna TA, Starovoytova MN, et al. Chronic stress and mental disorders in patients with systemic scleroderma: Results of an interdisciplinary study. Ter Arkh 2017;89(5):26–32.
9. Thombs BD, Kwakkenbos L, Henry RS, et al. Changes in mental health symptoms from pre-COVID-19 to COVID-19 among participants with systemic sclerosis from four countries: a Scleroderma Patient-centered Intervention Network (SPIN) Cohort study. J Psychosom Res 2020;139. 110262.
10. Amaral TN, Peres FA, Lapa AT, et al. Neurologic involvement in scleroderma: a systematic review. Semin Arthritis Rheum 2013;43(3):335–47.
11. Jha A, Danda D, Gojer AR, et al. Common mental disorders in South Asian patients with systemic sclerosis: a CIS-R-based cross-sectional study. Rheumatol Int 2022;42(8):1383–91.
12. Faezi ST, Paragomi P, Shahali A, et al. Prevalence and severity of depression and anxiety in patients with systemic sclerosis: an epidemiologic survey and investigation of clinical correlates. J Clin Rheumatol 2017;23(2):80–6.
13. Legendre C, Allanore Y, Ferrand I, et al. Evaluation of depression and anxiety in patients with systemic sclerosis. Joint Bone Spine 2005;72(5):408–11.
14. CSDH. Closing the gap in a generation: health equity through action on the social determinants of health. Final. 2008. Available at: apps.who.int/iris/bitstream/handle/10665/43943/9789241563703_eng.pdf. Accessed March 2, 2022.
15. Braveman P, Gottlieb L. The social determinants of health: It's time to consider the causes of the causes. Publ Health Rep 2014;129(2):19–31.
16. Hood C, Gennuso K, Swain G, et al. County health rankings relationships between determinant factors and health outcomes. Am J Prev Med 2016;50(2): 129–35.
17. Beech BM, Ford C, Thorpe RJ, et al. Poverty, racism, and the public health crisis in America. Front Public Health 2021;9(9). 699049.
18. Berkowitz SA, Basu S, Gundersen C, et al. State-level and county-level estimates of health care costs associated with food insecurity. Prev Chronic Dis 2019; 16(16). 180549.
19. FlinT KL, Davis GM, Umpiorroz GE. Emerging trends and the clinical impact of food insecurity in patients with diabetes. J Diabetes 2019;12(3):187–96.
20. Food insecurity and poverty in the United States. 2018. Available at: https://hungerandhealth.feedingamerica.org/wp-content/uploads/2018/10/Food-Insecurity-Poverty-Brief_2018.pdf. Accessed March 28, 2022.
21. Leonard T, Hughes AE, Donegan C, et al. Overlapping geographic clusters of food security and health: where do social determinants and health outcomes converge in the U.S? SSM Popul Health 2018;5(5):160–70.

22. Barnidge E, Stenmark S, Seligman H. Clinic-to-community models to address food insecurity. JAMA Pediatr 2017;171(6):507.
23. Fraze TK, Brewster AL, Lewis VA, et al. Prevalence of screening for food insecurity, housing instability, utility needs, transportation needs, and interpersonal violence by US physician practices and hospitals. JAMA Netw Open 2019;2(9). e1911514.
24. Eldred D, Kameg BN. Addressing food insecurity in primary care. J Nurse Pract 2021;17(7):799–802.
25. Mouthon L, Alami S, Boisard AS, et al. Patients' views and needs about systemic sclerosis and its management: a qualitative interview study. BMC Musculoskelet Disord 2017;18(1):230.
26. Arat S, Verschueren P, De Langhe E, et al. The association of illness perceptions with physical and mental health in systemic sclerosis patients: an exploratory study. Musculoskeletal Care 2011;10(1):18–28.
27. Henry RS, Kwakkenbos L, Carrier ME, et al. Mental health before and during the pandemic in people with systemic sclerosis. The Lancet Rheumatology 2022; 4(2):e82–5.
28. Herrera PA, Campos-Romero S, Szabo W, et al. Understanding the relationship between depression and chronic diseases such as diabetes and hypertension: a grounded theory study. Int J Environ Res Publ Health 2021;18(22). 12130.
29. White CA. Cognitive behavioral principles in managing chronic disease. West J Med 2001;175(5):338–42.
30. Sudak DM. CBT in patients with chronic illness. Psychiatr News 2017;52(11):1.
31. Andersson G, Cuijpers P, Carlbring P, et al. Guided internet-based vs. face-to-face cognitive behavior therapy for psychiatric and somatic disorders: a systematic review and meta-analysis. World Psychiatr 2014;13(3):288–95.
32. Beugen S van, Ferwerda M, Hoeve D, et al. Internet-based cognitive behavioral therapy for patients with chronic somatic conditions: a meta-analytic review. J Med Internet Res 2014;16(3):e88.
33. Yanguas J, Pinazo-Henandis S, Tarazona-Santabalbina F. The complexity of loneliness. Acta Biomed 2018;89(2):302–14.
34. Turner KA, Rice DB, Carboni-Jiménez A, et al. Effects of training and support programs for leaders of illness-based support groups: commentary and updated evidence. Syst Rev 2019;8(1):67.
35. Rice DB, Thombs BD. Support groups in scleroderma. Curr Rheumatol Rep 2019; 21(4):9.
36. Nordlund J, Henry R, Kwakkenbos L, et al. The Scleroderma Patient-centered Intervention Network Self-Management (SPIN-SELF) Program: protocol for a twoarm parallel partially nested randomized controlled feasibility trial with progression to full-scale trial. Trials 2021;22(1):856.
37. Carrier ME, Kwakkenbos L, Nielson WR, et al. The scleroderma patient-centered intervention network self-management program: protocol for a randomized feasibility trial. JMIR Res Protoc 2020;9(4). e16799.

22. Bandolie E, Shewmaker S, Balgobin H, et al. Consumerism leads to India food insecurity. JAMA Pediatr 2013;(216):67.

23. Frace TK, Biewalet AL, Lewis VA, et al. Prevalence of screening for food insecurity, housing instability, utility needs, transportation needs, and interpersonal violence by US physician practices and hospitals. JAMA Netw Open 2019.

24. [illegible reference] 466(7704):249.

25. [illegible reference] Blood 2019(29):10.

Preventative Care in Scleroderma

What Is the Best Approach to Vaccination?

Leonardo Martin Calderon, MD[a], Janet E. Pope, MD[a,b],
Ami A. Shah, MD, MS[c], Robyn T. Domsic, MD, MPH[d,*]

KEYWORDS

- Systemic sclerosis • Scleroderma • Vaccination • Vaccines • SARS-CoV-2
- Prevention • Preventative medicine

KEY POINTS

- Patients with systemic sclerosis should be encouraged to have age-appropriate vaccinations.
- Immunosuppressive medications commonly used for disease modulation, such as methotrexate and rituximab, can reduce the efficacy of influenza, pneumococcal, and SARS-CoV-2 vaccines.
- Temporary suspension of immunosuppressants may be warranted to improve seroconversion following vaccination.

INTRODUCTION

Systemic sclerosis (scleroderma, SSc) is a rare multisystem autoimmune disease characterized by vasculopathy, autoimmunity, and fibrosis of the internal organs and skin.[1] SSc is divided into 2 subtypes, which include limited cutaneous and diffuse cutaneous SSc.[1] There are multiple complications associated with SSc, which include interstitial lung disease (ILD), pulmonary arterial hypertension, and digital ulcers that decrease patients' quality of life and increase their morbidity and mortality.[2,3] SSc can also affect other aspects of health that cause morbidity and mortality such as increased risk for infections coupled with decreased vaccination uptake and seroconversion. The purpose

This article has not been submitted and is not simultaneously being submitted elsewhere.
[a] Department of Medicine, Schulich School of Medicine and Dentistry, University of Western Ontario, London, Ontario, Canada; [b] Division of Rheumatology, St. Joseph's Health Care, London, Ontario, Canada; [c] Division of Rheumatology, Johns Hopkins University School of Medicine, Johns Hopkins Scleroderma Center, Baltimore, MD, USA; [d] Division of Rheumatology and Clinical Immunology, University of Pittsburgh School of Medicine, 3500 Terrace Street, Pittsburgh, PA 15261, USA
* Corresponding author.
E-mail address: rtd4@pitt.edu

of this review is to provide an update and "points to consider" regarding vaccinations for patients with SSc.

Vaccine Use

Patients with autoimmune diseases are at risk for infections and associated poor outcomes due to the underlying autoimmune disease itself, associated medical comorbidities, and the use of immunosuppressive medications. These immunosuppressive medications include glucocorticoids and disease-modifying antirheumatic drugs composed of conventional synthetic, biological, and targeted synthetic drugs. Most of the disease-modifying drugs currently used in SSc, with the exception of hydroxychloroquine, nintedanib, and intravenous immunoglobulin, are immunosuppressive in nature, such as mycophenolate mofetil, methotrexate, cyclophosphamide, rituximab, tocilizumab, and azathioprine.

Vaccination is of particular importance, as it is thought to translate into less emergency room visits, hospitalizations, and death. Infections were the most common diagnosis in SSc patient hospitalizations (18%) and in-hospital deaths (33%) before the SARS-CoV-2 pandemic.[4] The SARS-CoV-2 pandemic has highlighted the increased risk of severe infections and hospitalization in patients with autoimmune disease, particularly those who are immunocompromised. The lower vaccination seroconversion rate among the frail and immunosuppressed to vaccines has been highlighted, as multiple countries are recommending additional doses of SARS-CoV-2 vaccines for this patient population. Although this was previously addressed in several publications for influenza and pneumococcal vaccines among rheumatology patients, this reduced vaccine response was previously not broadly discussed in the media.[5–8]

The pandemic has clearly demonstrated the link between vaccination and reduction of severe illness and death for the general public.[9] The importance of vaccines as a preventative measure to disease in patients with autoimmune disease, particularly the immunocompromised, seems self-evident. Disturbingly, studies published predominantly before the pandemic had demonstrated poor vaccine uptake among patients with rheumatic diseases and patients with SSc specifically, where rates before 2020 ranged from 28% to 69% for influenza and 28% to 78% for pneumococcal vaccines.[10–14] The care gap with respect to vaccination uptake in SSc has not been thoroughly studied.

It remains unknown if the SARS-CoV-2 pandemic has altered or accentuated this disconnect between vaccine need and use across the rheumatology population. Interestingly, the one small study published in SSc since the pandemic reported on 91 Italian patients with SSc who had higher influenza vaccination rates than the general population.[15] However, influenza coverage was still only 84% among those immunosuppressed, and 89% in the elderly, leaving many patients uncovered. A survey of vaccine attitudes specific to SARS-CoV-2 vaccines published in 2021 showed 72% of patients with SSc (n = 104) had positive attitudes toward the vaccine, compared with 87% of patients with inflammatory arthritis (n = 111).[16]

There are no SSc-specific guidelines for vaccinations published. However, there are society recommendations (**Box 1**) that can be consulted, in combination with national recommendations, to aid the SSc patient provider in determining an individual patient's risk profile and vaccine counseling.

Vaccine recommendations and schedules: at the time of this writing, American College of Rheumatology (ACR) is developing a new clinical practice guideline for vaccinations in patients with rheumatic diseases, with an anticipated publication date of late 2022. The European League Against Rheumatism (EULAR) published updated

---

Box 1
Vaccination recommendations in systemic sclerosis

Recommendations
1. Seasonal flu vaccine should be actively recommended to all patients with SSc every year in the United States (per national guidelines) and to most of the patients with SSc per age- and risk-based national guidelines in multiple other countries (CRA, BSR, EULAR). [Influenza vaccine]
2. SARS-CoV-2 vaccination status should be assessed for each individual patient by the rheumatology health care provider. Recommendations for timing of vaccinations should be based on current immunosuppressive therapy use, individual patient risk factors, and current national societal recommendations for timing and specific vaccine use. [SARS-CoV2 vaccination]
3. The "prime-boost" approach to administering PCV13 or PCV15 followed at least 8 weeks later by PPSV23 should be provided to all patients receiving immunosuppression and who fit age and comorbidity criteria per the Advisory Committee on Immunization Practices guidelines.[50] It is not known if PCV20 alone is adequate in immunocompromised patients.
4. Rituximab and methotrexate reduce the efficacy of influenza, pneumococcal, and SARS-CoV-2 vaccine. Vaccine administration should be before rituximab dosing, if possible (at least 2 weeks), or delayed until more than or equal to 5 months after dosing, if possible, according to multiple societal recommendations. Studies suggest holding methotrexate for 2 weeks after influenza improves efficacy, and current ACR guidance suggests holding 1 to 2 weeks after SARS-CoV-2 vaccination if disease activity permits. No other society recommendations specifically address methotrexate cessation around the time of vaccine administration.
5. Mycophenolate mofetil is known to decrease the immunogenicity of SARS-CoV-2 vaccination.[24–26] ACR guidance suggests holding for 1 to 2 weeks following each vaccine dose.
6. Evaluate vaccine status and encourage patients with SSc to have age-appropriate (according to current recommendations) vaccinations including HPV and herpes zoster vaccinations.

---

recommendations for vaccination in adult patients with autoimmune inflammatory rheumatic diseases, which are cited throughout this article.[17] The Canadian Rheumatology Association (CRA) published guidance in 2019.[18] In the United States, the adult immunization schedule is updated annually by the Advisory Committee on Immunization Practices in the United States, which can be found at cdc.gov. These guidelines address vaccination for 10 preventable infectious diseases and include influenza, varicella, zoster, human papillomavirus (HPV), tetanus/diphtheria/pertussis (Tdap), measles/mumps/rubella, pneumococcal, hepatitis A, hepatitis B, meningococcal A, C, W, Y, meningococcal B, and haemophilus influenzae type b.

General principles endorsed by all societies include that vaccination status and indications for vaccination should be assessed yearly by the rheumatology team.[17] These indications include age, autoimmune disease, underlying immunosuppressive therapy, occupation or high-risk exposure profile, and level of endemic disease in their area. There are thorough reviews of the safety and timing of vaccinations (other than SARS-CoV2 vaccines) for patients with immune-mediated diseases and timing of holding immune suppressive therapy, which can be used for guidance.[17–19]

SSc experience with vaccine immunogenicity is limited: there are relatively few articles dedicated to exploring vaccine immunogenicity in patients with SSc. Most literature focuses on patients with rheumatoid arthritis (RA), inflammatory arthritis, or lupus. A small study in 26 patients with SSc and 16 controls investigated response to the seasonal influenza vaccine.[20] The investigators reported a satisfactory response, not different from controls, was seen in patients with SSc following trivalent influenza vaccination. Furthermore, a study of 69 patients with mixed connective tissue disease and age- and gender-matched controls showed similar rates of seroprotection, seroconversion, and geometric mean titer with the influenza vaccine.[21] One study of 51 patients with SSc receiving the CoronaVac (Sinovac) vaccine, a whole inactivated vaccine, for SARS-CoV-2 were compared with 153 healthy controls in Brazil.[22] Patients with SSc had moderately lower immunogenicity response compared with controls, with vaccine response clearly affected by mycophenolate use. In a large study of 502 patients with autoimmune disease, which included 265 patients with SSc, a higher rate of SARS-CoV-2 vaccine nonresponse was observed in those with ILD, or treated with glucocorticoids, mycophenolate mofetil, and rituximab.[23] Findings of decreased immunogenicity were observed in 1 or 2 vaccine dose patients with autoimmune diseases, and specifically with SSc, on rituximab or mycophenolate mofetil.[24–26] A very recent study of 100 patients with SSc demonstrated a 70% response rate to SARS-CoV-2 vaccination with 2 doses of messenger RNA (mRNA) vaccine or 1 J&J vaccine. Higher doses of mycophenolate and history of rituximab use was found in those with a negative seroconversion with the initial vaccine doses.[26] Although the data limit definitive conclusions, the findings fail to suggest a reduction in vaccine efficacy associated with SSc alone. However, use of immunosuppressive therapy and SSc complicated by ILD have reported associations with reduced vaccine immunogenicity.

Immunosuppressive medications: immunosuppressive medications may affect vaccine immunogenicity, in combination with the effect of aging. In the following section the authors cover the knowledge by medication and drug class for those commonly used in SSc management.

Rituximab: rituximab has been demonstrated to impair vaccine immunogenetic response across multiple vaccines in both patients with autoimmune disease and malignancies. Patients with RA with rituximab demonstrated impaired response to hepatitis B vaccination compared with controls; and use of high-dose hepatitis B vaccine did not increase vaccine response rate in patients on antitumor necrosis factor agents.[27,28] Prime-boost vaccination with the 13-valent pneumococcal vaccine followed by the 23-valent was not effective in rituximab patients. Furthermore, regarding SARS-CoV-2 vaccination, the well-designed RituxiVac study of 96 patients and 29 immunocompetent controls found that antispike immunoglobulin G antibodies were found in just half the patients compared with 100% of controls after the second mRNA vaccine dose.[29] Regression modeling identified time since last anti-CD20 therapy, peripheral CD19+ cell count, and CD4+ lymphocyte count as predictive of humoral vaccine response. In addition, a meta-analysis in SARS-CoV-2 confirmed low rates of seroconversion for humoral (41%) and cell-mediated responses (73%) with anti-CD20 therapies after 2-dose regimens.[30] Rates seemed lowest in those within 6 months of therapy, low circulating B-cell counts, and in transplant patients on multiple immunosuppressants. Ultimately, an assessment of vaccine-induced seroconversion may be a consideration, particularly for those within 6 months of last dose of anti-CD20 therapy. In a study of 404 patients with autoimmune disease receiving 2 doses of a mRNA SARS-CoV-2 vaccine, the antibody response rate was 94%, but patents on rituximab had only a 26% conversion rate after the second dose.[25] Overall, the data support considering timing of vaccine before rituximab administration, ideally, as covered by multiple guidelines[14,15] (https://www.rheumatology.org/Portals/0/Files/COVID-19-Vaccine-Clinical-Guidance-Rheumatic-Diseases-Summary.pdf).

Methotrexate: there are conflicting results among the studies published on methotrexate that suggest reduced responses to the influenza vaccine in patients with inflammatory arthropathies. However, recent studies, including a randomized controlled trial, show improved influenza vaccine response if methotrexate is held for 2 weeks after vaccination.[31,32] Methotrexate was found to have a negative influence on diphtheria antibody responses, but not tetanus, in the Tdap vaccine in patients with inflammatory arthritides and vasculitis compared with healthy controls.[33] Several studies have shown an impaired response in patients with RA treated with methotrexate for the pneumococcal vaccines, and a meta-analysis suggests that conventional disease-modifying antirheumatic drugs (methotrexate was the most common) were associated with reduced immunogenicity.[34,35] Recent ACR guidelines for SARs-CoV-2 vaccine administration recommend holding methotrexate for 1 to 2 weeks after booster vaccination (https://www.rheumatology.org/Portals/0/Files/COVID-19-Vaccine-Clinical-Guidance-Rheumatic-Diseases-Summary.pdf). The British Society of Rheumatology (BSR) and CRA SARs-CoV-2 recommendations do not suggest holding methotrexate after the COVID vaccination. EULAR recommendations stress that despite the reduced efficacy, vaccination for influenza, pneumococcal, and SARS-CoV-2 be addressed with patients by the rheumatology provider.[17,36] No current recommendations from rheumatology organizations suggest holding methotrexate for inactivated vaccines other than SARS-CoV-2.

Mycophenolate mofetil: much of the literature on vaccine immunogenicity and mycophenolate mofetil comes from studies in organ transplant recipients. A recent meta-analysis pooling data from 8 trials reported a significantly lower response rate to influenza vaccination than those on other types of immunosuppression.[37] In renal transplant patients given the PCV13 vaccine, immunogenic response was adequate. However, lower antibody titers correlated with mycophenolate use.[38] A report from the Global Rheumatology Alliance found that more than half of fully vaccinated individuals with breakthrough SARS-CoV-2 infections requiring hospitalization were on mycophenolate or B-cell depleting therapies.[39] The study of 404 patients with autoimmune disease showed a seroconversion rate of 73% after 2 doses of mRNA vaccine in patients on mycophenolate, whereas the overall seroconversion rate in all patients studied was 94%.[25] Current EULAR recommendations encourage addressing vaccine use in patients using mycophenolate mofetil. The ACR guidance summary recommends holding mycophenolate for 1 to 2 weeks (as disease activity allows) after each SARS-CoV-2 vaccine dose, with recommendations regarding other vaccines expected in 2023 (https://rheum.ca/wp-content/uploads/2021/11/V3_Nov_23_2021_EN.pdf). The BSR and CRA currently recommend patients on immunosuppression continue immunosuppressive therapy uninterrupted for inactivated vaccines.

Glucocorticoids: although glucocorticoids need to be used with caution in patients with SSc due to their association with renal crisis, studies show they are used frequently still in Europe.[40,41] Multiple studies across rheumatic diseases have been performed. For influenza, no reduction in immunogenicity has been appreciated in doses less than 10 mg/day and generally for mean doses less than 20 mg/day in pneumococcal vaccines and no effect on immunogenicity seen for the herpes vaccines.[17,19,36] The Infectious Diseases Society of America guidelines for vaccination in the immunocompromised host do not consider patients on prednisone less than 20 mg/day to be immunocompromised. No societal guidelines recommend holding glucocorticoids around the time of vaccination, but it is generally encouraged to vaccinate when patients are at their lowest tolerable dose.[42] Regarding SARS-CoV-2, patients with autoimmune diseases who were exposed to glucocorticoids were found to be at higher risk of infection.[43]

Tocilizumab: a handful of studies have evaluated antibody response to various vaccines. A small study in patients with RA and Castleman disease demonstrated high efficacy for both influenza and pneumococcal vaccines.[44] A larger study in 194 patients with RA showed that tocilizumab did not hamper influenza vaccine response, with a third study reporting similar results.[45,46] As of this writing, none of the ACR, BSR, CRA, and EULAR had specific guidelines or recommendations specific to tocilizumab and any vaccination.

Human papillomavirus and herpes zoster vaccination: there are some infections that may be increased in SSc where prevention with vaccination is important. These infections include viral reactivation with HPV infection and Varicella zoster (Shingles). HPV infection is increased in other connective tissue diseases such as systemic lupus erythematosus (SLE) and Sjogren syndrome.[47] Precancerous Pap tests were increased nearly 8-fold in a large population study of 1043 patients with SSc compared with age-matched women in Taiwan.[48] Shingles is increased in SLE and likely also in SSc due to the disease itself where interferon is altered, increasing the risk of herpes zoster reactivation and the use of immune suppressive drugs.[49] Assessment and recommendation of the inactivated form of herpes zoster vaccination is encouraged in rheumatic diseases.[17,18]

SUMMARY

There are some complications associated with SSc that can be prevented or attenuated with appropriate screening and treatment, which may not be consistently performed such as preventing infections with routine vaccinations. Patients with SSc can be at risk of decreased seroconversion due to immunosuppressants, and temporary DMARD suspension around vaccinations may be warranted. In addition, patients may benefit from the "prime-boost" approach to influenza vaccination.

CONFLICT OF INTEREST

There are no conflicts of interest to disclose.

AUTHOR CONTRIBUTIONS

L.M. Calderon, R.T. Domsic, A.A. Shah, and J.E. Pope were involved in study design, review of literature, and article writing. All authors reviewed the article and approved the final version.

FUNDING

No specific funding was received from any bodies in the public, commercial, or not-for-profit sectors to carry out the work described in this article. A.A. Shah is supported by NIH, United States/NIAMS, United States K24AR080217. R.T. Domsicis supported by NIH/NIAMS R01 AR080356.

FUNDING AND COMPETING INTERESTS

There are no conflicts of interest. A.A. Shah is supported by NIH/NIAMS K24AR080217.

CONTRIBUTION

L.M. Calderon, R.T. Domsic, A.A. Shah, and J.E. Pope were involved in study design, analysis, and article writing. All authors reviewed the article and approved the final version.

CLINICS CARE POINTS

- Patients with systemic sclerosis should be encouraged to have age-appropriate vaccinations.

- Temporay suspensio fo immunosuppressants may be warranted to improve seroconversion following vaccination. Clinicians are encouraged to reference the latest guidelines for their region.

REFERENCES

1. Hughes M, Herrick AL. Systemic sclerosis. Br J Hosp Med 2019;80(9):530–6.
2. Hudson M, Thombs BD, Steele R, et al. Health-related quality of life in systemic sclerosis: a systematic review. Arthritis Rheum 2009;61(8):1112–20.
3. Al-Dhaher FF, Pope JE, Ouimet JM. Determinants of morbidity and mortality of systemic sclerosis in Canada. Semin Arthritis Rheum 2010;39(4):269–77.
4. Ram Poudel D, George M, Dhital R, et al. Mortality, length of stay and cost of hospitalization among patients with systemic sclerosis: results from the National Inpatient Sample. Rheumatology 2018;57(9):1611–22.
5. Elkayam O, Bashkin A, Mandelboim M, et al. The effect of infliximab and timing of vaccination on the humoral response to influenza vaccination in patients with rheumatoid arthritis and ankylosing spondylitis. Semin Arthritis Rheum 2010; 39(6):442–7.
6. Fischer L, Gerstel PF, Poncet A, et al. Pneumococcal polysaccharide vaccination in adults undergoing immunosuppressive treatment for inflammatory diseases–a longitudinal study. Arthritis Res Ther 2015;17:151.
7. Hua C, Barnetche T, Combe B, et al. Effect of methotrexate, anti-tumor necrosis factor α, and rituximab on the immune response to influenza and pneumococcal vaccines in patients with rheumatoid arthritis: a systematic review and meta-analysis. Arthritis Care Res 2014;66(7):1016–26.
8. Arad U, Tzadok S, Amir S, et al. The cellular immune response to influenza vaccination is preserved in rheumatoid arthritis patients treated with rituximab. Vaccine 2011;29(8):1643–8.
9. Lauring AS, Tenforde MW, Chappell JD, et al. Clinical severity of, and effectiveness of mRNA vaccines against, covid-19 from omicron, delta, and alpha SARS-CoV-2 variants in the United States: prospective observational study. BMJ 2022;376:e069761.
10. Costello R, Winthrop KL, Pye SR, et al. Influenza and pneumococcal vaccination uptake in patients with rheumatoid arthritis treated with immunosuppressive therapy in the UK: a retrospective cohort study using data from the clinical practice research datalink. PLoS One 2016;11(4):e0153848.
11. McCarthy EM, de Barra E, Bergin C, et al. Influenza and pneumococcal vaccination and varicella status in inflammatory arthritis patients. Ir Med J 2011;104(7):208–11.
12. Brocq O, Acquacalda E, Berthier F, et al. Influenza and pneumococcal vaccine coverage in 584 patients taking biological therapy for chronic inflammatory joint: a retrospective study. Joint Bone Spine 2016;83(2):155–9.
13. Hmamouchi I, Winthrop K, Launay O, et al. Low rate of influenza and pneumococcal vaccine coverage in rheumatoid arthritis: Data from the international CO-MORA cohort. Vaccine 2015;33(12):1446–52.
14. Rosamilia F, Noberasco G, Olobardi D, et al. Flu and pneumococcal vaccine coverage in scleroderma patients still need to be prompted: a systematic review. Vaccines (Basel) 2021;9(11):1330.

15. Murdaca G, Noberasco G, Olobardi D, et al., Systemic sclerosis and vaccinations: a three-year register-based cohort study about vaccination rate and uptake from Liguria referral center, northwest Italy, Hum Vaccines Immunother, 2022;18(1):2025732.

16. Ciaffi J, Giuggioli D, Mari A, et al. COVID-19 vaccine hesitancy in systemic sclerosis. Clin Exp Rheumatol 2021;39(4):165–6.

17. Furer V, Rondaan C, Heijstek MW, et al. 2019 update of EULAR recommendations for vaccination in adult patients with autoimmune inflammatory rheumatic diseases. Ann Rheum Dis 2020;79(1):39–52.

18. Papp KA, Haraoui B, Kumar D, et al. Vaccination guidelines for patients with immune-mediated disorders taking immunosuppressive therapies: executive summary. J Rheumatol 2019;46(7):751–4.

19. Calabrese C. Vaccinations in patients with rheumatic disease: consider disease and therapy. Med Clin North Am 2021;105(2):213–25.

20. Litinsky I, Balbir A, Zisman D, et al. Vaccination against influenza in patients with systemic sclerosis. Clin Exp Rheumatol 2012;30(2 Suppl 71):S7–11.

21. Miossi R, Fuller R, Moraes J, et al. Immunogenicity of influenza H1N1 vaccination in mixed connective tissue disease: effect of disease and therapy. Clinics 2013; 68(2):129–33.

22. Sampaio-Barros PD, Medeiros-Ribeiro AC, Luppino-Assad AP. et al. SARS-CoV-2 vaccine in patients with systemic sclerosis: Impact of disease subtype and therapy, Rheumatology, 2022;61(SI2):SI169-SI174.

23. Ferri C, Ursini F, Gragnani L, et al. Impaired immunogenicity to COVID-19 vaccines in autoimmune systemic diseases. High prevalence of non-response in different patients' subgroups. J Autoimmun 2021;125:102744.

24. Boyarsky BJ, Ruddy JA, Connolly CM, et al. Antibody response to a single dose of SARS-CoV-2 mRNA vaccine in patients with rheumatic and musculoskeletal diseases. Ann Rheum Dis 2021;80(8):1098–9.

25. Ruddy JA, Connolly CM, Boyarsky BJ, et al. High antibody response to two-dose SARS-CoV-2 messenger RNA vaccination in patients with rheumatic and musculoskeletal diseases. Ann Rheum Dis 2021;80(10):1351–2.

26. Wallwork R., Connolly C.M., Shneyderman M., et al., Effect of mycophenolate mofetil dose on antibody response following initial SARS-CoV-2 vaccination in patients with systemic sclerosis, Lancet Rheumatology, 2022;4(7):e462-e464.

27. Intongkam S, Samakarnthai P, Pakchotanon R, et al. Efficacy and safety of hepatitis B vaccination in rheumatoid arthritis patients receiving disease-modifying antirheumatic drugs and/or biologics therapy. J Clin Rheumatol 2019;25(8): 329–34.

28. Haykir Solay A, Eser F. High dose hepatitis B vaccine is not effective in patients using immunomodulatory drugs: a pilot study. Hum Vaccines Immunother 2019; 15(5):1177–82.

29. Moor MB, Suter-Riniker F, Horn MP, et al. Humoral and cellular responses to mRNA vaccines against SARS CoV-2 in patients with a history of CD20 B-cell-depleting therapy (RituxiVac): an investigator-initiated, single-centre, open-label study. Lancet Rheumatology 2021;3(11):e789–97.

30. Schietzel S. Anderegg M. Limacher A. et al. Humoral and cellular immune responses on SARS-CoV-2 vaccines in patients with anti-CD20 therapies: a systematic review and meta-analysis of 1342 patients, RMD Open, 2022;8(1):e002036.

31. Kapetanovic MC, Roseman C, Jönsson G, et al. Antibody response is reduced following vaccination with 7-valent conjugate pneumococcal vaccine in adult

methotrexate-treated patients with established arthritis, but not those treated with tumor necrosis factor inhibitors. Arthritis Rheum 2011;63(12):3723–32.

32. Park JK, Lee YJ, Shin K, et al. Impact of temporary methotrexate discontinuation for 2 weeks on immunogenicity of seasonal influenza vaccination in patients with rheumatoid arthritis: a randomised clinical trial, Ann Rheum Dis 2018;77(6): 898–904.

33. Bühler S, Jaeger VK, Adler S, et al. Safety and immunogenicity of tetanus/diphtheria vaccination in patients with rheumatic diseases—a prospective multicentre cohort study. Rheumatology 2019;58(9):1585–96.

34. Subesinghe S, Bechman K, Rutherford AI, et al. A systematic review and meta-analysis of antirheumatic drugs and vaccine immunogenicity in rheumatoid arthritis. J Rheumatol 2018;45(6):733–44.

35. van Aalst M, Lötsch F, Spijker R, et al. Incidence of invasive pneumococcal disease in immunocompromised patients: a systematic review and meta-analysis. Trav Med Infect Dis 2018;24:89–100.

36. Papp KA, Haraoui B, Kumar D, et al. Vaccination guidelines for patients with immune-mediated disorders on immunosuppressive therapies. J Cutan Med Surg 2019;23(1):50–74.

37. Khedmat H, Karbasi-Afshar R, Izadi M, et al. Response of transplant recipients to influenza vaccination based on type of immunosuppression: a meta-analysis. Saudi Journal of Kidney Diseases and Transplantation 2015;26(5):877.

38. Oesterreich S, Lindemann M, Goldblatt D, et al. Humoral response to a 13-valent pneumococcal conjugate vaccine in kidney transplant recipients. Vaccine 2020; 38(17):3339–50.

39. Liew J, Gianfrancesco M, Harrison C, et al. SARS-CoV-2 breakthrough infections among vaccinated individuals with rheumatic disease: results from the COVID-19 Global Rheumatology Alliance provider registry. RMD Open 2022;8(1):e002187.

40. Steen VD, Medsger TA. Case-control study of corticosteroids and other drugs that either precipitate or protect from the development of scleroderma renal crisis. Arthritis Rheum 1998;41(9):1613–9.

41. Herrick AL. Controversies on the Use of Steroids in Systemic Sclerosis. Journal of Scleroderma and Related Disorders 2017;2(2):84–91.

42. Rubin LG, Levin MJ, Ljungman P, et al. 2013 IDSA clinical practice guideline for vaccination of the immunocompromised host. Clin Infect Dis 2014;58(3):309–18.

43. Fitzgerald KC, Mecoli CA, Douglas M, et al. Risk factors for infection and health impacts of the coronavirus disease 2019 (COVID-19) pandemic in people with autoimmune diseases. Clin Infect Dis 2022;74(3):427–36.

44. Tsuru T, Terao K, Murakami M, et al. Immune response to influenza vaccine and pneumococcal polysaccharide vaccine under IL-6 signal inhibition therapy with tocilizumab. Mod Rheumatol 2014;24(3):511–6.

45. Mori S, Ueki Y, Hirakata N, et al. Impact of tocilizumab therapy on antibody response to influenza vaccine in patients with rheumatoid arthritis. Ann Rheum Dis 2012;71(12):2006–10.

46. Crnkic Kapetanovic M, Saxne T, Jönsson G, et al. Rituximab and abatacept but not tocilizumab impair antibody response to pneumococcal conjugate vaccine in patients with rheumatoid arthritis. Arthritis Res Ther 2013;15(5):R171.

47. Ma KS. Human papillomavirus infection increases risk of primary sjogren's syndrome: a population-based cohort study over a 15-year follow-up, Arthritis Rheumatol, 73, 2021. Available at: https://acrabstracts.org/abstract/human-papillomavirus-infection-increases-risk-of-primary-sjogrens-syndrome-a-population-based-cohort-study-over-a-15-year-follow-up/.

48. Tsai PH, Kuo CF. OP0070 The risk of precancerous lesions of the breast and cervix uteri in patients with autoimmune rheumatic diseases: a nationwide population study in Taiwan. Ann Rheum Dis 2020;79(Suppl 1):47.1–7.

49. Pope JE, Goodwin JL, Ouimet JM, et al. Infections are not increased in scleroderma compared to non-inflammatory musculoskeletal disorders prior to disease onset. Open Rheumatol J 2007;1(1):12–7.

50. Nived P, Jönsson G, Settergren B, et al. Prime-boost vaccination strategy enhances immunogenicity compared to single pneumococcal conjugate vaccination in patients receiving conventional DMARDs, to some extent in abatacept but not in rituximab-treated patients. Arthritis Res Ther 2020;22(1):36.

Preventative Care in Scleroderma

What Is the Best Approach to Bone Health and Cancer Screening?

Leonardo Martin Calderon, MD[a], Robyn T. Domsic, MD, MPH[b], Ami A. Shah, MD, MHS[c],*, Janet E. Pope, MD[a,d],*

KEYWORDS

- Systemic sclerosis • Scleroderma • Osteoporosis • Fracture • Avascular necrosis
- Cancer screening • Prevention

KEY POINTS

- Patients with SSc may have unique risk factors for osteoporosis including very-low body mass index, malnutrition, early menopause, medication exposures (proton pump inhibitors or steroids), and possibly the presence of calcinosis.
- Patients with SSc have an increased risk of cancer with studies suggesting a high risk of lung, hematologic, liver, esophageal, oropharyngeal, stomach, pancreatic, thyroid, cervical, uterine, prostate, testicular, and skin (melanoma and non-melanoma) cancers.
- Patients with SSc who have anti-RNA polymerase III antibodies have an increased risk of cancer around the time of SSc onset, with particular concern for high breast cancer risk.

INTRODUCTION

Systemic sclerosis (scleroderma, SSc) is a complex autoimmune disease characterized by fibrosis of the internal organs and skin, autoimmunity with distinct autoantibodies, and vascular abnormalities.[1] SSc is classified into the subtypes of limited

This article has not been submitted and is not simultaneously being submitted elsewhere.
[a] Department of Medicine, Schulich School of Medicine and Dentistry, University of Western Ontario, London, Ontario, Canada; [b] Division of Rheumatology and Clinical Immunology, University of Pittsburgh School of Medicine, Pittsburgh, PA, USA; [c] Johns Hopkins Scleroderma Center, Division of Rheumatology, Johns Hopkins University School of Medicine, 5200 Eastern Avenue, Mason F. Lord Building Center Tower, Suite 4100, Baltimore, MD 21224, USA; [d] Division of Rheumatology, University of Western Ontario, St. Joseph's Health Care, 268 Grosvenor Street, London, Ontario N6A 4V2, Canada
* Corresponding authors. Johns Hopkins Scleroderma Center, Division of Rheumatology, Johns Hopkins University School of Medicine, 5200 Eastern Avenue, Mason F Lord Building Center Tower, Suite 4100, Baltimore, MD 21224.
E-mail addresses: Ami.Shah@jhmi.edu (A.A.S.); Janet.Pope@sjhc.london.on.ca (J.E.P.)

Rheum Dis Clin N Am 49 (2023) 411–423
https://doi.org/10.1016/j.rdc.2023.01.011
0889-857X/23/© 2023 Elsevier Inc. All rights reserved.

rheumatic.theclinics.com

cutaneous (lcSSc) and diffuse cutaneous SSc (dcSSc).[1] SSc can affect various aspects of health, which cause morbidity and mortality, including increased rates of osteopenia and osteoporosis (OP), and increased malignancy risk. The purpose of this review is to provide an update regarding bone health and cancer screening in patients with SSc and to provide "points to consider" when addressing these domains with a preventative care approach.

Bone Health, Osteoporosis, and Fractures

OP is a disease characterized by microarchitectural disruption of bone, decreased bone mass, and general skeletal fragility with a resulting increased risk of fracture. OP leads to increased morbidity and mortality, with as high as 47% of women and 22% of men over the age of 50 years estimated to experience an OP-related fracture in their lifetime.[2] OP poses a large economic burden on society, as OP-related fractures cost approximately $17.9 billion per year in the United States.[3,4] OP is a common disease with a prevalence of 23.1% for women and 11.7% for men globally.[5] The risk of developing OP is influenced by multiple factors, including advanced age, race, obesity, postmenopausal status, family history, smoking, alcohol use, and systemic diseases, such as rheumatoid arthritis (RA), diabetes, chronic kidney and liver disease, and diseases of malnutrition and malabsorption.[6,7]

Traditionally, OP is diagnosed when a fragility fracture occurs at the wrist, spine, hip, humerus, rib, and pelvis, or when a T-score equal to or less than −2.5 standard deviations at any site based on bone mineral density (BMD) testing via dual-energy X-ray absorptiometry.[8,9] In addition, OP can be diagnosed if a patient is deemed to have an elevated 10-year fracture risk as determined by the fracture risk assessment tool.[8–10]

Despite the high frequency of OP in the general population, OP prevalence in SSc has been observed to be higher.[11–13] Theoretically, there are multiple factors inherent in SSc that may contribute to the development of OP, including chronic inflammation from autoimmunity, decreased skeletal calcium stores from subcutaneous calcinosis deposits, malabsorption, malnutrition, chronic ischemia from vasculopathy, corticosteroid use, frequent use of high chronic dosing of proton-pump inhibitors (PPIs), and early menopause.[14,15] Previous reviews tried to elucidate a relationship between SSc and OP, but heterogeneity in and between studies, and small sample sizes yielded no clear associations between SSc and OP.[16] However, more recent studies have illuminated the relationship between SSc and the development, risk factors, and fractures associated with OP which support the authors' bone health recommendations (**Box 1**).

Lai and colleagues[17] conducted a cohort study of 1712 patients with SSc, compared with age- and gender-matched controls without SSc, to determine the incidence and risk factors of OP-related fractures. The investigators observed an overall OP fracture incidence rate ratio of 1.69 for patients with SSc, which was driven by vertebral and hip fractures in female patients. Furthermore, patients with SSc were significantly younger than controls with hip fractures. Independent risk factors for OP fractures in patients with SSc were older age, female gender, more than 7.5 mg of daily oral prednisolone, and bowel dysmotility treated with intravenous metoclopramide.

These findings are further corroborated by Avouac and colleagues,[18] who investigated the prevalence of OP and fractures in female patients with SSc compared with age-matched women with RA and matched controls without these diseases. Patients with SSc had a higher prevalence of OP compared with controls, and a similar prevalence compared with RA patients, 30%, 11%, and 32%, respectively. Likewise, patients with SSc had a higher fracture prevalence compared with controls, and

---

Box 1
Bone health recommendations in systemic sclerosis

Recommendations
1. Follow local guidelines for bone density monitoring in SSc, especially in postmenopausal women and others with OP risk factors (very-low body mass index (BMI), malnutrition, early menopause, use of certain medications such as PPIs or steroids, and possibly the presence of calcinosis).
2. OP is increased in both diffuse and limited cutaneous SSc. Therefore, both subtypes require close monitoring of bone health parameters and appropriate interventions.[18,21,43]
3. Patients with SSc may be concerned with worsening of subcutaneous calcinosis from calcium (and possibly vitamin D supplementation), but there are not clear data that either will increase calcinosis. The authors recommend supplementation of calcium and vitamin D in patients, as this does not worsen calcinosis.
4. Given the prevalence of vitamin D deficiency in patients with SSc, higher than general population doses of vitamin D could be considered for supplementation in patients with SSc.[27] Serum vitamin D should be measured if there is a concern that it is low in patients with SSc at any age.
5. Usual investigations for OP in patients with SSc should be considered according to OP guidelines. These may include measurements of calcium, vitamin D, PTH, renal, liver, and thyroid function, and BMD. Tests are individualized when considering if a workup for secondary causes of OP is warranted. Some patients with SSc may also have concomitant primary biliary cholangitis or celiac disease, which are associated with OP.
6. In patients in whom there is moderate suspicion for osteopenia/OP development, more frequent OP risk factor assessments may be required.
7. BMI should be measured in patients with SSc, as those with very low BMI have an increased risk of OP.
8. Malnutrition should be screened for in patients with SSc at diagnosis and annually given the increased risk of malnutrition in a 12-month period.[44] Tools such as the Malnutrition Universal Screening Tool can aid clinicians in identifying patients at risk. Dietary interventions such as dietary counselling or artificial nutritional support may be required in patients with severe malnutrition.[33]
9. All available treatments for OP may be considered to treat OP in SSc. These include bisphosphonates (being cautious with the risk of erosive esophagitis with oral treatment in patients with esophageal dysmotility and reflux esophagitis), denosumab, PTH analogues, sclerostin inhibitor, and so forth.
10. Encourage regular exercise and healthy eating, including adequate dietary calcium where possible or supplemental calcium, limit alcohol and excessive caffeine. Target a normal BMI.

---

similar to RA at 35%, 10%, and 33%, respectively. Older age was a risk factor for OP and fractures in SSc, whereas low vitamin D level was associated with increased risk of fracture. In this study, prior corticosteroid use in SSc did not increase OP or fracture, but this may be due to short-duration and low-dose glucocorticoids. An association between previous steroid use in patients with SSc and BMD values was also not found, which is corroborated by a systematic review by Omair and colleagues.[19] This finding is consistent with an overall decreased cumulative dose of corticosteroids when compared with the RA patient population, where cumulative dose is associated with OP and decreased BMD.[18] The authors suspect that the known risk of glucocorticoid-induced OP would also be true in SSc, but the use of chronic prednisone/prednisolone is more common in RA.

Vitamin D deficiency may be more frequent in patients with SSc.[20] Vitamin D deficiency can lead to secondary hyperparathyroidism, mineralization defects, and low BMD, which can ultimately precipitate osteopenia, OP, and fractures.[2] Several studies have found increased prevalence of vitamin D deficiency in patients with SSc independent of geographic origin and despite regular supplementation.[21–25] Furthermore,

Atteritano and colleagues[26] observed a significant correlation for patients with SSc between 25-hydroxyvitamin D3 levels and parathyroid hormone (PTH) levels, BMD measurements in the lumbar spine, femoral neck, and total femur and bone turnover markers, such as osteocalcin and deoxy-pyridinoline. Therefore, vitamin D deficiency represents a modifiable risk factor of OP development in patients with SSc. Supplementation with 800 IU per day has been found insufficient to address deficiency in patients with SSc, and higher quantities could be required.[27] However, there is no consensus or guidelines on optimal dosing of vitamin D in SSc.

Another consideration for patients with SSc and their risk of developing OP is poor nutrition. Malnutrition in SSc confers increased morbidity and mortality.[28-30] Malnutrition in SSc can be secondary to microstomia, early satiety, fatigue, malabsorption, low caloric intake, small bowel overgrowth, and esophageal and other gut dysmotility.[28,31-33] Caimmi and colleagues[11] assessed the prevalence of malnutrition in an SSc cohort. They report 9.2% of patients with SSc met European Society of Clinical Nutrition and Metabolism malnutrition criteria.[34] Bone density measurements at the hip and spine were lower in malnourished patients, regardless of vitamin D status. Therefore, malnutrition contributes to OP in some patients with SSc.

Calcinosis in SSc, most commonly materializing through dystrophic calcification, occurs when there is subcutaneous calcium hydroxyapatite deposition in areas of trauma, such as fingertips and extensor surfaces. Calcinosis is more prevalent in the limited cutaneous subtype and is associated with normal serum calcium and phosphate levels.[35] Previous studies have been inconclusive in elucidating a relationship between the presence of calcinosis and decreased BMD in patients with SSc.[36,37] However, in a recent study, Valenzuela and colleagues[38] report a significant association between calcinosis and OP in a retrospective cohort of 5218 patients with SSc. Patients with SSc with calcinosis have been observed to have lower T scores compared with those without calcinosis.[39] Furthermore, vertebral fractures in patients with SSc were increased if calcinosis was present in nonvertebral regions.[40]

Chronic inflammation has been purported as a contributor to development of OP in SSc. Multiple studies have found no relationship between C-reactive protein and erythrocyte sedimentation rate levels and lower BMD, fragility fractures, or serum PTH levels.[18,26] However, active disease has been observed to be associated with OP. Vasculopathy in SSc may be associated with OP. Ruaro and colleagues[41] evaluated bone density (BMD) and trabecular bone analysis in SSc, RA, and controls. Patients with SSc with late or active nailfold videocapillaroscopic patterns were more likely to have low BMD. Marot and colleagues[42] described that digital ulcers were an independent risk factor for alterations in bone microarchitecture, which can lead to low bone mass.

Cancer Screening

Most epidemiologic studies have demonstrated that patients with SSc have an increased risk of cancer compared with the general population. Age- and sex-adjusted estimates suggest this may range from a 1.2- to 4.2-fold increased risk, with a wide variety of tumor types observed.[45-58] This heightened risk has consistently been demonstrated for lung and hematologic malignancies. In 3 recent meta-analyses, it was estimated that patients with SSc have a 3.1- to 4.4-fold increased risk of lung cancer and a 2.2- to 2.6-fold increased risk of hematologic malignancies.[45-47] Lung cancer may be increased, as the rate of smoking (ever) is higher in SSc than age- and sex-matched population controls; smoking increases lung cancer risk and may also be associated with worse SSc outcomes and organ complications, which may further increase lung cancer risk. Also, interstitial lung disease may increase lung cancer risk.[59]

Other studies have shown that patients with SSc may have an increased risk of liver, esophageal, oropharyngeal, stomach, pancreatic, thyroid, cervical, uterine, prostate, testicular, melanoma, and nonmelanoma skin cancers, and some cancers, including breast cancer, may be enriched in distinct autoantibody subgroups.[60–63] Abnormal Pap tests are increased in women with SSc compared with population controls, which can lead to precancerous changes and cancer of the cervix.[64] Skin cancer may be increased in the context of immunosupressive therapies or from cancers that may arise in diseased, fibrotic tissue.[65]

There is interest in identifying risk factors for cancer among patients with SSc to better target cancer screening efforts. Several demographic and clinical features have been identified as potential risk factors, including subtype (both dcSSc and lcSSc), older age at SSc onset, male sex, smoking, interstitial lung disease (for lung cancer, in particular), use of calcium channel blockers, and cyclophosphamide use (for bladder cancer), but these have not been consistently reproduced, which has limited their clinical utility.[46,50,51,54,59,66–69]

Recent work suggests autoantibody type may be a useful tool to identify patients with SSc who have an increased or decreased risk of cancer either around the time of SSc onset or during the disease course.[60,70,71] Many studies have demonstrated that patients with anti-RNA polymerase III antibodies have an increased risk of cancer within a few years of SSc onset, and recent mechanistic data suggest these patients may have a mechanism of cancer-induced autoimmunity.[60–62,66,67,70,72–74] Although most of these studies were within cohort analyses, Igusa and colleagues[60] investigated cancer risk in distinct autoantibody and phenotypic subgroups compared with the US Surveillance, Epidemiology, and End Results registry, adjusting for age, sex, race, ethnicity, and calendar time. Patients with anti-RNA polymerase III antibodies had a 2.8-fold increased risk of cancer (standardized incidence ratio [SIR], 2.84; 95% confidence interval [CI], 1.89–4.10) within 3 years of SSc symptom onset. Furthermore, patients with anti-RNA polymerase III antibodies were at high risk of different cancer types depending on their clinical phenotype. Patients with anti-RNA polymerase III and diffuse cutaneous SSc had a high risk of breast cancer (SIR, 5.14; 95% CI, 2.66–8.98), whereas those with anti-RNA polymerase III and limited cutaneous SSc had an increased risk of lung cancer (SIR, 10.4; 95%CI, 1.26–37.7). Patients with anti-RNA polymerase III antibodies also had an increased risk of prostate and tongue cancer around the time of SSc onset. Importantly, 80% to 85% of patients with anti-RNA polymerase III antibodies do not have a cancer diagnosed. Indeed, recent work has demonstrated that patients with RNA polymerase III antibodies who have greater breadth of the immune response, targeting the large subunit of RNA polymerase I or the Th/To complex, may be protected from cancer around the time of SSc onset.[75,76] In aggregate, these data suggest that cancer screening strategies could be targeted based on autoantibody type and clinical phenotype in patients with SSc, but this requires further study.

Although patients with RNA polymerase III antibodies had an increased risk of cancer around the time of SSc onset, the Igusa study suggested that patients with anticentromere antibodies have a decreased risk of cancer during the disease course, and those who were negative for centromere, topoisomerase I, and RNA polymerase III (referred to as CTP-negative) antibodies also have a high cancer risk around the time of SSc onset.[60] Individual cohort studies have shown that patients with anti-PM-Scl, antitopoisomerase I, anti-U1 RNP, and anti-RNPC3 antibodies may have an increased risk of cancer either during the disease course or around the time of SSc onset.[63,77–79] It is important to see if these findings are replicated in external cohorts and could be useful tools for cancer risk stratification.

Approach to cancer screening

Although there is strong evidence that patients with SSc have an increased risk of cancer and that subsets of patients with SSc may have cancer-induced autoimmunity, data are sparse with respect to the optimal approach to cancer detection in patients with SSc at the time of disease onset or during the disease course. Recognizing that data are lacking on cancer screening effectiveness or cost-effectiveness in patients with SSc, an approach to cancer detection reflecting a combination of age, sex, and risk factor-based recommendations seems appropriate.

All patients with SSc should have a comprehensive history and physical examination, with particular attention to personal and family history of cancer, tobacco, alcohol, and sun exposure, and prior or current immunosuppressive therapies, which may influence cancer screening strategies. In women, the authors recommend routine cervical cancer screening. Society guidelines vary. The American Cancer Society recently issued new guidance suggesting primary human papillomavirus (HPV) testing in samples taken from the cervix every 5 years beginning at the age of 25 years, with shorter intervals if there have been abnormal results.[80] Where primary HPV testing is unavailable, other acceptable screening methods include cotesting (cytology in combination with HPV testing) every 5 years or cytology only every 3 years. Other organizations, including the US Preventative Services Task Force and the American College of Obstetricians and Gynecologists, recommend initiating Pap screening at age 21 years with addition of HPV testing at age 30 years.[81] Although current guidelines recommend that Pap smears should be performed until the age of 65 years, the authors suggest performing a Pap smear once in women with new-onset SSc above 65 years. International recommendations vary as to the appropriate age at which to initiate breast cancer screening and the optimal screening interval. Given studies suggesting that women with SSc have an increased risk of breast cancer, particularly those with anti-RNA polymerase III antibodies, mammography may be initiated earlier, such as at age 40 years in high-risk patients, and continued annually.[60–62] Men younger than age 40 years should have a testicular examination, and in high-risk patients, this could be repeated at regular intervals. For older men, the risks and benefits of prostate cancer screening are discussed, including a digital rectal examination and prostate-specific antigen (PSA) testing. Given the controversies regarding the utilization of PSA testing, this test may be particularly valuable in men with new-onset SSc at an older age and/or RNA polymerase III antibodies. Colon cancer screening with colonoscopy starting at 45 years of age, based on updated guidance from the US Preventative Services Task Force, is recommended.[82] Testing should be repeated at 10-year intervals if the initial test is normal. In the general population, it is not recommended to perform colonoscopies above the age of 75 years based on life expectancy, but in older patients with new-onset SSc, the authors do recommend testing owing to concern for paraneoplastic disease at older ages. For patients who are reluctant to undergo colonoscopy, fecal occult blood testing plus flexible sigmoidoscopy or stool DNA testing may be considered. Additional cancer screening tests may be warranted for specific exposures or SSc characteristics (**Table 1**).

More intensive cancer detection strategies may be warranted in patients deemed to be at particularly high risk of having an underlying cancer. This includes patients with anti-RNA polymerase III antibodies, an older age of SSc onset, atypical, aggressive, or treatment unresponsive disease, profound weight loss or other constitutional features out of proportion with disease severity, unexplained anemia, hemoptysis, or patients with a personal or striking family history of cancer.[86] If SSc is rapidly progressive at onset in an elderly patient, a thorough search for cancer is performed especially for

Table 1
Risk factor-based cancer screening recommendations in systemic sclerosis[a]

Specific Risk Factor	Recommendation
Cigarette smoking 30+ pack-years AND active smoking or quit <15 years ago AND age 55–74 y	Annual low-dose chest CT[b] [83]
Neck mass, oral lesions, unexplained oropharyngeal dysphagia, or globus sensation	Otolaryngology referral for head and neck examination and appropriate investigations
Barrett esophagus	EGD every 1–3 y[84]
Refractory GERD	EGD[84]
Esophagitis	Repeat EGD per local gastroenterology specialist's practice[84]
Primary biliary cholangitis overlap	Liver ultrasound every 6–12 mo ± alpha-fetoprotein in known or suspected cirrhosis[85]
Cytopenias not explained by immunosuppression	SPEP/IFE, peripheral blood flow cytometry Workup of iron-deficient anemia, including upper and lower endoscopies
Cyclophosphamide exposure	Annual urinalysis, and urine cytology if unexplained microscopic or macroscopic hematuria or after long exposure to cyclophosphamide
Mycophenolate exposure	Annual full-body skin examination
All routine age and sex-based cancer screening recommendations	

Abbreviations: EGD, esophagogastroduodenoscopy; GERD, gastroesophageal reflux disease; SPEP/IFE, serum protein electrophoresis/immunofixation.
[a] All patients should also undergo age- and sex-based cancer screening measures as detailed above.
[b] Consider baseline high-resolution chest CT instead if risk factors for significant interstitial lung disease (such as African descent, diffuse cutaneous SSc, anti–topoisomerase I antibodies).

adenocarcinomas. Further testing with computed tomography (CT) scan of the chest, abdomen, and pelvis or whole-body PET/CT may be warranted in these patients. Given the significantly higher risk of breast cancer in women with new-onset diffuse cutaneous SSc and RNA polymerase III autoantibodies, breast MRI may be considered. The EUSTAR group conducted a Delphi exercise including 82 SSc experts to generate cancer screening recommendations for patients with anti-RNA polymerase III antibodies. The investigators suggested a specific focus on breast cancer with consideration of ultrasound or MRI when needed.[62] PSA testing in men, otolaryngology examination, and chest CT may also be warranted in patients with new-onset SSc and RNA polymerase III autoantibodies given recent epidemiologic studies demonstrating a higher risk of prostate, tongue, and lung cancers in these patients.[60] Tumor markers may also be considered, but these have not been well studied in SSc at this time. Additional studies are underway to test the utility of these cancer detection strategies in high-risk SSc subsets, as it is critical to maximize cancer detection and minimize the harms and costs of overscreening in this patient population.

Cancer prevention measures
There are data on healthy lifestyle choices that can reduce the risk of several cancers. Smoking cessation is strongly recommended. Aiming for a normal BMI, limiting red

meat and processed meat, considering a Mediterranean diet or a diet high in fruits and vegetables and plant proteins (lentils, bean, whole grains), regular exercise, avoiding excessive alcohol, using sunscreen and avoiding excessive sun exposure, and getting vaccinations (HPV, hepatitis B) are important preventative measures.[87] Regular screening, such as Pap tests, breast screening, colon cancer screening, and other recommended screening, in certain high-risk populations as detailed above are recommended.[83–85]

SUMMARY

A preventative care approach can help to ameliorate the effect of SSc-related complications, such as OP and malignancies. Clinicians are encouraged to ensure vitamin D levels are in the normal range, as some patients with SSc are at increased risk of deficiency despite supplementation. Furthermore, patients should be screened for malnutrition, and patients identified at risk should undergo appropriate dietary interventions. Bone densities should be ordered using OP guidelines, and treatment may be indicated in moderate- to high-risk patients. Last, given the increased risk of malignancies in SSc, patients should be regularly screened in accordance with their specific risk factors.

CONFLICT OF INTEREST

There are no conflicts of interest to disclose.

AUTHOR CONTRIBUTIONS

L.M. Calderon, R.T. Domsic, A.A. Shah, and J.E. Pope were involved in study design, review of literature, and article writing. All authors reviewed the article and approved the final version.

FUNDING

No specific funding was received from any bodies in the public, commercial, or not-for-profit sectors to carry out the work described in this article. A.A. Shah is supported by NIH/NIAMS K24AR080217.

CLINICS CARE POINTS

- Standard osteoporosis screening per local guidelines is recommended, which may include measurements of calcium, vitamin D, PTH, renal, liver, and thyroid function, and bone mineral density testing via dual-energy X-ray absorptiometry.
- Osteoporosis medications may be used for treatment in SSc including bisphosphonates, with caution being noted for the risk of erosive esophagitis with oral therapy in patients with esophageal dysmotility and reflux esophagitis.
- Age, sex and risk factor based cancer screening recommendations are appropriate, with consideration given to enhanced cancer detection strategies (such as computed tomography (CT) scan of the chest, abdomen, and pelvis, whole-body PET/CT, and/or breast ultrasound or MRI) in patients with new onset SSc with anti-RNA polymerase III antibodies, an older age of SSc onset, atypical, aggressive, or treatment unresponsive disease, profound weight loss or other constitutional features out of proportion with disease severity, or a personal or striking family history of cancer.

FUNDING AND COMPETING INTERESTS

There are no conflicts of interest. A.A. Shah is supported by NIH, United States/ NIAMS, United States K24AR080217. Contributions: L.M. Calderon, R.T. Domsic, A.A. Shah, and J.E. Pope were involved in study design, analysis, and article writing. All authors reviewed the article and approved the final version.

REFERENCES

1. Hughes M, Herrick AL. Systemic sclerosis. Br J Hosp Med 2019;80(9):530–6.
2. Holick MF. Vitamin D Deficiency. N Engl J Med 2007;357(3):266–81.
3. Clynes MA, Harvey NC, Curtis EM, et al. The epidemiology of osteoporosis. Br Med Bull 2020;133(1):105–17.
4. Bliuc D, Nguyen ND, Nguyen T v, et al. Compound risk of high mortality following osteoporotic fracture and refracture in elderly women and men. J Bone Miner Res 2013;28(11):2317–24.
5. Salari N, Ghasemi H, Mohammadi L, et al. The global prevalence of osteoporosis in the world: a comprehensive systematic review and meta-analysis. J Orthop Surg Res 2021;16(1):609.
6. Curtis EM, Moon RJ, Dennison EM, et al. Recent advances in the pathogenesis and treatment of osteoporosis. Clin Med 2015;15(Suppl 6):s92–6.
7. Pouresmaeili F, Kamali Dehghan B, Kamarehei M, et al. A comprehensive overview on osteoporosis and its risk factors. Therapeut Clin Risk Manag 2018;14: 2029–49.
8. Siris ES, Adler R, Bilezikian J, et al. The clinical diagnosis of osteoporosis: a position statement from the National Bone Health Alliance Working Group. Osteoporos Int 2014;25(5):1439–43.
9. Lorentzon M, Cummings SR. Osteoporosis: the evolution of a diagnosis. J Intern Med 2015;277(6):650–61.
10. Kanis JA, McCloskey E v, Johansson H, et al. Development and use of FRAX in osteoporosis. Osteoporos Int 2010;21(Suppl 2):S407–13.
11. Caimmi C, Caramaschi P, Barausse G, et al. Bone metabolism in a large cohort of patients with systemic sclerosis. Calcif Tissue Int 2016;99(1):23–9.
12. Chuealee W, Foocharoen C, Mahakkanukrauh A, et al. Prevalence and predictive factors of osteoporosis in Thai systemic sclerosis. Sci Rep 2021;11(1):9424.
13. Yuen SY, Rochwerg B, Ouimet J, et al. Patients with scleroderma may have increased risk of osteoporosis. A comparison to rheumatoid arthritis and noninflammatory musculoskeletal conditions. J Rheumatol 2008;35(6):1073–8.
14. la Montagna G, Vatti M, Valentini G, et al. Osteopenia in systemic sclerosis. Evidence of a participating role of earlier menopause. Clin Rheumatol 1991; 10(1):18–22.
15. Serup J, Hagdrup H, Tvedegaard E. Bone mineral content in systemic sclerosis measured by photonabsorptiometry. Acta Derm Venereol 1983;63(3):235–7.
16. Loucks J, Pope JE. Osteoporosis in scleroderma. Semin Arthritis Rheum 2005; 34(4):678–82.
17. Lai CC, Wang SH, Chen WS, et al. Increased risk of osteoporotic fractures in patients with systemic sclerosis: a nationwide population-based study. Ann Rheum Dis 2015;74(7):1347–52.
18. Avouac J, Koumakis E, Toth E, et al. Increased risk of osteoporosis and fracture in women with systemic sclerosis: a comparative study with rheumatoid arthritis. Arthritis Care Res 2012;64(12):1871–8.

19. Omair MA, Pagnoux C, McDonald-Blumer H, et al. Low bone density in systemic sclerosis. A systematic review. J Rheumatol 2013;40(11):1881–90.

20. Groseanu L, Bojinca V, Gudu T, et al. Low vitamin D status in systemic sclerosis and the impact on disease phenotype. Eur J Rheumatol 2016;3(2):50–5.

21. Vacca A, Cormier C, Piras M, et al. Vitamin D Deficiency and Insufficiency in 2 Independent Cohorts of Patients with Systemic Sclerosis. J Rheumatol 2009; 36(9):1924–9.

22. Fernández RR, Roldán CF, Rubio JLC, et al. Vitamin D Deficiency in a Cohort of Patients with Systemic Scleroderma from the South of Spain. J Rheumatol 2010; 37(6):1355.

23. Trombetta AC, Smith V, Gotelli E, et al. Vitamin D deficiency and clinical correlations in systemic sclerosis patients: a retrospective analysis for possible future developments. PLoS One 2017;12(6):e0179062.

24. Adami Fassio, Rossini Caimmi, Giollo Orsolini, et al. Osteoporosis in rheumatic diseases. Int J Mol Sci 2019;20(23):5867.

25. Giuggioli D, Colaci M, Cassone G, et al. Serum 25-OH vitamin D levels in systemic sclerosis: analysis of 140 patients and review of the literature. Clin Rheumatol 2017;36(3):583–90.

26. Atteritano M, Sorbara S, Bagnato G, et al. Bone mineral density, bone turnover markers and fractures in patients with systemic sclerosis: a case control study. PLoS One 2013;8(6):e66991.

27. Schneider L, Hax V, Monticielo O, et al. Dualities of the vitamin D in systemic sclerosis: a systematic literature review. Adv Rheumatol 2021;61(1):34.

28. Baron M, Hudson M, Steele R, Canadian Scleroderma Research Group. Malnutrition is common in systemic sclerosis: results from the Canadian scleroderma research group database. J Rheumatol 2009;36(12):2737–43.

29. Cruz-Domínguez MP, García-Collinot G, Saavedra MA, et al. Malnutrition is an independent risk factor for mortality in Mexican patients with systemic sclerosis: a cohort study. Rheumatol Int 2017;37(7):1101–9.

30. Krause L, Becker MO, Brueckner CS, et al. Nutritional status as marker for disease activity and severity predicting mortality in patients with systemic sclerosis. Ann Rheum Dis 2010;69(11):1951–7.

31. Mouthon L, Rannou F, Berezne A, et al. Development and validation of a scale for mouth handicap in systemic sclerosis: the Mouth Handicap in Systemic Sclerosis scale. Ann Rheum Dis 2007;66(12):1651–5.

32. de Carlan M, Lescoat A, Brochard C, et al. Association between Clinical Manifestations of Systemic Sclerosis and Esophageal Dysmotility Assessed by High-Resolution Manometry. Journal of Scleroderma and Related Disorders 2017; 2(1):50–6.

33. Harrison E, Herrick AL, McLaughlin JT, et al. Malnutrition in systemic sclerosis. Rheumatology 2012;51(10):1747–56.

34. Cederholm T, Bosaeus I, Barazzoni R, et al. Diagnostic criteria for malnutrition – an ESPEN Consensus Statement. Clinical Nutrition 2015;34(3):335–40.

35. Valenzuela A, Chung L. Calcinosis: pathophysiology and management. Curr Opin Rheumatol 2015;27(6):542–8.

36. di Munno O, Mazzantini M, Massei P, et al. Reduced bone mass and normal calcium metabolism in systemic sclerosis with and without calcinosis. Clin Rheumatol 1995;14(4):407–12.

37. da Silva HC, Szejnfeld VL, Assis LS, et al. [Study of bone density in systemic scleroderma]. Revista da Associacao Medica Brasileira (1992) 1997;43(1):40–6.

38. Valenzuela A, Baron M, Herrick AL, et al. Calcinosis is associated with digital ulcers and osteoporosis in patients with systemic sclerosis: a Scleroderma Clinical Trials Consortium study. Semin Arthritis Rheum 2016;46(3):344–9.

39. Valenzuela A, Baron M, Rodriguez-Reyna TS, et al. Calcinosis is associated with ischemic manifestations and increased disability in patients with systemic sclerosis. Semin Arthritis Rheum 2020;50(5):891–6.

40. Fauny M, Bauer E, Albuisson E, et al. Vertebral fracture prevalence and measurement of the scanographic bone attenuation coefficient on CT-scan in patients with systemic sclerosis. Rheumatol Int 2018;38(10):1901–10.

41. Ruaro B, Casabella A, Paolino S, et al. Correlation between bone quality and microvascular damage in systemic sclerosis patients. Rheumatology 2018; 57(9):1548–54.

42. Marot M, Valéry A, Esteve E, et al. Prevalence and predictive factors of osteoporosis in systemic sclerosis patients: a case-control study. Oncotarget 2015;6(17): 14865–73.

43. Sampaio-Barros PD, Costa-Paiva L, Filardi S, et al. Prognostic factors of low bone mineral density in systemic sclerosis. Clin Exp Rheumatol 2005;23(2):180–4.

44. Bagnato G, Pigatto E, Bitto A, et al. The PREdictor of MAlnutrition in Systemic Sclerosis (PREMASS) score: a combined index to predict 12 months onset of malnutrition in systemic sclerosis. Front Med (Lausanne) 2021;8:651748.

45. Zhang JQ, Wan YN, Peng WJ, et al. The risk of cancer development in systemic sclerosis: a meta-analysis. Cancer Epidemiol 2013;37(5):523–7.

46. Onishi A, Sugiyama D, Kumagai S, et al. Cancer incidence in systemic sclerosis: meta-analysis of population-based cohort studies. Arthritis Rheum 2013;65(7): 1913–21.

47. Bonifazi M, Tramacere I, Pomponio G, et al. Systemic sclerosis (scleroderma) and cancer risk: systematic review and meta-analysis of observational studies. Rheumatology 2013;52(1):143–54.

48. Kuo CF, Luo SF, Yu KH, et al. Cancer risk among patients with systemic sclerosis: a nationwide population study in Taiwan. Scand J Rheumatol 2012;41(1):44–9.

49. Hashimoto A, Arinuma Y, Nagai T, et al. Incidence and the risk factor of malignancy in Japanese patients with systemic sclerosis. Intern Med 2012;51(13): 1683–8.

50. Siau K, Laversuch CJ, Creamer P, et al. Malignancy in scleroderma patients from south west England: a population-based cohort study. Rheumatol Int 2011;31(5): 641–5.

51. Olesen AB, Svaerke C, Farkas DK, et al. Systemic sclerosis and the risk of cancer: a nationwide population-based cohort study. Br J Dermatol 2010;163(4): 800–6.

52. Kang KY, Yim HW, Kim IJ, et al. Incidence of cancer among patients with systemic sclerosis in Korea: results from a single centre. Scand J Rheumatol 2009;38(4):299–303.

53. Derk CT, Rasheed M, Artlett CM, et al. A cohort study of cancer incidence in systemic sclerosis. J Rheumatol 2006;33(6):1113–6.

54. Hill CL, Nguyen AM, Roder D, et al. Risk of cancer in patients with scleroderma: a population based cohort study. Ann Rheum Dis 2003;62(8):728–31.

55. Rosenthal AK, McLaughlin JK, Gridley G, et al. Incidence of cancer among patients with systemic sclerosis. Cancer 1995;76(5):910–4.

56. Rosenthal AK, McLaughlin JK, Linet MS, et al. Scleroderma and malignancy: an epidemiological study. Ann Rheum Dis 1993;52(7):531–3.

57. Abu-Shakra M, Guillemin F, Lee P. Cancer in systemic sclerosis. Arthritis Rheum 1993;36(4):460–4.

58. Roumm AD, Medsger TA. Cancer and systemic sclerosis. An epidemiologic study. Arthritis Rheum 1985;28(12):1336–40.

59. Morrisroe K, Hansen D, Huq M, et al. Incidence, Risk Factors, and Outcomes of Cancer in Systemic Sclerosis. Arthritis Care Res 2020;72(11):1625–35.

60. Igusa T, Hummers LK, Visvanathan K, et al. Autoantibodies and scleroderma phenotype define subgroups at high-risk and low-risk for cancer. Ann Rheum Dis 2018;77(8):1179–86.

61. Moinzadeh P, Fonseca C, Hellmich M, et al. Association of anti-RNA polymerase III autoantibodies and cancer in scleroderma. Arthritis Res Ther 2014;16(1):R53.

62. Lazzaroni MG, Cavazzana I, Colombo E, et al. Malignancies in Patients with Anti-RNA Polymerase III Antibodies and Systemic Sclerosis: Analysis of the EULAR Scleroderma Trials and Research Cohort and Possible Recommendations for Screening. J Rheumatol 2017;44(5):639–47.

63. Shah AA, Xu G, Rosen A, et al. Brief Report: Anti-RNPC-3 Antibodies As a Marker of Cancer-Associated Scleroderma. Arthritis Rheumatol 2017;69(6):1306–12.

64. Tsai PH, Kuo CF. OP0070 The risk of precancerous lesions of the breast and cervix uteri in patients with autoimmune rheumatic diseases: a nationwide population study in Taiwan. Ann Rheum Dis 2020;79(Suppl 1):47.1–7.

65. Boozalis E, Shah AA, Wigley F, et al. Morphea and systemic sclerosis are associated with an increased risk for melanoma and nonmelanoma skin cancer. J Am Acad Dermatol 2019;80(5):1449–51.

66. Shah AA, Hummers LK, Casciola-Rosen L, et al. Examination of autoantibody status and clinical features associated with cancer risk and cancer-associated scleroderma. Arthritis Rheumatol 2015;67(4):1053–61.

67. Nikpour M, Hissaria P, Byron J, et al. Prevalence, correlates and clinical usefulness of antibodies to RNA polymerase III in systemic sclerosis: a cross-sectional analysis of data from an Australian cohort. Arthritis Res Ther 2011; 13(6):R211.

68. Pontifex EK, Hill CL, Roberts-Thomson P. Risk factors for lung cancer in patients with scleroderma: a nested case-control study. Ann Rheum Dis 2007;66(4): 551–3.

69. Kaşifoğlu T, Bilge Ş Y, Yıldız F, et al. Risk factors for malignancy in systemic sclerosis patients. Clin Rheumatol 2016;35(6):1529–33.

70. Shah AA, Rosen A, Hummers L, et al. Close temporal relationship between onset of cancer and scleroderma in patients with RNA polymerase I/III antibodies. Arthritis Rheum 2010;62(9):2787–95.

71. Shah AA, Casciola-Rosen L, Rosen A. Review: cancer-induced autoimmunity in the rheumatic diseases. Arthritis Rheumatol 2015 Feb;67(2):317–26.

72. Airo' P, Ceribelli A, Cavazzana I, et al. Malignancies in Italian patients with systemic sclerosis positive for anti-RNA polymerase III antibodies. J Rheumatol 2011;38(7):1329–34.

73. Saigusa R, Asano Y, Nakamura K, et al. Association of anti-RNA polymerase III antibody and malignancy in Japanese patients with systemic sclerosis. J Dermatol 2015;42(5):524–7.

74. Joseph CG, Darrah E, Shah AA, et al. Association of the autoimmune disease scleroderma with an immunologic response to cancer. Science 2014; 343(6167):152–7.

75. Shah AA, Laiho M, Rosen A, et al. Protective Effect Against Cancer of Antibodies to the Large Subunits of Both RNA Polymerases I and III in Scleroderma. Arthritis Rheumatol 2019;71(9):1571–9.
76. Mecoli CA, Adler BL, Yang Q, et al. Cancer in Systemic Sclerosis: Analysis of Antibodies Against Components of the Th/To Complex. Arthritis Rheumatol 2021; 73(2):315–23.
77. Bernal-Bello D, de Tena JG, Guillén-Del Castillo A, et al. Novel risk factors related to cancer in scleroderma. Autoimmun Rev 2017;16(5):461–8.
78. Hoa S, Lazizi S, Baron M, et al. Association between autoantibodies in systemic sclerosis and cancer in a national registry. Rheumatology (Oxford) 2022;61(7): 2905–14.
79. Xu GJ, Shah AA, Li MZ, et al. Systematic autoantigen analysis identifies a distinct subtype of scleroderma with coincident cancer. Proc Natl Acad Sci U S A 2016; 113(47):E7526–34.
80. Fontham ETH, Wolf AMD, Church TR, et al. Cervical cancer screening for individuals at average risk: 2020 guideline update from the American Cancer Society. CA A Cancer Journal for Clinicians 2020;70(5):321–46.
81. Shami S, Coombs J. Cervical cancer screening guidelines. J Am Acad Physician Assistants 2021;34(9):21–4.
82. US Preventive Services Task Force, Davidson KW, Barry MJ, Mangione CM, et al. Screening for Colorectal Cancer: US Preventive Services Task Force Recommendation Statement. JAMA 2021;325(19):1965–77.
83. Shah AA, Casciola-Rosen L. Cancer and scleroderma: a paraneoplastic disease with implications for malignancy screening. Curr Opin Rheumatol 2015;27(6): 563–70.
84. Rock CL, Thomson C, Gansler T, et al. American Cancer Society guideline for diet and physical activity for cancer prevention. CA A Cancer J Clin 2020;70(4): 245–71.
85. Smith RA, Andrews KS, Brooks D, et al. Cancer screening in the United States, 2018: A review of current American Cancer Society guidelines and current issues in cancer screening. CA: A Cancer Journal for Clinicians 2018 Jul;68(4):297–316.
86. Shaheen NJ, Weinberg DS, Denberg TD, et al. Upper endoscopy for gastroesophageal reflux disease: best practice advice from the clinical guidelines committee of the American College of Physicians. Ann Intern Med 2012;157(11): 808–16.
87. Lindor KD, Bowlus CL, Boyer J, et al. Primary Biliary Cholangitis: 2018 Practice Guidance from the American Association for the Study of Liver Diseases. Hepatology 2019;69(1):394–419.

Training the Next Generation of Rheumatologists

What Is the Best Way to Teach Fellows About Scleroderma?

Tatiana S. Rodríguez-Reyna, MD, MSc[a], Faye N. Hant, DO, MSCR[b],
Maurizio Cutolo, MD[c], Vanessa Smith, MD[d,e,f],*

KEYWORDS

- Systemic sclerosis • Training • Capillaroscopy • mRSS

KEY POINTS

- Systemic sclerosis (SSc) training requires knowledge of the multisystemic nature of the disease, its clinical subsets and phases, and antibodies.
- SSc training should also include proficiency in special skills such as the performance of modified Rodnan skin score, capillaroscopy, and the detection of tendon friction rubs.
- National and international research and education networks participate in the formation of specialized professionals that will continue the care of patients with SSc and the basic and clinical research in this field.

 Video content accompanies this article at http://www.rheumatic.theclinics. com.

[a] Department of Immunology and Rheumatology, Instituto Nacional de Ciencias Médicas y Nutrición Salvador Zubirán, Vasco de Quiroga 15, Col. Belisario Domínguez Sección XVI, Tlalpan, Mexico City 14080, Mexico; [b] Department of Medicine, Division of Rheumatology and Immunology, Medical University of South Carolina, 96 Jonathan Lucas Street Suite 822, Charleston, SC 29425, USA; [c] Laboratory of Experimental Rheumatology and Academic Division of Clinical Rheumatology, Department of Internal Medicine and Medical Specialties, University of Genova, IRCCS San Martino Polyclinic Hospital, Viale Benedetto XV, 6, Genova 16132, Italy; [d] Department of Internal Medicine, Ghent University, Corneel Heymanslaan 10, Ghent 9000, Belgium; [e] Department of Rheumatology, Ghent University Hospital, Corneel Heymanslaan 10, Ghent 9000, Belgium; [f] Unit for Molecular Immunology and Inflammation, VIB Inflammation Research Center (IRC), Ghent, Belgium
* Corresponding author. Department of Internal Medicine, Ghent University, Corneel Heymanslaan 10, Ghent 9000, Belgium.
E-mail address: vanessa.smith@ugent.be

Rheum Dis Clin N Am 49 (2023) 425–444
https://doi.org/10.1016/j.rdc.2023.01.013
0889-857X/23/© 2023 Elsevier Inc. All rights reserved.

BACKGROUND

It is important for a fellow to be able to classify scleroderma into systemic sclerosis (SSc) and localized scleroderma (morphea), as these conditions vary in their presentation, management, and treatment (**Fig. 1**). In addition, the fellow must recognize that not all "thick skin" is scleroderma, and basic knowledge to recognize potential mimics of scleroderma (**Box 1**) is essential in training, to ensure that the correct diagnosis and management is made. The authors focus on SSc within this article, recognizing the importance of the basic knowledge learners should master during their fellowship training even if they do not train in a scleroderma specialty center.

SSc is a rare autoimmune connective tissue disease (CTD) of unknown cause, with an estimated annual incidence of 19.3 new cases per million adults per year.[1] SSc is characterized by 3 major processes: disease-specific autoantibodies and immune dysregulation, organ fibrosis, and small-vessel vasculopathy. It is vital that the fellow recognizes the evolution of the SSc classification criteria throughout the years. The initial American College of Rheumatology (ACR) classification criteria were published in 1980 (**Box 2**) but lacked sensitivity for early SSc and limited cutaneous SSc (lcSSc), and the updated ACR/European Alliance of Associations for Rheumatology (EULAR) classification for SSc published in 2013 served to update this classification[2] (**Table 1**). The ACR/EULAR classification determined that skin thickening of the fingers extending proximal to the metacarpophalangeal joints is sufficient for the patient to be classified as having SSc and that if that is not present, 7 additive items can be applied, with different weights for each: skin thickening of the fingers, fingertip lesions, telangiectasia, abnormal nailfold capillaries, interstitial lung disease or pulmonary arterial hypertension, Raynaud phenomenon (RP), and SSc-related autoantibodies. Classification criteria do not equal diagnostic criteria, so it is possible that some patients may be diagnosed with SSc but do not meet the ACR/EULAR SSc classification criteria.

SUBTYPES OF SYSTEMIC SCLEROSIS

The rheumatology fellow must recognize the differentiating features between the subtypes of systemic sclerosis: lcSSc (formerly known as CREST syndrome), diffuse cutaneous systemic sclerosis (dcSSc), systemic sclerosis sine scleroderma, and overlap syndromes. Patients with SSc sine scleroderma have features of lcSSc without the skin thickening, whereas overlap patients meet criteria for SSc along with another

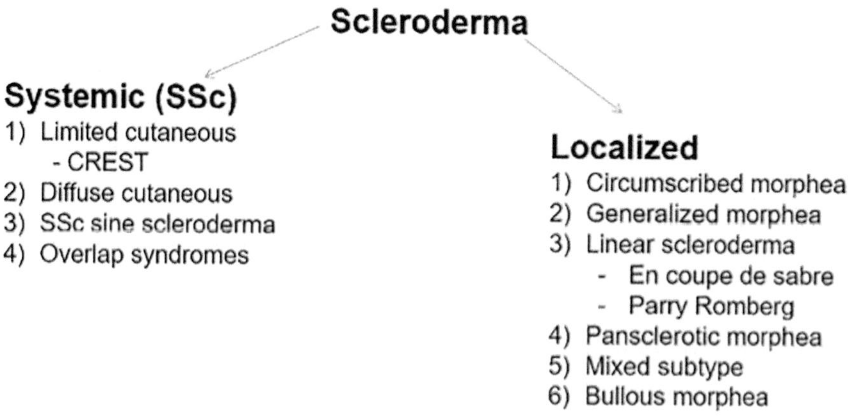

Scleroderma

Systemic (SSc)
1) Limited cutaneous
   - CREST
2) Diffuse cutaneous
3) SSc sine scleroderma
4) Overlap syndromes

Localized
1) Circumscribed morphea
2) Generalized morphea
3) Linear scleroderma
   - En coupe de sabre
   - Parry Romberg
4) Pansclerotic morphea
5) Mixed subtype
6) Bullous morphea

Fig. 1. Systemic sclerosis classification.

> **Box 1**
> **Differential diagnosis of thickened skin**
>
> - Scleredema
> - Scleromyxedema
> - Nephrogenic systemic fibrosis
> - Localized scleroderma
> - Eosinophilic fasciitis
> - Eosinophila myalgia syndrome
> - Toxic oil syndrome
> - Lipodermatosclerosis
> - Lichen sclerosus et atrophicans
> - Porphyria cutanea tarda
> - Sclerodermiform chronic graft versus host disease
> - POEMS syndrome
> - Environmentally or drug-induced systemic sclerosis–like disorders
> - Scleroderma-like lesions in endocrine disorders

CTD, including, but not limited to, systemic lupus erythematosus, rheumatoid arthritis, inflammatory myopathies, or mixed CTD. **Table 2** reviews key features associated with and that differentiate lcSSc and dcSSc. In addition, current knowledge of autoantibody associations has allowed rheumatologists to better phenotype patients with SSc.

Systemic Sclerosis–Specific and Associated Antibodies

Research in this field has advanced greatly. The association of the presence of autoantibodies with specific SSc phenotypes and target organs is crucial for the initial evaluation of patients with SSc; it is preserved along different ethnic groups, so rheumatology fellows should learn and understand these associations in order to standardize patient evaluation and follow-up according to their risk for internal organ involvement. Literature in this field is vast but excellent reviews can be found in recent articles.[3]

It is useful to have a practical visual tool to summarize these associations; the authors' proposal, based on the aforementioned reference and others that they recommend us to review, is depicted in **Table 3**.[4–18]

> **Box 2**
> **1980 American College of Rheumatology classification criteria for systemic sclerosis**
>
> Major
> - Proximal skin thickening or induration (proximal to the MCPs or MTPs)
>   (Usually bilateral, symmetrical, and almost always including sclerodactyly)
>
> Minor
> - Sclerodactyly
> - Digital pitting or loss of finger pad substance
> - Bibasilar pulmonary fibrosis on CXR (chest imaging) not attributable to primary lung disease
>
> SSc diagnosed when 1 major and 2 or more minor criteria are present*Abbreviations:* MCP, metacarpophalangeal; MTP, metatarsophalangeal.

Table 1
2013 ACR/EULAR systemic sclerosis classification criteria

Item	Subitem	Weighted Score
Skin thickening of the fingers of both hands extending to the metacarpophalangeal (MCP) joints		9
Skin thickening of the fingers	Puffy fingers	2
(only count the highest score)	Whole finger, distal to MCP	4
Finger tip lesions	Digital tip ulcers	2
(only count the highest score)	Pitting scars	3
Telangiectasias	—	2
Abnormal nailfold capillaries	—	2
Pulmonary arterial hypertensionS and/or interstitial lung disease	—	2
Raynaud phenomenon	—	3
Scleroderma-related antibodies (any of anticentromere, antitopoisomerase I (anti-SCL70), anti-RNA polymerase III)	—	3
—	Total score[a]	—

Patients with a total score of $\geq$ 9 are being classified as having definite systemic sclerosis.
[a] Add the maximum weight (score) in each category to calculate the total score.
Adapted from van den Hoogen F, Khanna D, Fransen J, et al. 2013 classification criteria for systemic sclerosis: an American college of rheumatology/European league against rheumatism collaborative initiative. Ann Rheum Dis. 2013;72(11):1747-1755.

History Taking in the Patient with Systemic Sclerosis

Given the multisystem involvement in SSc, it is imperative that the rheumatology fellow approaches the patient in a thorough and organized manner; this is necessary to avoid missing key items that require specific workup, laboratory investigations, radiologic

Table 2
Features associated with limited cutaneous systemic sclerosis and diffuse cutaneous systemic sclerosis

Limited Cutaneous SSc (lcSSc)	Diffuse Cutaneous SSc (dcSSc)
• Skin thickening distal to elbows & knees	• Skin thickening proximal to elbows & knees
• Skin involvement of face	• Truncal (chest and abdominal) involvement at any time during the course of the disease
• Low skin score	
• Calcinosis	• Skin involvement of face
• Long-standing Raynaud phenomenon even years before appearance of other symptoms	• High skin score (typically > 18 within 12 months of onset)
	• Abrupt new-onset Raynaud phenomenon
• Esophageal dysmotility	• Early, rapid visceral involvement
• Sclerodactyly (distal to MCPs)	• Tendon friction rubs
• Telangiectasias	• Scleroderma renal crisis
• Gastrointestinal involvement	• ILD
• ILD	• Antitopoisomerase (SCL-70) antibodies
• Late development of PAH	• Anti-RNA polymerase III antibodies
• Anticentromere antibodies	

Abbreviations: ILD, interstitial lung disease; PAH, pulmonary arterial hypertension.

Table 3
Autoantibodies in systemic sclerosis

Diffuse SSc	Overlap SSc	Limited SSc
Topoisomerase I • ILD (>60%) • Cardiac involvement • Early digital ulcers • Myopathy • Renal crisis	U1-RNP • Myositis (25%) • ILD • Joints • Trigeminal neuropathy	Centromere • Calcinosis • Digital ulcers • Pulmonary hypertension • ILD low frequency (20%–30%)
RNA polymerase III • Severe skin • Renal crisis • Gastric antral vascular ectasia (GAVE) • Cancer	PM/Scl • Myositis (>50%) • Calcinosis	Th/To • Pulmonary hypertension (25%) • ILD (>25%)
U3-RNP (Fibrillarin) • Myositis • Pulmonary hypertension • Cardiomyopathy • Severe Gastrointestinal	Ku • Myositis • Cardiac involvement	U11/U12-RNP • Severe ILD • Severe gastrointestinal
Ruv BL1/2 • Myositis • Diffuse or overlap		Bicaudal D2 • Myopathy • ILD

assessment, and specific treatments. An approach to consider is an "organ systems"–based approach similar to those taken while working in an intensive care setting that ensures "no organ system is left behind."

This approach focuses on the evaluation of the patient with SSc within 9 systems: skin/integument, ENT/dental/oral, vascular, cardiopulmonary, gastrointestinal, renal, musculoskeletal, neurological, and psychiatric. Performing a scleroderma-specific history and physical examination using this organized frame, with specific subitems within each organ, allows the rheumatology fellow to easily form assessments and management plans for these complicated patients. This approach is reviewed later.

Skin/integument
The following questions related to the history gathering of the integument system should be considered in patients with SSc. The presence, time of onset, progress, and speed of skin thickening should be elucidated. It should be noted if the patient has puffy hands and/or feet or sclerodactyly. If the skin changes involve or have involved the chest and/or abdomen, or if there are or were changes above the elbows or knees, then the patient has dcSSc.

A modified Rodnan skin score (mRSS) should be performed to quantify the skin thickening. Monitoring of the mRSS is essential over time especially in patients with dcSSc where rapid progression may be seen early in the inflammatory stage. Skin progression tends to occur over a 2- to 3-year course, wherein many patients will have skin softening or atrophy after this time frame.

The presence of telangiectasias and calcinosis should also be questioned. The existence of pruritis should be reviewed, as this can be an unrelenting, difficult-to-treat symptom, leading to significant mental anguish.

Ear, Nose and Throat (ENT)/dental/oral
The following questions related to the history gathering of the ENT/dental/oral system should be considered in patients with SSc. Patients with scleroderma can be affected

by sicca symptoms and secondary Sjögren syndrome; thus questioning the presence of dry eyes and mouth is essential. The oral cavity is often significantly affected in the patient with SSc. Reduction in oral aperture, dental caries, reflux-induced dental erosion, and difficulty brushing the teeth due to oral aperture or even related to inability to hold a toothbrush or other dental equipment can be an issue in patients with SSc and should be questioned. **Box 3** reviews the common oral considerations in SSc and provides a framework of questions to ask to these patients.

Vascular

Vascular manifestations in SSc can occur as a consequence of microvascular and macrovascular involvement. RP presence, frequency, date of onset, and associated symptoms should be discussed with the patient, as well as the time of onset of the patients' first non–Raynaud-associated scleroderma feature. The fellow should consider asking the following questions to make the diagnosis of RP: (1) are your fingers unusually sensitive to the cold? (2) do your fingers change color when they are exposed to the cold? and (3) do they turn white, blue, and red? The presence of RP is confirmed if positive response to all 3 questions and excluded if the response to # 2 and # 3 are negative.[19] A history of digital tip sensitivity, digital ulcerations, and gangrene should also be questioned. The fellow should inquire about a history of bleeding problems and blood clots that could affect future management and treatment.

Cardiopulmonary

As pulmonary manifestations have become the leading cause of morbidity and mortality in these patients,[20] it is imperative that this be reviewed with the patient. Lung involvement in scleroderma is common and can occur in all SSc subtypes. A rheumatology fellow should be prepared to screen patients for the presence of interstitial lung disease (ILD) and pulmonary arterial hypertension (PAH) both at diagnosis and periodically according to current guidelines and if new symptoms develop. Many patients may be asymptomatic in the early stages of SSc. In addition, if they are sedentary and inactive, they may not perceive a change in exercise capacity. Asking about the presence of shortness of breath, dyspnea on exertion (DOE), nonproductive cough, fatigue, and atypical chest pain is necessary, as this may occur in patients with ILD. Similarly,

---

Box 3
Oral manifestations in patients with systemic sclerosis

- Xerostomia
- Enamel erosion
- Microstomia
- Increased risk of periodontal disease and dental caries
- Mandibular reabsorption
- Fibrosis of the soft and hard palate
- Periodontal ligament space widening
- Frenulum shortening
- Mucosal telangiectasias
- Trigeminal neuralgia
- Dysphagia
- Osteonecrosis of the jaw (in relation to possible medication use)

patients with PAH may present with fatigue, DOE, dizziness, and/or syncope and may endorse symptoms and signs of right-sided heart failure.

Cardiac involvement (silent or evident) is also an underrecognized but frequently encountered association in patients with SSc (**Table 4**). The pericardium, myocardium, and conduction systems within the heart can be affected.[21] The astute rheumatology fellow will gather a history evaluating for the presence of chest pain (with and without exertion, and pleuritic), palpitations, lower extremity edema, and syncope and should be knowledgeable about cardiac involvement.

Gastrointestinal

Involvement of the gastrointestinal (GI) tract is second only to skin involvement and can affect the entire GI tract from the oral orifice to the anal sphincter. The most common organ involved is the esophagus and thus questioning about dysphagia (upper/lower) can elucidate the possible presence of dysmotility and esophageal stricture/web/ring, in addition to questions about reflux (timing, associations) and any history of an esophageal dilatation procedure. Small intestinal involvement can lead to postprandial bloating and cramping in patients with SSc. The presence of alternating constipation and diarrhea may raise the possibility of small intestine bacterial overgrowth and malabsorption and that of abdominal pain the presence of pseudo-obstruction. Patients may suffer from anal sphincter dysfunction, leading to soiling of clothing and increased morbidity. It is essential to evaluate any change in bowel habits such as dark tarry stools, or bright red blood per rectum, which would raise the concern for a GI bleed, the presence of gastric antral vascular ectasia, or a colorectal malignancy. It should be ensured that patients have had age-appropriate malignancy testing including colonoscopy. The questionnaire designed by Khanna and colleagues[22] (UCLA-GIT) is very useful to ensure all GI items are reviewed.

Renal

The diagnosis of scleroderma renal crisis (SRC) is a true rheumatologic emergency and was the leading cause of mortality before the use of angiotensin-converting enzyme inhibitors to treat this condition in the 1980s. A rheumatology fellow's knowledge of SRC and prompt recognition can mean the difference between full recovery and progression to end-stage renal disease and even death. SRC may be the presenting feature of SSc in some patients, most commonly seen in patients with dcSSc within the first 4 years of disease.[23] Because of the high renin state of SRC, the blood pressure of all patients with scleroderma should be closely monitored at visits and trainees should inquire about home monitoring of blood pressure. SRC can occur

Table 4	
Cardiac manifestations of systemic sclerosis	
Cardiac Area	**Presentation**
Pericardial	Acute pericarditis, chronic pericarditis, pericardial fibrosis, pericardial effusion, tamponade
Myocardial	Myocardial fibrosis, ventricular diastolic dysfunction, ventricular systolic dysfunction, myocarditis
Conduction system disease	Autonomic dysfunction, heart block, supraventricular dysrhythmia, ventricular dysrhythmia
Vascular	Mural fibrosis, intimal proliferation, platelet-fibrin clotting

From Parks JL, Taylor MH, Parks LP, Silver RM. Systemic sclerosis and the heart. Rheum Dis Clin North Am. 2014;40(1):87-102.

as hypertensive or normotensive SRC, so fellows should be aware of this possibility. History taking should include questions related to uncontrolled hypertension such as headache, vision disturbances, encephalopathy, and seizures. Changes in urine color or frequency can point to concerns about hematuria, proteinuria, and impending azotemia. Within history taking, it is important to inquire about possible precipitating factors leading to the development of SRC, such as anemia, recent cardiac involvement, recent use of corticosteroids (dose $\geq$ 15 mg daily), and presence of anti-RNA-polymerase III antibodies.[24,25]

Musculoskeletal

This system is frequently involved, and the rheumatology fellow needs to inquire about the presence of arthralgia and whether a true arthritis exists, as patients with SSc with and without overlap syndromes can develop an inflammatory arthropathy.[12,15] History taking should include the presence and duration of morning stiffness, alleviating and aggravating factors, and grip. The occurrence of muscle weakness is important, as patients with SSc can develop a bland or inflammatory myositis.[26] In addition, impairment of gait and fall risk should be assessed in history taking.

Neurological

Patients with scleroderma can develop some neurologic complications. The presence of dysesthesia should be reviewed with the patient, as this can be a common finding when the skin is tight. Peripheral nerve involvement in SSc is rare, but patients can develop a sensorimotor polyneuropathy, cranial neuropathies (especially trigeminal), and mononeuropathies (carpal tunnel, cubital tunnel).[27] The rheumatology fellow should inquire about the presence of pain and paresthesia along the face, numbness and tingling in the extremities, and in the distribution of the median and ulnar nerves.

Psychiatric

Symptoms of SSc, including fatigue, pain, pruritus, sleep problems, and sexual impairments, negatively influence quality of life in many patients and may lead to emotional consequences such as depression, anxiety, and body image distress caused by appearance changes. Patients with SSc experience high rates of anxiety, with 64% reporting at least one anxiety disorder in their lifetime and between 23% and 56% of patients with SSc meeting criteria for major depressive disorder at least once in their lifetime.[28,29]

Discussing these aspects during the office visit and providing accessible information regarding problems common to people living with the disease, as well as information regarding useful resources and services to address these problems, can help patients with SSc to cope with their disease and to seek for psychological help in a timely manner.

Physical Examination of the Patient with Systemic Sclerosis

It is imperative that rheumatology fellows get experience in performing a physical examination in patients with SSc (**Table 5**). There is no substitute to performing an in-person examination in order to be able to feel the unique skin changes, cardiopulmonary findings, and musculoskeletal findings unique to the patient with systemic sclerosis. An outline of key physical examination points can be found in **Box 4**.

Skin/integument

An mRSS should be performed to quantify the thickness of skin. This score measures 17 areas of the body, including the face, anterior abdomen, anterior chest, and the right and left sides of the following locations: upper arms, forearms, dorsum of

Table 5
Key features for the physical examination of patients with systemic sclerosis

System	Exam Evaluation/Finding
Skin	• mRSS • Telangiectasias • Calcinosis • Hypopigmentation/hyperpigmentation • Atrophy
ENT/Oral	• Change in facial features • Oral candidiasis • Oral cheilitis • Microstomia • Dental caries/erosion • Hyposalivation/dry mouth
Vascular	• Presence of Raynaud phenomenon • Digital pits • Digital ulcers (tip vs traumatic) • Gangrene (perform Allen testing)
Cardiopulmonary	• Bibasilar crackles • Jugular venous distension • Lower extremity edema • Arrythmia/murmur/gallop • Accentuated P2
GI	• Abdominal distension • Decreased bowel sounds • Abdominal pain
Renal	• Blood pressure assessments • Lower extremity edema
Musculoskeletal	• Presence of Arthritis • Tendon friction rubs • Acro-osteolysis • Joint contractures (small and large joints) • Muscle strength testing
Neurological	• Sensory and motor testing • Tinel and Phalen testing

hand, fingers, thighs, lower legs, and feet. Each area is scored for thickness as a 0, 1, 2, or 3, where 0 is normal/uninvolved skin, 1 is mildly thickened skin, 2 is moderately thickened skin, and 3 is severely thickened skin. A maximum score is 51.

There is some subjectivity to the performance of the mRSS, and this has been studied by several groups.[30,31] Training in the performance of mRSS has been standardized, and it is routinely used in clinical trials. Scleroderma Clinical Trials Consortium offers specific training recommendations[32] that have been reproduced with good results; these include the specific training in order to achieve uniformity among skin scorers and the fact that ideally the same scorer should perform a mRSS for any given subject throughout the trial.[33] It is logistically impossible to have this formal training in all centers, but an effort should be made to have at least formal theoretical teaching on the performance of this procedure with a lecture and review of the publicly available video on "Youtube" by Dr Daniel Furst on performing the mRSS (https://www.youtube.com/watch?v=BI3EX_2PaUc) and then to have hands-on training during the clinics, with the professors of the rheumatology courses. In addition, a skin scoring blank document can be completed in the clinic while performing in real time (**Fig. 2**).

Box 4
Manifestations of systemic sclerosis in the respiratory system

- ILD
  - Nonspecific interstitial pneumonia (NSIP)
  - Usual interstitial pneumonia (UIP)
  - Diffuse alveolar damage (DAD)
  - Cryptogenic organizing pneumonia (COP)

- Pulmonary hypertension

- Pleural involvement

- Aspiration pneumonia

- Alveolar hemorrhage

- Small airways disease

- Malignancy

- Respiratory muscle weakness

- Drug-induced toxicity

- Spontaneous pneumothorax

- Pneumoconiosis (silicosis)

- Telangiectasias (endobronchial)

The presence of digital pitting and/or ulcerations, calcinosis, hypopigmentation, hyperpigmentation, skin atrophy, telangiectasias, and poikiloderma should be assessed on examination. The number of digital pits and the location and size of digital ulcerations and presence of gangrene should be documented, so this can be monitored over time.

ENT/dental/oral
Most clinical oral manifestations in SSc commence with tongue rigidity and skin hardening, leading to the characteristic facial features. Patients with SSc are at an increased risk of developing several types of oral infections, such as periodontal disease, oral candidiasis, and angular cheilitis due to hyposalivation. Subcutaneous deposition of collagen in the perioral tissues results in varying degrees of microstomia. Evaluation of patients for this in clinic with an oral examination should be performed with appropriate treatment and dental evaluation/referral instituted.[34] Fellows in clinic can measure oral aperture (lip to lip distance < 3 cm and/or interdental distance <2.5 cm is considered decreased oral aperture); note the presence of oral telangiectasias, dental erosion/caries, tongue lesions, and hyposalivation.

Vascular
Trainees in rheumatology should perform nailfold capillary examination in all patients with RP and in those with SSc, using tools at their disposal; these may include an ophthalmoscope, dermatoscope, widefield nailfold microscopy, or video capillaroscopy. The presence of an abnormal capillaroscopy examination predicts the development of a CTD in patients with RP, and a positive antinuclear antibody further increases that risk.[35] Nailfold capillaroscopy is discussed further later. Examination should also assess for the presence of trophic skin changes, such as digital pits and digital tip ulcers as well as traumatic ulcerations at the proximal interphalangeal joints in addition to gangrene. The rheumatology fellow should perform Allen test of bilateral hands to evaluate for the presence of larger vessel involvement such as ulnar artery occlusion that can be seen in patients with SSc.[36]

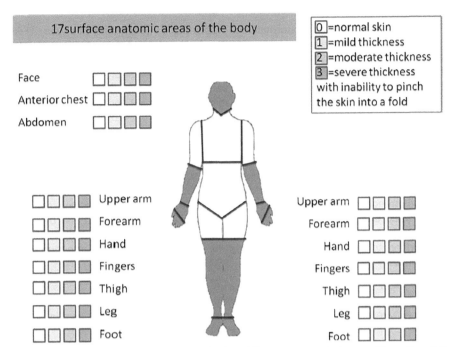

Fig. 2. Modified Rodnan skin score (mRSS) of 17 different anatomical areas. (*From* Ferreli C, Gasparini G, Parodi A, Cozzani E, Rongioletti F, Atzori L. Cutaneous Manifestations of Scleroderma and Scleroderma-Like Disorders: a Comprehensive Review. Clin Rev Allergy Immunol. 2017;53(3):306-336.)

Cardiopulmonary

The presence of fine, late inspiratory crackles will alert the rheumatology fellow of the presence of ILD. Evaluation for clubbing (rare) is also important. Measuring for the presence of jugular venous distention, hepatomegaly/right upper quadrant tenderness, and lower extremity edema can alert the fellow to the presence of right-sided heart failure (cor pulmonale) that can be seen in the setting of ILD and PAH. Auscultation of the heart may reveal arrythmia, murmur, gallop, or rub, alerting the fellow to a cardiac conduction or valvular abnormality. In addition, in pulmonary hypertension an accentuated pulmonic valve (P2) closure heart sound may be heard.

Gastrointestinal

An abdominal examination should be undertaken to evaluate for distention, reduced bowel sounds, and pain that can accompany constipation or more concerning pseudo-obstruction. The presence of organomegaly should also be noted.

Renal

The blood pressure of all patients with SSc should be taken during triage of patients. If sustained hypertension greater than or equal to 140/9010 mm Hg or 10 mm Hg higher than documented baseline is present, workup for SRC should be accomplished. If SRC is suspected, the presence of pallor, lower extremity edema, and petechiae should be evaluated for as clinical signs of anemia, proteinuria, and thrombocytopenia, respectively.

Musculoskeletal

The existence of tendon abnormalities, presenting as tendon friction rubs (TFRs) should be evaluated; they are described as leathery crepitus on palpation of the tendon sheaths and overlying fascia at shoulders, elbows (olecranon bursae), wrist extensors, wrist flexors, finger extensors, finger flexors, knees (suprarotulian tendon), and anterior tibial and Achilles tendons, related to fibrinous deposits and inflammation. The presence of 2 or more TFRs has been independently associated to dcSSc and decreased survival.[37]

The presence of acro-osteolysis (AO) can be assessed on physical examination of both hands and feet and can also be seen radiographically. AO is present if there is shortening of the digit or a tapered look to the digit from the sides and/or tip.

A thorough swollen and tender joint count should be performed in all patients with SSc to evaluate for the presence of an inflammatory arthropathy. Also, a complete muscle strength examination should be performed to evaluate for muscle weakness. The presence of joint contractures of the small and large joints should also be examined, as this has particular importance when evaluating the patients' functionality and also underscores the importance of need for adjunct services such as occupational and physical therapy.

Neurological

Sensory and motor testing should be performed in patients with suspected sensorimotor polyneuropathy. In addition, Tinel test at the elbows and wrist should be performed to evaluate for cubital and carpal tunnel syndrome, respectively.

CAPILLAROSCOPY

Capillaroscopy is one of the cornerstones in "early" and "very early diagnosis (VEDOSS)" of SSc.[38,39] A high proportion of patients who meet the 2001 LeRoy and Medsger criteria for "early" SSc diagnosis (RP, SSc-specific antibodies, and "scleroderma-type" changes on capillaroscopy) will meet the 2013 ACR/EULAR SSc criteria.[2,35] Likewise, a large proportion of patients with RP meeting the VEDOSS criteria (which are similar to the Leroy's-Medsger 2001 criteria with the addition of "puffy fingers") will transition to meet the 2013 ACR/EULAR criteria for SSc over 5 years.[39,40] Also, capillaroscopy is relevant in the longitudinal evaluation of patients with SSc at risk of developing complications such as digital ulcers and interstitial lung disease.[41–44]

Large efforts have been made the last decade to standardize the interpretation and execution of capillaroscopy. First, the EULAR Study Group on Microcirculation in Rheumatic diseases has joint forces with the Scleroderma Clinical Trials Consortium (SCTC) and the Pan American League of Associations for Rheumatology (PANLAR) working group on capillaroscopy and published a consensus on how to describe in uniform standardized language the capillaroscopic findings.[45,46] This worldwide consensus is meant to be used unanimously in clinical practice and to avoid interpretational Babylonic language barriers between capillaroscopic studies. Second, the EULAR study group proposed and validated a "fast track" algorithm to discern a "scleroderma pattern" (**Fig. 3**A) from a "nonscleroderma pattern"[47] (**Fig. 3**B). This algorithm is internally and externally validated; is fastly, simply, and reliably applicable; and is usable by novices in capillaroscopy after merely one hour of training. Third, to step forward to US colleagues who more frequently use dermatoscopy instead of videocapillaroscopy, a consensus on what steps to take in evaluating nailfolds with dermatoscopy has been published.[48,49]

Per expert opinion training of capillaroscopy is to be performed on micro, meso, and macro level. The microlevel comprises hands-on training, ideally one half-day per

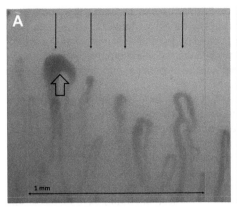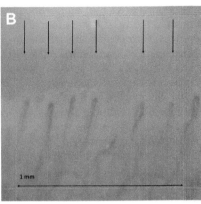

Fig. 3. Fast-track algorithm to distinguish "scleroderma pattern" from "normal pattern" in capillaroscopy. (*A*) Scleroderma pattern. Magnification 200x; density: 4 capillaries per linear mm (↓); dimensión: giant capillary present (⇧); morphology: no abnormal shapes present; microhemorrhages: absent. (*B*). Normal capillaroscopic pattern. Magnification: 200x; density: 7 capillaries per linear mm (↓); dimension: no giants present; morphology: no abnormal shapes present; microhemorrhages: absent. (*Courtesy of* V Smith, MD, Ghent, Belgium.)

week during 6 months. Besides hands-on training, meso-level efforts exist such as EULAR, PANLAR, EUSTAR, and local training courses on capillaroscopy in which a trainee can attend yearly or biannual courses. In these courses, knowledge is refreshed, updated, and challenged. Importantly, solely attending a capillaroscopic course is not sufficient for a trainee to be ready to perform and report capillaroscopy. Hands-on training should be executed by anyone who is to execute the technique in the future. Last, but not least, macrolevel standardization efforts, such as the recently published EULAR/SCTC consensus on what capillaroscopic parameters to describe and how to uniformly standardly interpret, are paramount in streamlining the use and utility of capillaroscopy.

Despite its relevance, capillaroscopy is not routinely performed in some centers in the United States and Latin America, but efforts have been carried out to increase awareness and availability of the technique in our region.[50,51] In Latin American Countries, the local Rheumatology Societies and PANLAR have organized regular short courses and workshops during their annual meetings, to train Rheumatology fellows and certified rheumatologists in this technique. Also, PANLAR researchers, through their Capillaroscopy Group, and EULAR researchers have determined that a short training can improve the identification of major abnormalities[50,52] and have agreed upon uniform nomenclature in Spanish and Portuguese for reporting this study.[46] This effort was later coordinated with EULAR microvascular study group, as previously mentioned.

International Teaching, Research, and Patient Networks and Foundations

United States of America and Canada

The Scleroderma Clinical Trials Consortium (SCTC) is an international organization that represents a large number of researchers and clinicians globally who have a particular interest and expertise in the care of, and research in, SSc. Each institution constitutes an individual member of the SCTC, and the researchers within that institution are invited to attend the SCTC Annual General Meetings and may participate in various working groups. Member Institutions have a dedicated clinic for the care of persons with scleroderma or a large number of patients with scleroderma under the direct care of the Member. The SCTC offers formal training in the mRSS performance over a half day, which leads to a certificate and can be applied to ongoing clinical trials. Additional information can be found at https://sclerodermaclinicaltrialsconsortium.org/. Also, the American College of Rheumatology offers a wide range of periodic and yearly courses with hands-on learning opportunities.

The National Scleroderma Foundation (NSF) was founded in 1998 to advance medical research, promote disease awareness, and provide support and education to people with scleroderma, their families, and support networks. The NSF has many opportunities for rheumatology fellows to get involved through membership, advocacy, fund-raising, and sponsorship, and it provides educational tools to teach patients with scleroderma about the disease.

In Canada, the Canadian Scleroderma Research Group and the Scleroderma Patient-Centered Investigation Network have organized international research groups that collaborate with SCTC and Latin American and European networks; they promote research and training of Rheumatology Fellows and clinical, epidemiological, and basic researchers. On the patients' perspective, Scleroderma Canada is the National Scleroderma Patient organization that provides educational tools for patients, advocacy, fund-raising, sponsorship, and membership opportunities.

Latin America

Countries in Latin America face many challenges in the education of Rheumatologists, particularly in relation to uncommon diseases. Institutions affiliated to international Rheumatology or Immunology societies such as the FOCIS (Federation of Clinical Immunology Society), SCTC, and PANLAR have the opportunity to offer their fellows access to specialized courses and training grants in Centers for Excellence in Immunology or in SCTC centers to acquire hands-on experience assessing patients with SSc. Rheumatology fellows should identify the attending physician who is responsible for that program in their center, in order to submit applications for specific trainings. Also, national Rheumatology Associations in Latin America are usually affiliated to PANLAR. These National associations usually offer periodical trainings for Rheumatology Fellows in the form of professor-fellow meetings, capillaroscopy courses, and monthly actualization meetings.

National and Local Patient associations in Latin America usually organize educational activities and network with international patient organizations to increase awareness of the disease and to connect patients with specialized medical centers.

Europe

The patterns of rheumatology health care are highly variable across different European countries. Furthermore, there is considerable diversity among European training centers in providing an adequate spectrum of experience to ensure the future specialists' competence and suitability.[53]

The European Alliance of Associations for Rheumatology (EULAR) School of Rheumatology (ESoR) is involved, in collaboration with the Union Européene des Médecins Specialist (UEMS), to create a common high-quality educational system. The first core curriculum in rheumatology was created in 1999 for undergraduate students by the EULAR Standing Committee on Education and Training (ESCET) and was successively developed in the UEMS European curriculum for young rheumatologists, which defined skills, attitudes, and knowledge that must be provided to trainees.[54,55] At present, in order to offer students integrated in the Emergent EULAR Network (EMEUNET) the best education on rheumatology, EULAR-ESoR offers 13 online courses: one of them about systemic sclerosis and one about Capillaroscopy and Microcirculation in rheumatic diseases (https://esor.eular.org–see catalog).[56]

Furthermore, there are 15 live courses available each year; for example, the EULAR live course on Capillaroscopy in Connective Tissue Diseases already had 11 editions from 2004 and has already instructed more than 1200 young rheumatologists from 80 Countries (see a practical video enclosed- Video 1). The ESoR offers EULAR scientific training grants for young fellows (short term 1–3 weeks or long term 1–6 months), a textbook dedicated to SSc, and free learning materials. Among the educational materials, several tools are available for patients (PARE group) and health professionals in rheumatology and in particular for systemic sclerosis, including the hormonal influences as risk factors for the development of systemic sclerosis (https://esor.eular.org/course/view.php?id=188). Finally, there is a new educational series of webinars by EULAR (from June 2022 https://esor.eular.org/enrol/index.php?id=262), which are organized every 2 months. In these webinars, experts in the field show presentations and have live discussions with the audience.

European Research efforts in SSc include the European Scleroderma Trials and Research group (EUSTAR) and the Capillaroscopy and Microcirculation in Rheumatic Diseases Study Group that offer cooperative research experiences that include opportunities for fellows and young investigators, connect young rheumatologists from all the Continents, and stimulate active cooperation and scientific production (https://www.eular.org/myUploadData/files/EULAR_Study_Group_Microcirculation_in_Rheumatic_Diseases_rebranded_6.02.18.pdf).

European reference networks on rare and complex connective tissue diseases
The European Reference Networks (ERNs) are virtual networks involving health care providers across Europe. The mission of the ERNs is to tackle low prevalence diseases that require highly specialized treatment and a concentration of knowledge and resources.

Twenty-four ERNs were launched in 2017, after approval by the Board of Member States, involving more than 900 highly specialized health care teams (located in more than 300 hospitals in 26 European countries). The ERN dealing with rare connective tissue and musculoskeletal diseases, such as SSc, more specifically the European Reference Network on Rare Connective Tissue and Musculoskeletal Diseases (ERN ReCONNET), is an infrastructure actually consisting of 64 health care providers covering 23 members states in Europe.[57,58]

Teaching and training of rheumatologists to manage appropriately rare CTD such as SSc has been executed in several ways by ReCONNET. First, on the ReCONNET Web site (https://reconnet.ern-net.eu), for each rare CTD, including SSc, a synopsis of the disease can be found, as well as useful references for optimal management of the patient affected by the rare CTD. Respective patients' organizations as well as centers recognized by the European Commission to manage the rare CTD are displayed as well. Lay versions of the disease that can be handed out to the patient for better understanding of the disease and well-informed co-decision-making with the rheumatologist are also available. For each rare CTD, including SSc, ReCONNET has published a state of the art on clinical practice guidelines (recommendations that are intended to optimize patient care that are informed of evidence by systematic reviews and assessment of harms and benefits of alternative options) gathered in a supplement in RMD Open, an official journal of EULAR.[58] Third, training of next generation of rheumatologists also means creating the awareness that clinical practice guidelines must be adapted to local health care systems, authorities, legislation, and specific needs. To this end, ReCONNET has started with SSc as pilot to adapt the existing SSc-related clinical practice guidelines to the context of different EU countries with a validated rigorous methodology[57–59] called ADAPTE. Fourth, dealing with SSc means need for education and availability of a cross-border problem-solving approach. To this end, ReCONNET foresees webinars (besides the already existing ones on the ReCONNET Web site) that are tailored to the needs of physicians and patients. Also, there is a clinical patient management form and a secure IT platform, developed by the European Commission in order to discuss clinical cases, cross-border with peers/experts, for the optimal treatment of the SSc patient.

In conclusion, altogether, SCTC, NSF, CSRG, SPIN, ACR, PANLAR, ESoR of EULAR, EUSTAR, the Microcirculation Study Group, and the ERN-ReCONNET offer some of the best armamentaria of educational tools for fellows with interest in scleroderma.

SUMMARY

This article focuses on an approach to training the next generation of rheumatologists to take care of patients with scleroderma. Given its multisystem presentation, fellows are faced with learning and mastering a complex disease process. The management and treatment of organ-specific processes in SSc is reviewed elsewhere in this book and is essential in training the next generation to be competent providers in taking care of patients with SSc. By using a systems-based approach to performing a complete history and physical examination, the trainees in rheumatology will remain organized in their approach to evaluate patients with SSc. In addition, gaining knowledge and expertise in the specific examination tools used in the care of patients with SSc such as nailfold capillary examination, the mRSS, and evaluation of TFR will allow the rheumatology fellow to master the care of patients with SSc.

CLINICS CARE POINTS

- Systemic sclerosis is a multisystemic autoimmune disease that requires a standardized clinical approach.
- Rheumatology residents are required to know and understand the relevance of the baseline and follow-up standardized evaluations required for systemic sclerosis patients, as well as the main causes of morbidity and mortality of SSc patients.
- Currently, these are several opportunities of face to face and online trainings for rheumatology residents to learn about systemic sclerosis. Residents benefit from the use of these resources and they should approach the dedicated sites for basic and advanced education in this field.

DISCLOSURE

T.S. Rodríguez-Reyna, F.N. Hant, and M. Cutolo have no commercial or financial conflicts of interest or funding sources related to the present article. V. Smith has received grant/research support to her institution from the Research Foundation Flanders, Belgian Fund for Scientific Research in Rheumatic Diseases, Janssen-Cilag, and Boehringer Ingelheim, Germany; consulting fees from Boehringer-Ingelheim (payments made to self and institution) and Janssen-Cilag (payments made to institution); speaker fees from UCB (payments made to institution), Boehringer-Ingelheim (payments made to self and institution), Janssen-Cilag (payments made to institution);

support for attending meetings and/or travel from Boehringer Ingelheim (payments made to institution). None of the authors has been paid to write this article by a pharmaceutical company or other agency.

ACKNOWLEDGMENTS

The authors thank our rheumatology fellows for all their daily feedback and enthusiasm that drive us to improve to find new ways to teach and to love our work.

SUPPLEMENTARY DATA

Supplementary data related to this article can be found online at https://doi.org/10.1016/j.rdc.2023.01.013.

REFERENCES

1. Mayes MD, Lacey JV, Beebe-Dimmer J, et al. Prevalence, incidence, survival, and disease characteristics of systemic sclerosis in a large US population. Arthritis Rheum 2003;48:2246–55.
2. van den Hoogen F, Khanna D, Fransen J, et al. 2013 classification criteria for systemic sclerosis: an American college of rheumatology/European league against rheumatism collaborative initiative. Ann Rheum Dis 2013;72:1747–55.
3. Domsic RT, Medsger TA. Disease Subsets in Clinical Practice. In: Varga J, Denton C, Wigley F, et al, editors. Scleroderma. Cham: Springer; 2017. p. 39–48.
4. Stochmal A, Czuwara J, Trojanoska M, et al. Antinuclear antibodies in systemic sclerosis: an update. Clin Rev Allergy Immunol 2020;58:40–51.
5. Hamaguchi Y, Takehara K. Anti-nuclear autoantibodies in systemic sclerosis: news and perspectives. J Scleroderma Relat Disord 2018;3:201–13.
6. Mecoli CA, Casciola-Rosen L. An update on autoantibodies in scleroderma. Curr Opin Rheumatol 2018;30:548–53.
7. Fritzler MJ, Hudson M, Choi MY, et al. Bicaudal D2 is a novel autoantibody target in systemic sclerosis that shares a key epitope with CENP-A but has a distinct clinical phenotype. Autoimmun Rev 2018;17:267–75.
8. McMahan ZH, Domsic RT, Zhu L, et al. Anti-RNPC-3 (U11/U12) antibodies in systemic sclerosis in patients with moderate-to-severe gastrointestinal dysmotility. Arthritis Care Res (Hoboken) 2019;71:1164–70.
9. Kaji K, Fertig N, Medsger TA Jr, et al. Autoantibodies to RuvBL1 and RuvBL2: a novel systemic sclerosis related antibody associated with diffuse cutaneous and skeletal muscle involvement. Arthritis Care Res 2014;66:575–84.
10. Koschik RW 2nd, Fertig N, Lucas MR, et al. Anti-PM-Scl antibody in patients with systemic sclerosis. Clin Exp Rheumatol 2012;30(2Suppl71):S12–6.
11. Sharif R, Fritzler MJ, Mayes MD, et al. Anti-fibrillarin antibody in African American patients with systemic sclerosis: immunogenetics, clinical features and survival analysis. J Rheumatol 2011;38:1622–30.
12. Rodriguez-Reyna TS, Hinojosa-Azaola A, Martinez-Reyes C, et al. Distinctive autoantibody profile in Mexican Mestizo Systemic Sclerosis Patients. Autoimmunity 2011;44:576–84.
13. Fertig N, Domsic RT, Rodriguez-Reyna T, et al. Anti-U11/U12 RNP antibodies in systemic sclerosis: a new serologic marker associated with pulmonary fibrosis. Arthritis Rheum 2009;61:958–65.
14. Aggarwal R, Lucas M, Fertig N, et al. Anti-U3 RNP autoantibodies in systemic sclerosis. Arthritis Rheum 2009;60:112–8.

15. Meyer OC, Fertig N, Lucas M, et al. Disease subsets, antinuclear antibody profile, and clinical features in 127 French and 247 US adult patients with systemic sclerosis. J Rheumatol 2007;34:104–9.

16. Mitri GM, Lucas M, Fertig N, et al. A comparison between anti-Th/To and anticentromere antibody-positive systemic sclerosis patients with limited cutaneous involvement. Arthritis Rheum 2003;48:203–9.

17. Sacks DG, Okano Y, Steen VD, et al. Isolated pulmonary hypertension in systemic sclerosis with diffuse cutaneous involvement: association with serum anti-U3-RNP antibody. J Rheumatol 1996;23:639–42.

18. Okano Y, Steen VD, Medsger TA Jr. Autoantibody reactive with RNA polymerase III in systemic sclerosis. Ann Intern Med 1993;119:1005–13.

19. McMahan ZH, Wigley FM. Raynaud's phenomenon and digital ischemia: a practical approach to risk stratification, diagnosis and management. Int J Clin Rheumtol 2010;5:355–70.

20. Steen VD, Medsger TA. Changes in causes of death in systemic sclerosis, 1972-2002. Ann Rheum Dis 2007;66:940–4.

21. Rodriguez-Reyna TS, Rosales-Uvera SG, Kimura-Hayama E, et al. Myocardial fibrosis detected by magnetic resonance imaging, elevated U-CRP and higher mRSS are predictors of cardiovascular complications in systemic sclerosis patients. Semin Arthritis Rheum 2019;49:273–8.

22. Khanna D, Hays RD, Maranian P, et al. Reliability and validity of the University of California, Los Angeles Scleroderma Clinical Trial Consortium Gastrointestinal Tract Instrument. Arthritis Rheum 2009;61:1257–63.

23. Steen VD, Medsger TA Jr, Osial TA Jr, et al. Factors predicting development of renal involvement in progressive systemic sclerosis. Am J Med 1984;76:779–86.

24. Steen VD, Medsger TA. Case-control study of corticosteroids and other drugs that either precipitate or protect from the development of scleroderma renal crisis. Arthritis Rheum 1998;41:1613–9.

25. Guillevin L, Mouthon L. Scleroderma Renal Crisis. Rheum Dis Clin North Am 2015;41:475–88.

26. Matas-García A, Guillén-Del-Castillo A, Kisluk B, et al. Clinico-pathological phenotypes of Systemic Sclerosis related myopathy: analysis of a multicenter larger cohort. Rheumatology (Oxford) 2022;keac361. https://doi.org/10.1093/rheumatology/keac361.

27. Gwathmey Kelly G, Satkowiak Kelsey. Peripheral nervous system manifestations of rheumatological diseases. J Neurol Sci 2021;424:117421.

28. Thombs BD, van Lankveld W, Bassel M, et al. Psychological health and wellbeing in systemic sclerosis: State of the science and consensus research agenda. Arthritis Care Res 2010;62:1181–9.

29. Kwakkenbos L, Delisle VC, Fox RS, et al. Psychosocial aspects of scleroderma. Rheum Dis Clin North Am 2015;41:519–28.

30. Showalter K, Merkel PA, Khanna D, et al. Assessment of skin disease in scleroderma: practices and opinions of investigators studying scleroderma. J Scleroderma Relat Disord 2020;5:167–71.

31. Gordon JK, Girish G, Berrocal VJ, et al. Reliability and validity of the tender and swollen joint counts and the modified rodnan skin score in early diffuse cutaneous systemic sclerosis: analysis from the prospective registry of early systemic sclerosis cohort. J Rheumatol 2017;44:791–4.

32. Khanna D, Furst DE, Clements PJ, et al. J Scleroderma Relat Disord 2017;2:11–8. https://doi.org/10.5301/jsrd.5000231.

33. Low AHL, Ng SA, Berrocal V, et al. Evaluation of Scleroderma Clinical Trials consortium training recommendations on modified Rodnan skin scores assessment in scleroderma. Int J Rheum Dis 2019;22:1036–40.
34. Hant FN, Ravenel M. Chapter 32: a dentist inquires about his patient with systemic sclerosis. In: Silver RM, Denton P, editors. Case studies in systemic sclerosis. 1st edition. London: Springer; 2011. p. 299–315.
35. Koenig M, Joyal F, Fritzler MJ, et al. Autoantibodies and microvascular damage are independent predictive factors for the progression of Raynaud's phenomenon to systemic sclerosis: a twenty-year prospective study of 586 patients, with validation of proposed criteria for early systemic sclerosis. Arthritis Rheum 2008;58:3902–12.
36. Taylor MH, McFadden JA, Bolster MB, et al. Ulnar artery involvement in systemic sclerosis (scleroderma). J Rheumatol 2002;29:102–6.
37. Steen VD, Medsger TA Jr. The palpable tendón friction rub: an important physical examination finding in patients with systemic sclerosis. Arthritis Rheum 1997;40:1146–51.
38. LeRoy EC, Medsger TA. Criteria for the classification of early Systemic Sclerosis. J Rheumatol 2001;28:1573–6.
39. Avouac J, Fransen J, Walker UA, et al. Preliminary criteria for the very early diagnosis of systemic sclerosis: results of a Delphi Consensus Study from EULAR Scleroderma Trials and Research Group. Ann Rheum Dis 2011;70:476–81.
40. Bellando-Randone S, Del Galdo F, Lepri G, et al. Progression of patients with Raynaud's Phenomenon to systemic sclerosis: a five-year analysis of the European Scleroderma Trial and Research group multicentre, longitudinal registry study for Very Early Diagnosis of Systemic Sclerosis (VEDOSS). Lancet Rheumatol 2021;3:e834–43.
41. Silva-Viela V, Vanhaecke A, Rangel-Antunes-da Silva B, et al. Is there a link between nailfold videocapillaroscopy and pulmonary function tests in systemic sclerosis patients? A 24-month follow-up monocentric study. J Clin Rheumatol 2021. https://doi.org/10.1097/RHU.0000000000001798. epub ahead of print.
42. Castellvi I, Simeón-Aznar CP, Sarmiento M, et al. Association between nailfold capillaroscopy findings and pulmonary function tests in patients with Systemic Sclerosis. J Rheumatol 2015;42:222–7.
43. Cutolo M, Herrick AL, Distler O, et al. Nailfold videocapillaroscopic features and other clinical risk factors for digital ulcers in Systemic sclerosis. Arthritis Rheum 2016;68:2527–39.
44. Sebastiani M, Manfredi A, Colaci M, et al. Capillaroscopic skin ulcer risk index: a new prognostic tool for digital skin ulcer development in systemic sclerosis patients. Arthritis Rheum (Arthritis Care Research) 2009;621:688–94.
45. Smith V, Herrick AL, Ingegnoli F, et al. Standardisation of nailfold capillaroscopy for the assessment of patients with Raynaud's phenomenon and systemic sclerosis. Autoimmun Rev 2020;19:102458.
46. Bertolazzi C, Vargas Guerrero A, Rodríguez-Reyna TS, et al. Pan-American League of Associations for Rheumatology (PANLAR) capillaroscopy study group consensus for the format and content of the report in capillaroscopy in rheumatology. Clin Rheumatol 2019;38:2327–37.
47. Smith V, Vanhaecke A, Herrick AL, et al. Fast track algorithm: how to differentiate a "scleroderma pattern" from a "non-scleroderma pattern". Autoimmun Rev 2019;18:102394.
48. Radic M, Snow M, Frech TM, et al. Consensus-based evaluation of dermatoscopy versus nailfold videocapillaroscopy in Raynaud's phenomenon linking USA and

Europe: a European League against Rheumatism study group on microcirculation in rheumatic diseases Project. Clin Exp Rheumatol 2020;38(Suppl 125): 132–6.

49. Ingegnoli F, Herrick AL, Schioppo T, et al. Reporting items for capillaroscopy in clinical research on musculoskeletal diseases: a systematic review and international Delphi consensus. Rheumatology (Oxford) 2021;60:1410–8.

50. Hatzis C, Lemer D, Paget S, et al. Integration of capillary microscopy and dermoscopy into the rheumatology fellow curriculum. Clin Exp Rheumatol 2017;35: 850–2.

51. Snow MH, Saketkoo LA, Frech TM, et al. Results from an American pilot survey among Scleroderma Clinical Trials consortium members on capillaroscopy use and how to best implement nailfold capillaroscopy training. Clin Exp Rheumatol 2019;37(S119):151.

52. Rodriguez-Reyna TS, Bertolazzi C, Vargas-Guerrero A, et al, PANLAR Capillaroscopy Group. Can nailfold videocapillaroscopy images be interpreted reliably by different observers? Results of an inter-reader and intra-reader exercise among rheumatologists with different experience in this field. Clin Rheumatol 2019;38: 205–10.

53. Bandinelli F, Bijlsma JWJ, Ramiro MS, et al. Rheumatology education in Europe: results of a survey of young rheumatologists. Clin Exp Rheumatol 2011;29:843–5.

54. Doherti M, Woolf AD. Guidelines for rheumatology undergraduate core curriculum. Ann Rheum Dis 1999;58:133–5.

55. Da Silva JAP, Faarvang KJ, Bandila K, et al. UEMS charter on the training of rheumatologists in Europe. Ann Rheum Dis 2008;67:555–8.

56. Cutolo M, Smith V. Detection of microvascular changes in systemic sclerosis and other rheumatic diseases. Nat Rev Rheumatol 2021;17:665–77.

57. Smith V, Scire CA, Talarico R, et al. Systemic sclerosis: state of the art on clinical practice guidelines. RMD open 2018;4:e000782.

58. Talarico R, Aguilera S, Alexander T, et al. The added value of a European Reference Network on rare and complex connective tissue and musculoskeletal diseases: insights after the first 5 years of the ERN ReCONNET. Clin Exp Rheumatol 2022;40(Suppl 134):3–11.

59. Mosca M, Cutolo M. Clinical practice guidelines: the first year of activity of the European Reference Network on Rare and Complex Connective Tissue and Musculoskeletal Diseases (ERN ReCONNET). RMD Open 2018;4(Suppl 1):e000791.

The Exciting Future for Scleroderma

What Therapeutic Pathways Are on the Horizon?

Jörg H.W. Distler, MD[a], Gabriela Riemekasten, MD[b],
Christopher P. Denton, PhD, FRCP[c],*

KEYWORDS

- Scleroderma • Extracellular matrix • Cytokine • Antibody • Clinical trial

KEY POINTS

- The characterization of functionally distinct subpopulations of fibroblasts and myofibro-blast precursors may have therapeutic implications.
- Several members of the nuclear receptor family have been implicated in the pathogenesis of SSc and have future potential as therapeutic targets.
- Epigenetic modifications establish self-sustaining activation loops to promote chronic fibroblast activation and progressive fibrotic tissue remodeling in SSc.
- SSc represents dysfunction or dysregulated connective tissue repair, and this may be normalized by modifying the cellular microenvironment through binding to extracellular proteins that are important regulators of fibroblast activation and differentiation, as outlined previously in this article.
- There are a number or promising future candidates for targeting extracellular proteins and ligands.

INTRODUCTION

There has been major progress in understanding pathogenic mechanisms in systemic sclerosis (SSc) at a molecular and cellular level. This has permitted key pathways, mediators, and cell types that may be central to the disease to be better characterized.

[a] Department of Internal Medicine 3 - Rheumatology and Immunology, Friedrich–Alexander University Erlangen–Nuremberg (FAU) and University Hospital Erlangen, Erlangen, Germany; [b] Department of Rheumatology, University Medical Center Schleswig-Holstein, Campus Lübeck, Ratzeburger Allee 160, Lübeck 23562, Germany; [c] Division of Medicine, Department of Inflammation, Centre for Rheumatology, University College London, London, UK
* Corresponding author. Centre for Rheumatology and Connective Tissue Diseases, UCL Division of Medicine, London NW3 2PF, United Kingdom.
E-mail address: c.denton@ucl.ac.uk

Rheum Dis Clin N Am 49 (2023) 445–462
https://doi.org/10.1016/j.rdc.2023.01.014
0889-857X/23/© 2023 Elsevier Inc. All rights reserved.

rheumatic.theclinics.com

The disease is regarded conceptually as one of dysfunctional connective tissue repair. This may arise because of ongoing injurious mechanisms or could reflect inability to harness the physiologic regulators of tissue repair and growth. It seems likely that most of the mechanisms and pathways involved in disease progression are also implicated in normal growth and repair of connective tissue. This adds extra challenges for therapeutics that modify the disease because they might also impair normal wound healing or connective tissue homeostasis. Because SSc is an autoimmune disease a key mechanism that drives the pathology is likely to be immune-mediated damage or cellular stimulation. The emerging biology and targets that could be exploited therapeutically are summarized in this article.

PATHWAYS AND MECHANISMS WITH CENTRAL ROLES IN FIBROBLAST ACTIVATION
Fibroblasts as Key Effector Cells of Fibrotic Tissue Remodeling in Systemic Sclerosis

Single-cell OMIC techniques demonstrated that fibroblasts are a highly heterogeneous population of cells composed of several subpopulations with distinct gene expression profiles and functional roles. Recent work from the Lafyatis laboratory identified 10 subpopulations of fibroblasts in SSc skin.[1] Fibrotic tissues in SSc are characterized by shifts from resting and homeostatic fibroblast subpopulations to inflammatory and profibrotic subpopulations. The proportions of several profibrotic and proinflammatory subpopulations, such as COL11A1+, COMP+, PRSS23/SFRP2+, SFRP4/SFRP2+ fibroblasts, and CCL19+ fibroblasts, positively correlated with clinical and histopathologic parameters of skin fibrosis, whereas immature, homeostatic populations, such as CXCL12+ and PI16+ fibroblasts, inversely correlated with progression of skin fibrosis (Honglin Zhu and colleagues, manuscript submitted). The profibrotic pathogenic subpopulations include so-called myofibroblasts. Myofibroblasts are defined by the expression of contractile proteins, such as α-smooth muscle actin (α-SMA), with the ability to contract tissue. Myofibroblasts release abundant amounts of extracellular matrix (ECM) and numerous soluble mediators that maintain a local profibrotic milieu. A variety of different cell types can acquire at least a partial myofibroblast phenotype and may thus contribute to the accumulation of myofibroblasts in fibrotic tissues. These precursor cells include resident fibroblasts (eg, a subpopulation of resident fibroblasts with high mRNA levels of SFRP2[1]) and cells of the vascular wall, such as pericytes, endothelial cells, and smooth muscle cells, but also epithelial cells, tissue-resident progenitor populations, and bone marrow–derived fibrocytes that reach fibrotic tissues via the bloodstream.[2]

The characterization of functionally distinct subpopulations of fibroblasts and myofibroblast precursors may have therapeutic implications. Specific targeting of pathogenic subpopulations may not only provide increased antifibrotic efficacy, but may also limit adverse events of antifibrotic therapies because they would not affect homeostatic subpopulations required for homeostasis. However, the molecular mechanisms that promote the expansion of these pathogenic fibroblast subpopulations in SSc require further studies. Researchers are just beginning to understand the transcriptional networks that are active in individual fibroblast subpopulations.

The transcription factor PU.1, a member of the ETS family of transcription factors encoded by the SPI1 gene, coordinates profibrotic gene expression programs in fibroblasts required for differentiation into profibrotic fibroblast subsets.[3] The expression of PU.1 is upregulated in a subset of profibrotic fibroblasts in SSc, but not in resting fibroblasts. Forced overexpression of PU.1 in proinflammatory and resting fibroblasts converts them into profibrotic fibroblasts with increased expression of contractile proteins and enhanced release of ECM. Vice versa, genetic inactivation of PU.1 or pharmacologic targeting with heterocyclic diamidines enables reprogramming of fibrotic fibroblasts into homeostatic fibroblasts with antifibrotic effects across different organs.[3] Although heterocyclic diamidines effectively inhibit PU.1 in vitro and ameliorate fibrosis in murine models, further pharmacologic refinement is required to yield candidates for clinical trials.

The transcription factor Engrailed 1 (EN1), a member of the family of homeodomain-containing transcription factors, is also involved in the differentiation of resting fibroblasts into profibrotic fibroblast subsets in SSc. A subset of fibroblasts in the skin that expressed EN1 during development can give rise to a subpopulation of fibroblasts with high capacity for ECM production that is required for scar formation.[4,5] Moreover, EN1 amplifies the profibrotic effects of transforming growth factor (TGF)-β in the skin of patients with SSc. EN1 is induced in certain fibroblast subpopulations in a TGF-β/SMAD3-dependent manner, and in turn facilitates the transcription of a subset of profibrotic TGF-β target genes to promote ROCK activation, cytoskeleton organization, and fibroblast-to-myofibroblast transition. Knockdown of EN1 inhibited fibroblast-to-myofibroblast transition and ameliorated experimental skin fibrosis in murine models and human models of skin fibrosis. Pharmaceutical targeting of EN1 has not been investigated so far but might be achieved by cell-permeable peptides.[6]

Nuclear receptors as potential targets for antifibrotic therapies

Nuclear receptors compose a superfamily of transcriptional regulators with 48 members. Several members of the nuclear receptor family have been implicated in the pathogenesis of SSc because they may regulate inflammatory processes, facilitate metabolic adaptation, or regulate fibroblast activation. The role of selected nuclear receptors with future potential as therapeutic targets in SSc is discussed next.

NR4A1 (also referred to as Nur77, TR3) signaling is repressed by epigenetic and posttranslational mechanisms in SSc.[7] Under physiologic conditions with short-term upregulation of TGF-β, NR4A1 expression is induced and recruits a repressor complex comprising SP1, SIN3A, CoREST, LSD1, and HDAC1 to limit the transcription of profibrotic genes downstream of TGF-β.[7] However, in SSc and other fibrotic diseases, persistently high levels of TGF-β deactivate this feedback loop; prolonged stimulation of fibroblasts with TGF-β represses NR4A1 signaling by histone deacetylase–induced silencing and phosphorylation-induced inactivation of NR4A1 via AKT kinases.[7,8] NR4A1 agonists prevent the inactivation of NR4A1 signaling, limit TGF-β-dependent fibroblast activation, and exert antifibrotic effects in mouse models of SSc and other fibrotic diseases.[7] However, the pharmacologic profile of the NR4A1 agonist used in these studies (cytosporone B, a natural product) is not suitable for use in humans and the development of potent and selective agonists of NR4A1 remains challenging to date.

Vitamin D receptor (VDR, NR1I1) is also an antifibrotic receptor that could serve as a potential target for antifibrotic therapies. Activated VDR binds to phosphorylated SMAD3 to inhibit TGF-β-SMAD-signaling and fibroblast-to-myofibroblast transition.[9] In SSc, however, the expression of VDR is decreased in the skin of patients with SSc[9] and additionally vitamin D deficiency is common in SSc and other chronic diseases. The resulting downregulation of VDR signaling fosters fibroblast activation. VDR signaling is activated by synthetic VDR agonists, which ameliorate TGF-β-induced fibroblast activation and tissue fibrosis. Multiple highly potent agonists of VDR are approved for clinical use and could be tested in SSc.

Other nuclear receptors that have been implicated into the pathogenesis of SSc include the constitutive androstane receptor (CAR)/NR1I3, the liver X receptors

(LXRs), and the pregnane X receptor (PXR)/NR1I2. CAR is thought to directly regulate fibroblast activation, whereas LXR and PXR may regulate the release of profibrotic mediators from macrophages or T cells, respectively. CAR is a profibrotic nuclear receptor. Its activation by treatment with CAR agonists fosters activation of canonical TGF-β signaling and exacerbates experimental fibrosis.[10] In contrast, LXRs limit macrophage activation and cytokine release and treatment with LXR agonists reduces macrophage influx and interleukin (IL)-6 release in murine models of SSc.[11] As for LXR, PXR activation also did not demonstrate direct inhibitory effects on fibroblasts, but inhibited the release of IL-13 from Th2 cells to ameliorate fibrosis in inflammatory mouse models of SSc.[12]

Targeting the reactivation of developmental pathways in systemic sclerosis

Several lines of evidence in complementary models demonstrate that hedgehog- and WNT signaling are central pathways of fibroblast activation in SSc and other fibrotic diseases.[13–22] These pathways are essentially required for embryonic development and are thus referred to as developmental pathways. After embryonic development, these pathways are silenced in most cell types except rapidly cycling stem cells. However, hedgehog signaling and WNT signaling are reactivated on injury to promote proliferation and differentiation of target cells. Persistent activation of those pathways in fibroblasts drives fibroblast-to-myofibroblast differentiation and fibrotic tissue remodeling.

The expression of the ligand sonic hedgehog (SHH) is upregulated in the skin of patients with SSc with consistent accumulation of the downstream transcription factor GLI2.[15,23] Moreover, SHH levels are increased in the blood of patients with SSc.[23] This upregulation might at least in part be mediated by TGF-β because TGF-β induces the expression of SHH and of GLI2 in fibroblasts.[15] Activation of hedgehog signaling stimulates fibroblast-to-myofibroblast transition and promotes experimental skin fibrosis,[15] whereas pharmacologic or genetic inactivation of hedgehog signaling (eg, by selective genetic or pharmacologic inactivation of GLI2 or by treatment with inhibitors of the receptor Smoothened) ameliorates experimental fibrosis in murine models of SSc.[24]

β-catenin-dependent WNT signaling, also referred to as canonical WNT signaling, is active in SSC and multiple other fibrotic diseases. Activation of canonical WNT signaling occurs as a consequence of deregulation on multiple levels with upregulation of WNT proteins, downregulation of endogenous WNT inhibitors, and by transcriptional synergism with other profibrotic mediators.[17,18,25–29] As for hedgehog signaling, TGF-β can activate canonical WNT signaling, intraperitoneal by epigenetic downregulation of the expression of endogenous WNT antagonists, such as dickkopf-1 (DKK1) or secreted frizzled-related protein-1 (SFRP1).[30–32] Canonical WNT signaling is sufficient and required for fibrotic tissue remodeling and targeted inhibition of WNT signaling exerts potent antifibrotic effects in various preclinical models of SSc and other fibrotic diseases.[3,17,21,22,25,27,30,33–39]

Despite their crucial role in embryonic development and stem cell maintenance, hedgehog and WNT signaling are both assessable for pharmacologic intervention. For hedgehog signaling, Smoothened inhibitors are already in clinical use for neoplastic diseases and GLI2 inhibitors are in clinical development.[40] Compounds with WNT inhibitory activity, such as pyrvinium, are also in clinical use and more selective and potent WNT inhibitors, such as porcupine or tankyrase inhibitors, are in clinical development. Indeed, clinical trials with WNT-targeting strategies are currently in preparation for interstitial lung diseases and are also discussed for sclerodermatous chronic graft-versus-host diseases. However, potential concerns of these approaches may include toxicity associated with impaired regeneration of stem cells on long-term treatment. Given the crucial roles of WNT and hedgehog signaling in stem cell regeneration, specific strategies might be required to minimize the effects on the stem cell compartment associated with long-term use.

Epigenetic Changes and the Establishment of a Profibrotic Tissue Memory

The chronic profibrotic milieu in affected tissues of patients with SSc induces epigenetic modifications in fibroblasts.[41–43] These epigenetic modifications consolidate an activated myofibroblast phenotype and render them at least in part independent of external stimuli. Epigenetic modifications establish self-sustaining activation loops to promote chronic fibroblast activation and progressive fibrotic tissue remodeling in SSc. This is best evidenced by the activated phenotype of SSc fibroblasts even on long-term culture: fibroblasts explanted from fibrotic skin of patients with SSc exert a myofibroblast-like phenotype with increased expression of contractile proteins and enhanced release of collagen, which persists for several passages in vitro. Epigenetic modifications are critical to maintain the profibrotic phenotype of SSc fibroblasts. This stabilization of an activated phenotype by epigenetic modifications is often referred to as profibrotic tissue memory. The tissue memory is encoded by a complex pattern of different epigenetic alterations. Epigenetic alterations including DNA methylation, histone acetylation, histone methylation, bromodomain (BRD)-dependent regulation, and noncoding RNAs, such as microRNAs (miRNAs) or long noncoding RNAs, are well established as drivers of progressive fibrotic tissue remodeling in SSc, but also in other fibrotic diseases.[44–52] Selected examples and potential approaches for therapeutic intervention are discussed next.

DNA methylation

DNA is methylated at position C5 of the pyrimidine ring of cytosine by a family of three DNA methyltransferases (DNMTs): DNMT1, DNMT3A, and DNMT3B.[53] Methylation of cytosine residues generates binding sites for methyl-CpG-binding domain (MBD) proteins, in particular when methylated cytosine residues are clustered in so-called CpG islands. Binding of MBD proteins promotes the recruitment of repressor complexes to silence transcription of the associated genes.[54] Several studies demonstrated a role of altered DNA methylation in fibrotic diseases including SSc.[34,47,55–57] The first and best studied target regulated by DNA methylation in SSc is the Friend leukemia integration factor 1 (FLI1) gene, which encodes for a transcription factor of the ETS family.[47,58,59] FLI1 limits TGF-β signaling to inhibit fibroblast activation under homeostatic conditions.[60] However, in the profibrotic milieu of SSc, FLI1 expression and activity are repressed by epigenetic and posttranslational mechanisms. TGF-β induces DNA methylation of the FLI1 promoter to silence its expression and also promotes FLI1 degradation via PKCδ-mediated phosphorylation.[61] Moreover, DNMT-induced silencing of the suppressor of cytokine signaling 3 (SOCS3) facilitates prolonged activation of JAK2/STAT3 signaling to facilitate TGF-β-induced fibroblast activation (PMID: 31990678). Aberrant DNA methylation also facilitates activation of canonical WNT signaling by silencing of the endogenous WNT antagonists Dickkopf-1 (DKK1) and secreted frizzled-related protein 1 (SFRP1).[34] Treatment with the DNMT inhibitor 5-aza-2'-deoxycytidine (5aza), which is in clinical use for myelodysplastic syndromes, has exerted antifibrotic effects in murine models of SSc and other fibrotic diseases.[34,45,62] Because treatment with 5aza is well tolerated, 5aza may offer potential for testing in clinical trials in SSc.

Histone acetylation

Histone modifications include acetylation and methylation at various sites. First evidence for a role of histone modulations in the pathogenesis of SSc was provided by the observation that treatment with histone deacetylation inhibitors reduced the activation of SSc fibroblasts and ameliorated bleomycin-induced skin fibrosis.[63] Because HDAC inhibitors, such as SAHA, are in clinical use for malignant diseases, targeting of HDACs may offer therapeutic potential for SSc.

Follow-up studies revealed that the expression of the profibrotic transcription factor PU.1 (discussed previously) is also controlled by a complex network of epigenetic mechanisms that include histone modifications.[3] In resting fibroblasts, PU.1 expression is silenced and the promoter and the upstream regulatory element of the PU.1 locus is dominated by repressive H3K9me3 and H3K27me3 marks. In fibrotic environments, however, the upstream regulatory element of the PU.1 locus becomes permissive with increased H3K27 acetylation and loss of H3K9me3 and H3K27me3. These epigenetic alterations at the PU.1 locus promote expression of PU.1 protein in fibrotic fibroblasts. As discussed previously, PU.1 inhibitors with improved pharmacologic profile are currently in development.

Moreover, histone acetylation at H4K16 has recently been shown to modulate the outcome of fibrotic diseases by fine-tuning autophagy.[64] Autophagy describes the catabolic cellular process of degradation of unnecessary or dysfunctional cellular organelles in particular during starvation or in response to cellular stress.[65] However, components of the autophagy machinery are also involved in unconventional secretion of proteins.[66–68] Autophagy is activated in a TGF-β-dependent manner in SSc fibroblasts.[64] TGF-β represses the expression of the H4K16 histone acetyltransferase MYST1 via SMAD3-dependent mechanisms to promote the expression of core components of the autophagy machinery. The resulting increase the autophagic flux induces activation of human dermal fibroblasts and fibrosis in murine skin and lungs. Re-establishment of the epigenetic control of autophagy by forced expression of MYST1 in fibroblasts impairs myofibroblast differentiation and ameliorates experimental dermal and pulmonary fibrosis. However, pharmaceutical approaches to selectively promote MYST1 activation are currently not available and further studies are required how to best transfer these findings from bench to bedside.

Other epigenetic modifications: microRNAs and bromodomain proteins

miRNAs are small noncoding RNAs. Binding of miRNAs to their respective target mRNAs promotes degradation of target mRNAs.[69] More than 50 miRNAs have been implicated in the pathogenesis of fibrotic diseases.[69] Most of these miRNAs are expressed in a highly cell-specific and/or context-specific manner. However, miR-21 and miR-29 are broadly expressed miRNAs that have been implicated in fibrotic remodeling of multiple organs and might thus be particularly relevant for a multisystemic disease, such as SSc. TGF-β induces the expression of miR-21, which in turn downregulates SMAD7 to promote canonical TGF-β signaling.[70] Antagomirs against miR-21 attenuated experimental pulmonary, myocardial, and renal fibrosis.[70–72] In contrast to miR-21, miR-29 is an antifibrotic miRNA that is downregulated in fibrotic diseases including SSc. miR-29 inhibits the translation of multiple collagen genes and of several enzymes involved in ECM turnover.[73] miR-29 mimics may thus offer potential for the treatment of SSc and other fibrotic diseases. Of note, miRNA-based therapies are currently evaluated for the treatment of cardiac fibrosis.

BRDs bind acetylated lysines in histone tails and regulate gene transcription by the recruitment of molecular partners. BRDs have recently been implicated in aberrant fibroblast activation in SSc. Chromatin accessibility and transcriptome profiling revealed constitutive activation of a TGF-β2 enhancer in SSc fibroblasts.[74] The constitutive activation of this enhancer required BRD4 and targeted inhibition of BRD4 reduced the TGF-β2 enhancer activity and the expression of profibrotic TGF-β2 target genes. Moreover, small molecule inhibitors of BRD2/4 ameliorated experimental fibrosis in preclinical models of SSc (unpublished data). BRD inhibitors are actively investigated in multiple clinical programs for malignant diseases. Although these studies faced obstacles including toxicity, modified application schemes (eg, with intermittent dosing) may limit concerns and offer opportunities for BRD inhibitors in fibrotic diseases.

EXTRACELLULAR LIGAND-RECEPTOR TARGETING OF FIBROSIS IN SYSTEMIC SCLEROSIS
Targeting the Extracellular Space in Systemic Sclerosis

Biologic therapies have transformed outcomes in immune-mediated inflammatory diseases by harnessing the specificity and binding affinity of antibody molecules or soluble receptors to trap or block the biologic effects of pathogenic cytokines. This was first demonstrated in rheumatoid arthritis using monoclonal antibodies that bound to tumor necrosis factor (TNF)-α and later with recombinant receptors fused to IgG heavy chains or other molecules. This approach has proven safe and effective and has been applied to many different clinical settings for TNF-α and other ligands. In addition to providing effective therapeutics this has provided important insight into pathogenesis and permitted exciting reverse translational studies.

Some of the established biologic agents have been applied to different diseases including SSc and have demonstrated some efficacy. This has included targeting cell types and cytokines and growth factors.

In addition to targeting cells and cytokines or growth factors through binding to ligand or receptor there is the possibility to bind other extracellular or matricellular proteins and this is an area of current investigations. SSc represents dysfunction or dysregulated connective tissue repair, and this may be normalized by modifying the cellular microenvironment through binding to extracellular proteins that are important regulators of fibroblast activation and differentiation, as outlined previously in this article.

Cytokines, Growth Factors, and Matrix Proteins in Systemic Sclerosis Pathogenesis

Cellular networks and fibroblasts activation by cytokines and extracellular matrix proteins

The hallmark pathologic processes in SSc are fibrosis and structural vasculopathy. These are likely to reflect the processes that are normally recruited for tissue repair and wound healing. A plausible explanation for the detrimental changes that develop and persist in SSc is that these usually coordinated and self-limiting biologic processes occur excessively and are not appropriately resolved. This is likely to reflect imbalance between profibrotic and proresolution pathways and mediators. Much of this regulation is likely to occur in the extracellular space and involve cytokines, growth factors, their receptors, and associated matricellular proteins. It is notable that many of these entities are identified as hallmarks of the SSc disease phenotype in recent gene and protein expression studies.[75,76] It is therefore logical to target these extracellular proteins using biologic therapeutics or small-molecule inhibitors. Some of the candidates that have been tested or are emerging in SSc are summarized next.

Targeting cytokines and receptors
Tumor necrosis factor-α. Although targeting TNF-α was enormously effective as a treatment of inflammatory disease including rheumatoid arthritis, seronegative

spondylarthritis, and inflammatory bowel disease it has not been shown to be effective in fibrotic disease.[77] This may reflect that it is a less critical driver in diseases that are less characterized by persistent inflammation or that pathways are redundant. A review of use did not suggest major benefit and a small open label clinical trial pointed toward only modest improvements that did not reach statistical significance.[78]

Interleukin-6. Although also considered a proinflammatory mediator, IL-6 was first defined as a lymphocyte regulator especially important for B cells.[79] It seems to have a much broader role and it was reported that patients with elevated IL-6 levels in the circulation had a worse outcome.[80] In addition, the markers for elevated IL-6 activity including acute phase markers seemed to predict poor outcome in several observational studies.[81] The availability of tocilizumab as an inhibitor of cis and trans signaling was attractive for clinical evaluation and a phase 2 trials (faSScinate) was supportive.[82] The subsequent phase 3 trial that included milder skin disease showed only a trend of benefit for skin but a convincing signal for clinically meaningful impact on lung fibrosis.[83] Indeed, the worsening of lung function over 48 weeks was essentially prevented at a group level in the trial. This led to Food and Drug Administration approval for tocilizumab as a treatment to reduce worsening of lung function in SSc. Parallel mechanistic studies from the phase 2 trial highlighted that the activated phenotype of explant cultured fibroblasts could be almost entirely reversed after 6 months treatment with tocilizumab.[84] This is notable because the clinical impact on skin was just a trend of benefit suggesting that other mechanisms or fibroblast populations may be important in determining the outcome and progression of skin fibrosis but that the population of fibroblasts attenuated by tocilizumab are critical in early stage lung fibrosis in SSc.

Interleukin-4/interleukin-13. There are multiple ways in which IL-4 and IL-13 may be implicated in pathogenesis of SSc.[85] This includes effects on fibroblast, perhaps in concert with TGF-β and driven by IL-13 and key roles related to immune cell activation.[86] In addition, these cytokines are critical for macrophage polarization an in vitro can induce and M2-like phenotype that is considered profibrotic.[87] It is encouraging that a phase 2 trial of romilkimab, a novel bispecific antibody targeting IL-4 and IL-13 was positive with greater improvement in mRSS and some encouraging signals in other relevant end points.[88] This requires further confirmation.

TARGETING THE ADAPTIVE IMMUNE SYSTEM

Autologous stem cell transplantation as maximal immunosuppressive therapy has shown to improve skin sclerosis and quality of life, and predicted forced vital capacity, a surrogate marker for interstitial lung disease and/or lung fibrosis, and 5-year survival rate. So far, this is the most effective therapy in SSc as shown by three different studies. However, as recently elucidated for patients fulfilling the criteria to be eligible for autologous stem cell transplantation, overall, 10-year survival by autologous stem cell transplantation is nowadays equivalent to the current best clinical practice indicating that less aggressive therapies are currently successfully applied.[89] Transfer of peripheral blood mononuclear cells from patients with SSc induces interstitial lung disease and inflammation of other organs, which is not present when peripheral blood mononuclear cells were transferred from rituximab-treated patients.[90] Those studies indicate an important role of B cells at least in the early inflammatory part of SSc. In line with this, a recent placebo-controlled phase II study on patients with early diffuse SSc revealed improvement of the predicted forced vital capacity (FVC) and skin fibrosis as assessed by the modified Rodnan skin score (mRSS).[91]

In addition to the attenuation of agonist antibodies that may be pathogenic, there is now convincing support for targeting B cells in SSc. This is based on biologic studies of the disease that highlight the potential role of abnormal B cells, especially transitional cell populations that may demonstrate a failure of peripheral tolerance.[92]

The putative role of agonistic autoantibodies in pathogenesis has now been further appreciated, having first been suggested some years previously.[93] Transfer for IgG purified from patients with SSc induced interstitial lung disease and obliterative vasculopathy in mice suggesting the potent role of antibodies in the development of inflammation and vasculopathy in SSc.[94] In vitro, purified IgG from patients with SSc induced an inflammatory and fibrotic proteome in monocytic cells lines and induced proteins show associations with the mRSS of the corresponding donors. Specifically, antibodies induced several cytokines and chemokines known to be important biomarkers for interstitial lung disease (ILD) in SSc.[95] The transfer of fibrotic signals by IgG from patients with SSc also induced a fibrotic transcriptome and proteome in fibroblasts also supporting the ability of IgG to induce disease mechanisms.[96] Indeed, recent studies identified antibodies directed to the angiotensin receptor type-1 (AT1R) as causative factors for interstitial lung disease and skin fibrosis.[97] The generation of these antibodies requires T-cell help also supporting the use of immunosuppressive therapies in the therapy for SSc. In vitro, these antibodies induced TGF-ß ad adhesion molecules in endothelial cells, collagen-1 in fibroblasts, and CCL18 or other cytokines in monocytes. AT1R antibodies often correlate with antibodies directed to the endothelin receptor type-1 (ETAR).

Other natural regulatory antibodies, such as antibodies against the thrombin receptor 1 (PAR-1), were recently shown to biologic activity, which further supports the potential for targeting antibodies therapeutically.

The use of B-cell-depleting treatments is further supported by a multicenter cohort analysis[98] and by a recent meta-analysis.[99]

Costimulatory Molecules

Abatacept, a fusion protein composed of the Fc region of IgG1 fused to the extracellular domain of CTLA-4, has been tested in a small phase 2 trial and showed only a trend of benefit at a group level.[100] However, certain subgroups of patients seemed to be driving the effect of abatacept on mRSS, especially in those patients with an inflammatory gene expression signature in their skin biopsy.[101] More encouragingly, all patients showed a meaningful impact on HAQ-DI. This was a phase 2 study, but it seems likely that if a phase 3 trial confirmed the results for HAQ-DI that this is a treatment that might be helpful for some patients with SSc.

Future candidates for targeted therapy in the extracellular compartment
There are several promising future candidates for targeting extracellular proteins and ligands. These are likely to emerge based on current studies and preclinical and supportive translational data.

OSM. Despite strong theoretic rationale,[102] a well conducted phase IIa trial of anti-OSM has recently been completed and unfortunately did not show evidence of benefit in SSc based on prespecified markers of biologic or clinical effect. This was an early stage study that was primarily testing the safety of the antibody and there was meaningful impact on hematologic parameters including anemia and thrombocytopenia in some cases. On this basis it is not being pursued further as a treatment of SSc (unpublished data).[103]

CTGF. This prototypic member of the CCN family of matricellular proteins has long been a hallmark marker of the profibrotic SSc fibroblast phenotype.[104] It seems to promote or augment fibrosis and may work as a downstream mediator or cofactor related to TGF-β.[105] There have been encouraging phase 2 data for targeting CTGF in idiopathic pulmonary fibrosis (IPF) and in the future it may be a promising target in SSc.[106]

S100A4. This protein was originally identified as a fibroblast expressed protein marker (FSP-1) based on differential display data for cells undergoing epithelial-mesenchymal transition.[107] It is now clear that this protein is a member of the S100 protein family,[108] is expressed by several cell types, and that it is an important ECM protein that can activate innate immune pathways.[109] Promising preclinical data support its potential as a target for treatment of fibrosis and in SSc.[110]

Interferon. An elevated interferon signature is seen in SSc and many other rheumatic diseases.[111] Although not present in all patients it seems to be associated with poor outcome and with an overlap phenotype.[112] Because targeting interferon using anifrolumab is now an approved treatment of systemic lupus erythematosus (SLE)[113] and because early phase studies showed attenuation often interferon signature in patients with SSc is a potential treatment for evaluation in SSc.[114]

Transforming growth factor-β. This profibrotic master regulator is an obvious candidate for ligand-directed therapy in SSc and other form of fibrosis.[115] However, the broad roles in connective tissue and immunologic development and homeostasis together with potential roles in protecting for neoplastic transformation have raised legitimate concerns about targeting TGF-β and the balance between risk and benefit.[116] The first trials using weak monospecific antibody against TGF-β1 suggested safety but showed no signal of efficacy.[117] An open-label study of fresolimumab was more encouraging.[118] There are several ongoing trials evaluating TGF-β-directed antibodies or ligand traps. The recent promising data for pulmonary arterial hypertension (PAH) targeting active pathways provide support for the potential of this approach[119] and the results of ongoing trials are eagerly awaited.

Reverse Translation and Insights into Pathogenesis

Trials of targeted treatment offers a unique platform for experimental medicine studies as was shown for tocilizumab and these give real insights into treatment mechanism, target engagement, and biology of SSc. There have been exciting results from studies and insights that may allow more targeted or stratified approaches in future trials to advance clinical trial development and pave the way for a more stratified approach to clinical practice.

Preclinical Models

It has proven challenging to use preclinical models to conform treatment benefit, but they are valuable in highlighting clinical potential and identifying the stage and type of SSc that may be most informative in a subsequent clinical trial.

SUMMARY

It is an exciting time for SSc therapeutics because the benefits of background treatments are being established and it is possible to design trials that add more targeted approaches on top of standard immunosuppression. The trials of nintedanib and romilkimab are excellent examples of this approach and it has been helpful in confirming the benefits from standard treatments and additive value of new drugs. The powerful effect of hematopoietic stem cell transplantation provides a gold standard of what can be achieved therapeutically, albeit with a mortality that has high morbidity and treatment-related mortality. In addition, it is unsuitable for many cases and indeed those most in need are excluded from current trial protocols despite having a demonstrably worse outcome than those that are eligible. In the future it is a legitimate goal to achieve the therapeutic impact of hematopoietic stem cell transplantation through combination targeted therapies with much less treatment-related toxicity. Emerging data suggest that an individual approach may be rewired and that tools, such as skin subset, disease duration, and antinuclear antibody (ANA) profile, and skin biopsy intrinsic subset or peripheral blood interferon signature may be valuable tools in developing an optimal approach to treatment of SSc.

CLINICS CARE POINTS

- Systematic screening for organ based complications ensures timely diagnosis and treatment of pulmonary complications in systemic sclerosis.
- Current treatment with immunosuppression has modest benefit for skin and lung firosis and severe or progressive cases shoudl be considered for autologous haematopoietic stem cell transplantation.
- Combination therapies targeting different mechanisms or mediators are effective in treating pulmonary arterial hyperetnsion in systemic sclerosis.
- Autoantibodies and skin subset are helpful in stratifying systemic sclerosis patiensts for risk of future complications.

DISCLOSURE

The authors have nothing to disclose.

REFERENCES

1. Tabib T, Huang M, Morse N, et al. Myofibroblast transcriptome indicates SFRP2(hi) fibroblast progenitors in systemic sclerosis skin. Nat Commun 2021;12(1):4384.
2. McAnulty RJ. Fibroblasts and myofibroblasts: their source, function and role in disease. Int J Biochem Cell Biol 2007;39(4):666–71.
3. Wohlfahrt T, Rauber S, Uebe S, et al. 1 controls fibroblast polarization and tissue fibrosis. Nature 2019;566(7744):344–9.
4. Rinkevich Y, Walmsley GG, Hu MS, et al. Skin fibrosis. Identification and isolation of a dermal lineage with intrinsic fibrogenic potential. Science 2015;348(6232): aaa2151.
5. Jiang D, Correa-Gallegos D, Christ S, et al. Two succeeding fibroblastic lineages drive dermal development and the transition from regeneration to scarring. Nat Cell Biol 2018;20(4):422–31.
6. Beltran AS, Graves LM, Blancafort P. Novel role of Engrailed 1 as a prosurvival transcription factor in basal-like breast cancer and engineering of interference peptides block its oncogenic function. Oncogene 2014;33(39):4767–77.
7. Palumbo-Zerr K, Zerr P, Distler A, et al. Orphan nuclear receptor NR4A1 regulates transforming growth factor-beta signaling and fibrosis. Nature medicine 2015;21(2):62–70.

8. Chen HZ, Liu QF, Li L, et al. The orphan receptor TR3 suppresses intestinal tumorigenesis in mice by downregulating Wnt signalling. Gut 2012;61(5): 714–24.

9. Zerr P, Vollath S, Palumbo-Zerr K, et al. Vitamin D receptor regulates TGF-beta signalling in systemic sclerosis. Ann Rheum Dis 2015;74(3):e20.

10. Avouac J, Palumbo-Zerr K, Ruzehaji N, et al. The nuclear receptor constitutive androstane receptor/NR1I3 enhances the profibrotic effects of transforming growth factor beta and contributes to the development of experimental dermal fibrosis. Arthritis Rheum 2014;66(11):3140–50.

11. Beyer C, Huang J, Beer J, et al. Activation of liver X receptors inhibits experimental fibrosis by interfering with interleukin-6 release from macrophages. Ann Rheum Dis 2015;74(6):1317–24.

12. Beyer C, Skapenko A, Distler A, et al. Activation of pregnane X receptor inhibits experimental dermal fibrosis. Ann Rheum Dis 2013;72(4):621–5.

13. Horn A, Kireva T, Palumbo-Zerr K, et al. Inhibition of hedgehog signalling prevents experimental fibrosis and induces regression of established fibrosis. Ann Rheum Dis 2012;71(5):785–9.

14. Lam AP, Flozak AS, Russell S, et al. Nuclear beta-catenin is increased in systemic sclerosis pulmonary fibrosis and promotes lung fibroblast migration and proliferation. Am J Respir Cell Mol Biol 2011;45(5):915–22.

15. Horn A, Palumbo K, Cordazzo C, et al. Hedgehog signaling controls fibroblast activation and tissue fibrosis in systemic sclerosis. Arthritis Rheum 2012;64(8): 2724–33.

16. Dees C, Tomcik M, Zerr P, et al. Notch signalling regulates fibroblast activation and collagen release in systemic sclerosis. Ann Rheum Dis 2011;70(7):1304–10.

17. He W, Dai C, Li Y, et al. Wnt/beta-catenin signaling promotes renal interstitial fibrosis. J Am Soc Nephrol 2009;20(4):765–76.

18. Konigshoff M, Kramer M, Balsara N, et al. WNT1-inducible signaling protein-1 mediates pulmonary fibrosis in mice and is upregulated in humans with idiopathic pulmonary fibrosis. J Clin Invest 2009;119(4):772–87.

19. Guan S, Zhou J. Frizzled-7 mediates TGF-beta-induced pulmonary fibrosis by transmitting non-canonical Wnt signaling. Experimental cell research 2017; 359(1):226–34.

20. Saito A, Nagase T. Hippo and TGF-beta interplay in the lung field. Am J Physiol Lung Cell Mol Physiol 2015;309(8):L756–67.

21. Burgy O, Konigshoff M. The WNT signaling pathways in wound healing and fibrosis. Matrix Biol : journal of the International Society for Matrix Biology 2018;68-69:67–80.

22. Zhang Y, Shen L, Dreißigacker K, et al. Targeting of canonical WNT signaling ameliorates experimental sclerodermatous chronic graft-versus-host disease. Blood 2021;137(17):2403–16.

23. Beyer C, Huscher D, Ramming A, et al. Elevated serum levels of sonic hedgehog are associated with fibrotic and vascular manifestations in systemic sclerosis. Ann Rheum Dis 2017;77(4):626–8.

24. Liang R, Šumová B, Cordazzo C, et al. The transcription factor GLI2 as a downstream mediator of transforming growth factor-β-induced fibroblast activation in SSc. Ann Rheum Dis 2017;76(4):756–64.

25. Wei J, Melichian D, Komura K, et al. Canonical Wnt signaling induces skin fibrosis and subcutaneous lipoatrophy a novel mouse model for scleroderma? Arthritis Rheum 2011;63(6):1707–17.

26. Konigshoff M, Balsara N, Pfaff EM, et al. Functional Wnt signaling is increased in idiopathic pulmonary fibrosis. PLoS One 2008;3(5):e2142.

27. Cheng JH, She HY, Han YP, et al. Wnt antagonism inhibits hepatic stellate cell activation and liver fibrosis. Am J Physiol Gastrointest Liver Physiol 2008; 294(1):G39–49.

28. He W, Zhang LN, Ni AG, et al. Exogenously administered secreted frizzled related protein 2 (Sfrp2) reduces fibrosis and improves cardiac function in a rat model of myocardial infarction. Proc Natl Acad Sci U S A 2010;107(49): 21110–5.

29. Trensz F, Haroun S, Cloutier A, et al. A muscle resident cell population promotes fibrosis in hindlimb skeletal muscles of mdx mice through the Wnt canonical pathway. Am J Physiol Cell Physiol 2010;299(5):C939–47.

30. Akhmetshina A, Palumbo K, Dees C, et al. Activation of canonical Wnt signalling is required for TGF-beta-mediated fibrosis. Nat Commun 2012;3:735.

31. Chen JH, Chen WLK, Sider KL, et al. Beta-catenin mediates mechanically regulated, transforming growth factor-beta 1-induced myofibroblast differentiation of aortic valve interstitial cells. Arterioscler Thromb Vasc Biol 2011;31(3):590–7.

32. Sato M. Upregulation of the Wnt/beta-catenin pathway induced by transforming growth factor-beta in hypertrophic scars and keloids. Acta Derm Venereol 2006; 86(4):300–7.

33. Chen CW, Beyer C, Liu J, et al. Pharmacological inhibition of porcupine induces regression of experimental skin fibrosis by targeting Wnt signalling. Ann Rheum Dis 2017;76(4):773–8.

34. Dees C, Schlottmann I, Funke R, et al. The Wnt antagonists DKK1 and SFRP1 are downregulated by promoter hypermethylation in systemic sclerosis. Ann Rheum Dis 2014;73(6):1232–9.

35. Beyer C, Reichert H, Akan H, et al. Blockade of canonical Wnt signalling ameliorates experimental dermal fibrosis. Ann Rheum Dis 2013;72(7):1255–8.

36. Beyer C, Schramm A, Akhmetshina A, et al. Beta-catenin is a central mediator of pro-fibrotic Wnt signaling in systemic sclerosis. Ann Rheum Dis 2012;71(5): 761–7.

37. Bergmann C, Akhmetshina A, Dees C, et al. Inhibition of glycogen synthase kinase 3 beta induces dermal fibrosis by activation of the canonical Wnt pathway. Ann Rheum Dis 2011;70(12):2191–8.

38. Brack AS, Conboy MJ, Roy S, et al. Increased Wnt signaling during aging alters muscle stem cell fate and increases fibrosis. Science 2007;317(5839):807–10.

39. Wei J, Fang F, Lam AP, et al. Wnt/beta-catenin signaling is hyperactivated in systemic sclerosis and induces Smad-dependent fibrotic responses in mesenchymal cells. Arthritis Rheum 2012;64(8):2734–45.

40. Rimkus TK, Carpenter RL, Qasem S, et al. Targeting the sonic hedgehog signaling pathway: review of smoothened and GLI inhibitors. Cancers 2016; 8(2):22.

41. Watson CJ, Collier P, Tea I, et al. Hypoxia-induced epigenetic modifications are associated with cardiac tissue fibrosis and the development of a myofibroblast-like phenotype. Hum Mol Genet 2014;23(8):2176–88.

42. Beyer C, Schett G, Gay S, et al. Hypoxia. Hypoxia in the pathogenesis of systemic sclerosis. Arthritis Res Ther 2009;11(2):220.

43. Parker MW, Rossi D, Peterson M, et al. Fibrotic extracellular matrix activates a profibrotic positive feedback loop. J Clin Invest 2014;124(4):1622–35.

44. Mann J, Oakley F, Akiboye F, et al. Regulation of myofibroblast transdifferentiation by DNA methylation and MeCP2: implications for wound healing and fibrogenesis. Cell Death Differ 2007;14(2):275–85.

45. Bechtel W, McGoohan S, Zeisberg EM, et al. Methylation determines fibroblast activation and fibrogenesis in the kidney. Nat Med 2010;16(5):544–50.

46. King TE, Pardo A, Selman M. Idiopathic pulmonary fibrosis. Lancet 2011; 378(9807):1949–61.

47. Wang Y, Fan PS, Kahaleh B. Association between enhanced type I collagen expression and epigenetic repression of the FLI1 gene in scleroderma fibroblasts. Arthritis Rheum 2006;54(7):2271–9.

48. Kato M, Putta S, Wang M, et al. TGF-beta activates Akt kinase through a microRNA-dependent amplifying circuit targeting PTEN. Nat Cell Biol 2009; 11(7):881. U263.

49. Montgomery RL, Yu G, Latimer PA, et al. MicroRNA mimicry blocks pulmonary fibrosis. EMBO Mol Med 2014;6(10):1347–56.

50. Zeisberg EM, Zeisberg M. The role of promoter hypermethylation in fibroblast activation and fibrogenesis. J Pathol 2013;229(2):264–73.

51. Mann J, Mann DA. Epigenetic regulation of wound healing and fibrosis. Curr Opin Rheumatol 2013;25(1):101–7.

52. Altorok N, Tsou PS, Coit P, et al. Genome-wide DNA methylation analysis in dermal fibroblasts from patients with diffuse and limited systemic sclerosis reveals common and subset-specific DNA methylation aberrancies. Ann Rheum Dis 2015 Aug;74(8):1612–20.

53. Razin A, Riggs AD. DNA methylation and gene function. Science 1980; 210(4470):604–10.

54. Nan X, Ng HH, Johnson CA, et al. Transcriptional repression by the methyl-CpG-binding protein MeCP2 involves a histone deacetylase complex. Nature 1998; 393(6683):386–9.

55. Chen X, Li WX, Chen Y, et al. Suppression of SUN2 by DNA methylation is associated with HSCs activation and hepatic fibrosis. Cell Death Dis 2018;9(10): 1021.

56. Sanders YY, Pardo A, Selman M, et al. Thy-1 promoter hypermethylation: a novel epigenetic pathogenic mechanism in pulmonary fibrosis. Am J Respir Cell Mol Biol 2008;39(5):610–8.

57. Zhang Y, Potter S, Chen CW, et al. Poly(ADP-ribose) polymerase-1 regulates fibroblast activation in systemic sclerosis. Ann Rheum Dis 2018;77(5):744–51.

58. Noda S, Asano Y, Nishimura S, et al. Simultaneous downregulation of KLF5 and Fli1 is a key feature underlying systemic sclerosis. Nat Commun 2014;5:5797.

59. Asano Y, Bujor AM, Trojanowska M. The impact of Fli1 deficiency on the pathogenesis of systemic sclerosis. J Dermatol Sci 2010;59(3):153–62.

60. Asano Y, Trojanowska M. Fli1 represses transcription of the human alpha2(I) collagen gene by recruitment of the HDAC1/p300 complex. PLoS One 2013; 8(9):e74930.

61. Asano Y, Czuwara J, Trojanowska M. Transforming growth factor-beta regulates DNA binding activity of transcription factor fli1 by p300/CREB-binding protein-associated factor-dependent acetylation. J Biol Chem 2007;282(48):34672–83.

62. Zhao S, Cao M, Wu H, et al. 5-aza-2'-deoxycytidine inhibits the proliferation of lung fibroblasts in neonatal rats exposed to hyperoxia. Pediatrics and neonatology 2017;58(2):122–7.

63. Huber LC, Distler JH, Moritz F, et al. Trichostatin A prevents the accumulation of extracellular matrix in a mouse model of bleomycin-induced skin fibrosis. Arthritis Rheum 2007;56(8):2755–64.
64. Zehender A, Li YN, Lin NY, et al. TGFβ promotes fibrosis by MYST1-dependent epigenetic regulation of autophagy. Nat Commun 2021;12(1):4404.
65. Wang CW, Klionsky DJ. The molecular mechanism of autophagy. Mol Med 2003; 9(3–4):65–76.
66. Deretic V, Jiang S, Dupont N. Autophagy intersections with conventional and unconventional secretion in tissue development, remodeling and inflammation. Trends Cell Biol 2012;22(8):397–406.
67. Ponpuak M, Mandell MA, Kimura T, et al. Secretory autophagy. Curr Opin Cell Biol 2015;35:106–16.
68. Guo H, Chitiprolu M, Roncevic L, et al. Atg5 disassociates the V(1)V(0)-ATPase to promote exosome production and tumor metastasis independent of canonical macroautophagy. Dev Cell 2017;43(6):716–30, e717.
69. Vettori S, Gay S, Distler O. Role of microRNAs in fibrosis. Open Rheumatol J 2012;6:130–9.
70. Liu G, Friggeri A, Yang YP, et al. miR-21 mediates fibrogenic activation of pulmonary fibroblasts and lung fibrosis. J Exp Med 2010;207(8):1589–97.
71. Thum T, Gross C, Fiedler J, et al. MicroRNA-21 contributes to myocardial disease by stimulating MAP kinase signalling in fibroblasts. Nature 2008; 456(7224):980–U983.
72. Zhong X, Chung ACK, Chen HY, et al. Smad3-mediated upregulation of miR-21 promotes renal fibrosis. J Am Soc Nephrol 2011;22(9):1668–81.
73. Maurer B, Stanczyk J, Jungel A, et al. MicroRNA-29, a key regulator of collagen expression in systemic sclerosis. Arthritis Rheum 2010;62(6):1733–43.
74. Shin JY, Beckett JD, Bagirzadeh R, et al. Epigenetic activation and memory at a TGFB2 enhancer in systemic sclerosis. Sci Transl Med 2019;11(497):eaaw0790.
75. Clark KEN, Campochiaro C, Csomor E, et al. Molecular basis for clinical diversity between autoantibody subsets in diffuse cutaneous systemic sclerosis. Ann Rheum Dis 2021;80(12):1584–93.
76. Jang DI, Lee AH, Shin HY, et al. The role of tumor necrosis factor alpha (TNF-α) in autoimmune disease and current TNF-α inhibitors in therapeutics. Int J Mol Sci 2021;22(5):2719.
77. Denton CP, Engelhart M, Tvede N, et al. An open-label pilot study of infliximab therapy in diffuse cutaneous systemic sclerosis. Ann Rheum Dis 2009;68(9): 1433–9.
78. Choy EH, De Benedetti F, Takeuchi T, et al. Translating IL-6 biology into effective treatments. Nat Rev Rheumatol 2020;16(6):335–45.
79. O'Reilly S, Cant R, Ciechomska M, et al. Interleukin-6: a new therapeutic target in systemic sclerosis? Clin Transl Immunology 2013;2(4):e4.
80. Khan K, Xu S, Nihtyanova S, et al. Clinical and pathological significance of interleukin 6 overexpression in systemic sclerosis. Ann Rheum Dis 2012;71(7): 1235–42.
81. Muangchant C, Pope JE. The significance of interleukin-6 and C-reactive protein in systemic sclerosis: a systematic literature review. Clin Exp Rheumatol 2013; 31(2 Suppl 76):122–34.
82. Khanna D, Denton CP, Jahreis A, et al. Safety and efficacy of subcutaneous tocilizumab in adults with systemic sclerosis (faSScinate): a phase 2, randomised, controlled trial. Lancet 2016;387(10038):2630–40.

83. Khanna D, Lin CJF, Furst DE, et al. Tocilizumab in systemic sclerosis: a randomised, double-blind, placebo-controlled, phase 3 trial. Lancet Respir Med 2020;8(10):963–74. Erratum in: Lancet Respir Med. 2020 Oct;8(10):e75.

84. Denton CP, Ong VH, Xu S, et al. Therapeutic interleukin-6 blockade reverses transforming growth factor-beta pathway activation in dermal fibroblasts: insights from the faSScinate clinical trial in systemic sclerosis. Ann Rheum Dis 2018;77(9):1362–71.

85. Nguyen JK, Austin E, Huang A, et al. The IL-4/IL-13 axis in skin fibrosis and scarring: mechanistic concepts and therapeutic targets. Arch Dermatol Res 2020; 312(2):81–92.

86. O'Reilly S. Role of interleukin-13 in fibrosis, particularly systemic sclerosis. Biofactors 2013;39(6):593–6.

87. Lescoat A, Lecureur V, Varga J. Contribution of monocytes and macrophages to the pathogenesis of systemic sclerosis: recent insights and therapeutic implications. Curr Opin Rheumatol 2021;33(6):463–70.

88. Allanore Y, Wung P, Soubrane C, et al. A randomised, double-blind, placebo-controlled, 24-week, phase II, proof-of-concept study of romilkimab (SAR156597) in early diffuse cutaneous systemic sclerosis. Ann Rheum Dis 2020;79(12):1600–7.

89. Spierings J, Nihtyanova SI, Derrett-Smith E, et al. Outcomes linked to eligibility for stem cell transplantation trials in diffuse cutaneous systemic sclerosis. Rheumatology 2022;61(5):1948–56.

90. Yue X, Petersen F, Shu Y, et al. Transfer of PBMC from SSc patients induces autoantibodies and systemic inflammation in Rag2-/-/IL2rg-/- mice. Front Immunol 2021;12:677970.

91. Ebata S, Yoshizaki A, Oba K, et al. Safety and efficacy of rituximab in systemic sclerosis (DESIRES): a double-blind, investigator-initiated, randomised, placebo-controlled trial. Lancet Rheumatology 2021;3(7):e489–97.

92. Taher TE, Ong VH, Bystrom J, et al. Association of defective regulation of autoreactive interleukin-6-producing transitional B lymphocytes with disease in patients with systemic sclerosis. Arthritis Rheum 2018;70(3):450–61.

93. Baroni SS, Santillo M, Bevilacqua F, et al. Stimulatory autoantibodies to the PDGF receptor in systemic sclerosis. N Engl J Med 2006;354(25):2667–76.

94. Becker MO, Kill A, Kutsche M, et al. Vascular receptor autoantibodies in pulmonary arterial hypertension associated with systemic sclerosis. Am J Respir Crit Care Med 2014;190(7):808–17.

95. Prasse A, Müller-Quernheim J. Non-invasive biomarkers in pulmonary fibrosis. Respirology 2009;14(6):788–95.

96. Kill A, Riemekasten G. Functional autoantibodies in systemic sclerosis pathogenesis. Curr Rheumatol Rep 2015;17(5):34.

97. Yue X, Yin J, Wang X, et al. Induced antibodies directed to the angiotensin receptor type 1 provoke skin and lung inflammation, dermal fibrosis and act species overarching. Ann Rheum Dis 2022;81(9):1281–9.

98. Jordan S, Distler JH, Maurer B, et al. EUSTAR Rituximab study group. Effects and safety of rituximab in systemic sclerosis: an analysis from the European Scleroderma Trial and Research (EUSTAR) group. Ann Rheum Dis 2015;74(6): 1188–94.

99. Moradzadeh M, Aghaei M, Mehrbakhsh Z, et al. Efficacy and safety of rituximab therapy in patients with systemic sclerosis disease (SSc): systematic review and meta-analysis. Clin Rheumatol 2021;40(10):3897–918.

100. Khanna D, Spino C, Johnson S, et al. Abatacept in early diffuse cutaneous systemic sclerosis: results of a phase II investigator-initiated, multicenter, double-blind, randomized, placebo-controlled trial. Arthritis Rheum 2020;72(1):125–36.
101. Chung L, Spino C, McLain R, et al. Safety and efficacy of abatacept in early diffuse cutaneous systemic sclerosis (ASSET): open-label extension of a phase 2, double-blind randomised trial. Lancet Rheumatol 2020;2(12):e743–53.
102. Duncan MR, Hasan A, Berman B. Oncostatin M stimulates collagen and glycosaminoglycan production by cultured normal dermal fibroblasts: insensitivity of sclerodermal and keloidal fibroblasts. J Invest Dermatol 1995 Jan;104(1): 128–33.
103. Denton CP, Del Galdo F, Khanna D, et al. Biological and clinical insights from a randomized phase 2 study of an anti-oncostatin M monoclonal antibody in systemic sclerosis. Rheumatology (Oxford) 2022;62(1):234–42.
104. Abraham D. Connective tissue growth factor: growth factor, matricellular organizer, fibrotic biomarker or molecular target for anti-fibrotic therapy in SSc? Rheumatology 2008;47(Suppl 5):v8–9.
105. Parada C, Li J, Iwata J, et al. CTGF mediates Smad-dependent transforming growth factor β signaling to regulate mesenchymal cell proliferation during palate development. Mol Cell Biol 2013;33(17):3482–93.
106. Richeldi L, Fernández Pérez ER, Costabel U, et al. Pamrevlumab, an anti-connective tissuegrowth factor therapy, for idiopathic pulmonary fibrosis (PRAISE): a phase 2, randomised, double-blind, placebo-controlled trial. Lancet Respir Med 2020;8(1):25–33.
107. Rossini M, Cheunsuchon B, Donnert E, et al. Immunolocalization of fibroblast growth factor-1 (FGF-1), its receptor (FGFR-1), and fibroblast-specific protein-1 (FSP-1) in inflammatory renal disease. Kidney Int 2005;68(6):2621–8.
108. Schneider M, Hansen JL, Sheikh SP. S100A4: a common mediator of epithelial-mesenchymal transition, fibrosis and regeneration in diseases? J Mol Med (Berl) 2008;86(5):507–22.
109. Li Z, Li Y, Liu S, et al. Extracellular S100A4 as a key player in fibrotic diseases. J Cell Mol Med 2020;24(11):5973–83.
110. Tomcik M, Palumbo-Zerr K, Zerr P, et al. S100A4 amplifies TGF-β-induced fibroblast activation in systemic sclerosis. Ann Rheum Dis 2015;74(9):1748–55.
111. Wu M, Assassi S. The role of type 1 interferon in systemic sclerosis. Front Immunol 2013;4:266.
112. Moinzadeh P, Frommolt P, Franitza M, et al. Whole blood gene expression profiling distinguishes systemic sclerosis-overlap syndromes from other subsets. J Eur Acad Dermatol Venereol 2020;34(5):e236–8.
113. Koh JWH, Ng CH, Tay SH. Biologics targeting type I interferons in SLE: a meta-analysis and systematic review of randomised controlled trials. Lupus 2020; 29(14):1845–53.
114. Ciechomska M, Skalska U. Targeting interferons as a strategy for systemic sclerosis treatment. Immunol Lett 2018;195:45–54.
115. Lichtman MK, Otero-Vinas M, Falanga V. Transforming growth factor beta (TGF-β) isoforms in wound healing and fibrosis. Wound Repair Regen 2016;24(2): 215–22.
116. Peng D, Fu M, Wang M, et al. Targeting TGF-β signal transduction for fibrosis and cancer therapy. Mol Cancer 2022;21(1):104.
117. Denton CP, Merkel PA, Furst DE, et al. Cat-192 Study Group; Scleroderma Clinical Trials Consortium. Recombinant human anti-transforming growth factor beta1 antibody therapy in systemic sclerosis: a multicenter, randomized,

placebo-controlled phase I/II trial of CAT-192. Arthritis Rheum 2007;56(1): 323–33.

118. Rice LM, Padilla CM, McLaughlin SR, et al. Fresolimumab treatment decreases biomarkers and improves clinical symptoms in systemic sclerosis patients. J Clin Invest 2015;125(7):2795–807.

119. Humbert M, McLaughlin V, Gibbs JSR, et al. PULSAR Trial Investigators. Sotatercept for the treatment of pulmonary arterial hypertension. N Engl J Med 2021;384(13):1204–15.

Patient Experience of Systemic Sclerosis–Related Calcinosis

An International Study Informing Clinical Trials, Practice, and the Development of the Mawdsley Calcinosis Questionnaire

Lesley Ann Saketkoo, MD, MPH[a,b,c,d,*], Jessica K. Gordon, MD, MSc[e],
Kim Fligelstone[f,g], Anne Mawdsley[h], Humza A. Chaudhry, BS[a,d],
Antonia Valenzuela, MD, MS[i], Angela Christensen, MD[j],
Samara M. Khalique, MD[k], Kelly Jensen, MD, MPH[a,d,l],
Sophia C. Weinmann, MD[m], Evan Busman[n],
Lorinda Chung, MD, MS[o,p], Vivien M. Hsu, MD[q],
Anne-Marie Russell, PhD, APRN[r,s], Virginia D. Steen, MD[t]

KEYWORDS

- Scleroderma • Calcinosis • Raynaud phenomenon • Digital ulcers
- Qualitative research • Patient-reported outcomes • Self-Management
- Qualtiy of LIfe

Continued

[a] New Orleans Scleroderma and Sarcoidosis Patient Care and Research Center, New Orleans, LA, USA; [b] University Medical Center–Comprehensive Pulmonary Hypertension Center and Interstitial Lung Disease Clinic Programs, New Orleans, LA, USA; [c] Section of Pulmonary Medicine, Louisiana State University School of Medicine, New Orleans, LA, USA; [d] Tulane University School of Medicine, New Orleans, LA, USA; [e] Department of Rheumatology, Hospital for Special Surgery, New York, NY, USA; [f] Scleroderma & Raynaud Society, UK (SRUK); [g] Federation of European Scleroderma Associations, UK; [h] Raynaud's & Scleroderma Association–Care and Support, London, UK; [i] Department of Rheumatology and Clinical Immunology, Pontificia Universidad Católica de Chile, Santiago, Chile; [j] Doctors Hospital, Renaissance, TX, USA; [k] Department of Rheumatology, Virginia Tech Carilion Clinic School of Medicine, Roanoke, VA, USA; [l] University of Colorado School of Medicine, Denver, CO, USA; [m] Department of Medicine, Division of Rheumatology and Immunology, Duke University Hospital, Durham, NC, USA; [n] Healthcare Patient Advocate, Atlanta, GA, USA; [o] Department of Medicine, Division of Immunology and Rheumatology, Stanford University School of Medicine and Palo Alto VA Healthcare System, Palo Alto, CA, USA; [p] Department of Dermatology, Division of Immunology and Rheumatology, Stanford University School of Medicine and Palo Alto VA Healthcare System, Palo Alto, CA, USA; [q] RWJ–Scleroderma Program, Rutgers Robert Wood Johnson Medical School, New Brunswick, NJ, USA; [r] Respiratory Institute, University of Exeter, Exeter, UK; [s] Respiratory Medicine, Royal Devon University Healthcare NHS Foundation Trust, UK; [t] Division of Rheumatology, Department of Medicine, Georgetown University, Washington, DC, USA
* Corresponding author.
E-mail address: lsaketk@tulane.edu

Rheum Dis Clin N Am 49 (2023) 463–481
https://doi.org/10.1016/j.rdc.2023.01.017
0889-857X/23/© 2023 Elsevier Inc. All rights reserved.

rheumatic.theclinics.com

Continued

KEY POINTS

- Calcinosis can be a debilitating, constantly painful vascular manifestation of systemic sclerosis (SSc) that severely impairs engagement and completion of routine life activities.
- SSc-calcinosis generates significant psychosocial stress related to pain, loss of hand function or mobility as well as fearfulness of and being able to predict complications, such as infection, digital ulceration, and finger loss.
- People living with SSc provided insight into the natural history of SSc-calcinosis, which includes affirming association with trauma, repetitive pressure, Raynaud phenomenon, and cold exposure.
- Management behavior of patients coping with SSc-calcinosis routinely included self-extrusion with soaking and use of instruments to relieve calcinosis that are often not communicated to health providers.
- The Mawdsley Calcinosis Questionnaire is the first patient-reported outcome measure for use in clinical practice and clinical trials to evaluate and monitor SSc-calcinosis.

BACKGROUND

Systemic sclerosis (SSc) -related calcinosis is often a debilitating, constantly painful, and poorly understood vascular complication resulting from calcium hydroxyapatite deposition in soft tissue structures, such as fat pads, muscles, tendons, and ligaments, that occurs in the presence of normal calcium and phosphorus metabolism. SSc-calcinosis affects approximately 40% of both limited cutaneous SSc and diffuse cutaneous SSc subtypes[1,2] and can occur in amorphic, tumoral, or sheetlike deposition. SSc-calcinosis most commonly affects areas of local trauma or vasoconstrictive injuries, such as areas vulnerable to pressure exposures, friction, or repetitive use, including extensor areas of elbows, fingertips, and thumbs.[3,4] Although considered a late-onset vascular manifestation,[5] it has also been described as occurring earlier for some patients.[1,6] SSc-calcinosis is highly associated with other vascular complications, such as digital ulcers (DUs), acro-osteolysis, telangiectasias, and pulmonary hypertension.[7–9] Although various imaging modalities can provide fairly reliable visualization and measurement of SSc-calcinosis in its solid, rock-like phase, calcinosis also occurs in liquid and pastelike phases. Calcinotic lesions can be asymptomatic, but for many patients, calcinosis results in disabling symptoms that result in poor health-related quality of life (HRQoL) owing to fairly constant pain and functional impairment and are frequently further complicated by ulceration and infection. No agreed-upon treatment exists for SSc-calcinosis, and there are no standardized measures to assess potential therapeutic responsiveness in clinical trials.

Furthermore, patients often rely on self-report and self-management.[6] Patients' insight into SSc-calcinosis is essential for clinician education, optimal patient self-care, and informing clinical study designs, which require patient-reported outcome measures (PROM) that capture clinically relevant changes in the severity and impact of experiential concepts.[10,11]

No studies to date have investigated a conceptual framework or domains relevant to the patient perspective of SSc-calcinosis. This international qualitative research study aims to comprehensively explore the patient experience of SSc-calcinosis and identify concept items for PROM development in future clinical research and clinical care. Reported here are the conceptual framework and patient-driven concepts informing the Mawdsley Calcinosis Questionnaire (MCQ) development.

METHODS
Study Design

An international multicenter study, aiming for broad geographical, cultural, and ethnic inclusion, obtained initial qualitative data collection via in-person focus groups (FG) in New York City; Salt Lake City; Washington, DC; New Orleans; and the United Kingdom; interviews were planned in the United Kingdom and Europe, with an intention to undertake additional FGs and interviews until "thematic saturation" was achieved[12-14] through inductive analysis. Concepts were anticipated to inform the understanding of SSc-calcinosis and drive the development of an SSc-calcinosis PROM under Food and Drug Administration (FDA) guidance, engaging patient partners to form question-item options from relevant concepts and then field-tested with patients from nationalities as wide-ranging as possible for patient preferences of language and formatting. Participants for field testing (FT) will be recruited through outreach to patient organizations.

Participants

Participants were ≥18 years of age, satisfied American College of Rheumatology/European League Against Rheumatism classification criteria,[15] had a history of calcinosis confirmed by their local rheumatologist, and had fluent English language skills with the capacity to provide informed consent. Participants provided informed consent according to institutional review board–approved protocol.

Study Team

The study team was overseen by a steering committee composed of 4 SSc experts (J.G., L.A.S., T.F., V.S.), 3 patient research partners (PRPs) in SSc (A.M., E.B., K.F.), a researcher trained in psychometrics (A.M.R.), and experienced PROM developers (A.M.R., L.A.S., T.F., V.S.). The study team included qualitative research trainees (A.C., A.V., H.C., J.K., S.K., S.W.).

Data Collection

FGs and semi-structured interviews were conducted globally, using a topic guide comprising open-ended questions and probes enquiring how patients would describe their calcinosis experiences. This was followed by more focused discussions, sometimes targeting incompletely explored emergent themes from earlier FGs and interviews, ensuring thematic saturation was achieved. FGs lasted approximately 90 minutes, led by L.A.S., and supported by at least 1 other research group member. Groups were audio-recorded, transcribed, and anonymized.

To capture both pathophysiologic and life impact, the following 2 questions were asked:

1. Since developing calcinosis, how has your life changed over time?
2. How has the calcinosis changed over time?

Patients were also asked to frame questions that would help a physician gauge if calcinosis was better, worse, or the same.

Data Analysis

Inductive thematic analysis was implemented iteratively to each anonymized transcript to ensure the findings were grounded in shared patient experiences rather than externally imposed pre-existing concepts.[16,17] At least 5 research team members, including at least 1 member with SSc and 1 experienced qualitative researcher (A.M.R., L.A.S., T.F., J.G.) read each transcript multiple times with extraction of discrete patient-expressed experiences. Ongoing analyses, cumulative notes, and the consistent presence of the lead FG facilitator (L.A.S.) informed thematic saturation and coding. Concepts were triangulated among team members to identify a comprehensive set of meaningful concepts with occurrences quantified per participant[16] with the subsequent agreement of conceptual framework and final analysis. The process allowed emerging themes to be explored and challenged, with amendments made if new concepts emerged.

Patient-Reported Outcome Measures Development

The map for developing question items anchored the overarching themes as domains that progressed to developing question options for each relevant concept as directed by PRP guidance. Questions evolved further after subsequent participant interviewing and FT. FT rigorously evaluated preferences for time reference, vocabulary, contextualization, language, importance, and relevance. In addition, the FT process also explored response scale and formatting preferences. During the FT process, preferences were rated using a 0 to 5 Likert scale anchored in the perceived ability of each variable to be "useful" in indicating improvement, worsening, or no change of SSc-calcinosis, with "Not applicable to me" also being an option.

RESULTS (1366)
Initial Data Collection

A total of 40 people with SSc-calcinosis participated, representing Brazil, Canada, France, Germany, Hungary, New Zealand, the United Kingdom, and the United States; 31 participants (96% women, 13% black, 6% Hispanic) generated the initial data (**Table 1**). Six FGs in New Orleans; New York City; Salt Lake City; the United Kingdom; Washington, DC; plus an Atlanta FG at the Scleroderma Foundation Patient Conference generated 78 original nonoverlapping concepts. Seven major themes, expanded upon in later discussion, emerged that encapsulated the patient experience of SSc-calcinosis. Frequencies of the most common concepts are found in **Tables 2–7**.

Mawdsley Calcinosis Questionnaire Development

Of the 78 items, all items considered "actionable" within the patient experience of body structure, function, or HRQoL (including work, family, and social activities) were extracted by iterative analyses and consolidated into 21 potential PROM concepts—17 question items with scalable responses and 4 items that elicit open-ended responses. Four PROM domains harbored all concept items: Quantity/Frequency of Calcinosis (4 items), Pain/Sensation (5 items), Physical Function/Functional Impairment (4 items), and Psychological Impact (6 items).

FT of potential question items and variables required the participation of 9 people with SSc-calcinosis in face-to-face interviews to reach a clear trend of preferences

Table 1	
Characteristics of 31 interview subjects in data collection	
Raynaud	100%
Gender (female)	93%
Race and ethnicity (black/Hispanic/white)	13%/6%/81%
Time from diagnosis (mean)	18.05 y
Cold exposure decreases core body temperature with sensation of systemic symptoms: "it's like intense—it racks your whole body."	26% (6/23 participants)

Table 2
Locations Where Calcinosis was Experienced in 31 Participants

	% of participants
Fingers	90
Palms	26
Wrists	19
Elbows	45
Arms	10
Scalp	19
Face, lips, eyelids, or ears	26
Lips	3
Eyelids	10
Ears	6
Face, other	10
Trunk (back, chest, buttock, armpit)	22
Thighs	6
Knees	6
Feet (including toes)	26

(**Table 8**) of time reference, each item in relation to language, vocabulary, and contextual variables, as well as verbiage, image, formatting, length, and degree of potential response scales.

Two of the 4 Quantity/Frequency items (50%) were rated greater than 4 by greater than 80%. Thirteen of the 17 scaled items (77%) were rated greater than 4 by greater than 80% of FT participants and greater than 4 by 100% for the remaining 4 items. Two question items that pertained strictly to Raynaud phenomenon (RP) and DUs may be reincorporated as "stabilization" questions, potentially to be scored separately for comparative reference. The Scleroderma Health Assessment Questionnaire (SHAQ) visual analogue scale (VAS) scales for RP and DU can also serve this purpose.[18] Only the 2 FT participants (22%, proportionately consistent with the FG participants) experiencing foot calcinosis rated the "walking" item highly, which led to the generation of a test question for future validation studies that combines upper- and lower-extremity physical function to ensure the possibility of a more uniformly weighted instrument.

Regarding response scale preferences, there was 100% selection of a 0 to 10 scale over other, for example, 0 to 5, 0 to 7, 0 to 9 point scales, greater than 90% selected Likert response over VAS, a reflective time reference of between 2 and 4 weeks with

Table 3
Calcinosis Properties Experienced by 31 Participants

	%
Rocklike/solid	90
Fluid/leaking	26
Calcinosis always recurrent, once appears in any site	19
Extrudes with warm soaking	45
Pastelike	10

Table 4
Calcinosis Related Effects and Sensations Experienced by 31 Participants

	% of Participants
Pain	96
Tender	94
Throbbing	52
Relief with extrusion	78
Tight w/ pressure	52
Impact causes pain for hours	84
Ulcer from calcinosis	52
Feel growth	48
Constant	84
Burning sensation	26 (6/23)
Sharp	22 (5/23)
Itchy	9 (2/23)

2 weeks being favored, and a reflective severity reference of "the worst degree" with 100% selection for single or brief word descriptors to cap scales, that is, "none" to "worst possible." The scoring/weighting of the question items is yet to be determined. The current prevalidation version of the instrument is presented in **Fig. 1**.

Qualitative Themes

Qualitative analysis from 31 participant interviews revealed insight into self-management, quality of life, mental/physical function, and natural history of SSc-calcinosis. Responses spanned broadly to include concepts of physical and emotional impact and insights into the natural history and management strategies of SSc-calcinosis. Selected participant quotes are populated in **Table 9**.

Theme 1: calcinosis qualities

This theme captures concepts relating to location, consistency, and some aspects of SSc-calcinosis behavior. The predominant location involved the hand, and the predominant consistency was rocklike, which is of interest when examining the latter themes related to functional impairment. Although SSc-calcinosis is typically considered a late finding in terms of disease duration, the timing of SSc-calcinosis onset, as reported in other studies, tended to present with variation. When SSc-calcinosis was reported to occur along with or soon after SSc diagnosis, it appeared to remain a potential manifestation throughout the disease duration. However, the correlation between SSc-calcinosis onset and time from first RP experience has not yet been investigated.

Properties of SSc-calcinosis were also subject to potential developments of complications that participants dreaded, such as infection or development of a deep DU, especially with larger-sized calcinosis.

Table 5
Functional Impact of Calcinosis as Described by 31 Participants

	% of Participants
Interferes with hand use	90
Interferes with activities of daily living	87
Interferes with walking	19

Table 6 Factors Perceived to Influence to Influence the Experience of Calcinosis	
Perceived Influencing Factors	**% of Participants**
Calcinosis occurs in areas of trauma or pressure	65
More frequent when Raynaud is worse	48
Trauma or banging interferes with healing	35
More frequent when cold or when not practicing cold prevention	35
Response to warmth or prevention against cold	39
Three patients conveyed positive effect to cyclophosphamide	13
Two patients conveyed positive effect to vasodilating medications	—
One patient conveyed positive effect of colchicine	—

Theme 2: physical sensation/pain quality

The physical symptoms of SSc-calcinosis were overwhelmingly consistent between participants. Pain was the predominant symptom to the extent that it became the key concept around which the theme revolved. Pain was most commonly described as "tender" or "throbbing" and "constant" when calcinosis was present by nearly all participants. SSc-calcinosis created pain that impeded sleep, reduced the ability to use hands and complete tasks, and created distractions that interfered with personal interactions and with work. Participants with areas of calcinosis and pre-existing baseline pain experience intensification of pain that is described as lasting hours on top of the baseline pain. Pain was relieved with calcinosis extrusion in most participants (78%).

Theme 3: functional impairment

SSc-calcinosis was reported by 90% of participants to involve the hand, and ~90% of participants reported interference with hand use and activities of daily living, likely owing to fingers being of central importance to accomplishing essential tasks at home and at work. Difficulty walking owing to SSc-calcinosis was reported by 22%.

There were stark impediments in self-care, family care, and complex and straightforward household tasks that participants previously described as being accomplished automatically and expeditiously throughout a day. Small routine tasks now required extended time with cautious execution or could not be accomplished at all.

Theme 4: influencing factors

Participants primarily conveyed antecedent physical trauma or repetitive pressure corresponding to locations for SSc-calcinosis. Cold exposure and Raynaud were perceived as associated with calcinosis severity—and controlling cold exposure

Table 7 Self Management Strategies Conveyed by 31 Participants	
	% of participants
Need self-management protocols for calcinosis	87 (20 of23 participants queired)
Cushioning (if material does not hurt)	65
Extrusion with pressure ± warm soak	45
Topical antibiotics	36
Extrusion with instruments at home	29

Table 8
Results of field testing

Item	Domain	Items Rating ≥4*	Scale
Geographical location	Reference only	*	None, report only
Hemisphere/season	Reference only	*	None, report only
Month	Reference only	*	None, report only
Number of calcinosis lesions (open or closed)	Quantity/frequency	*	Undetermined
Number of calcinosis lesions you FEEL that you have	Quantity/frequency	—	Undetermined
Number of digital ulcers	Quantity/frequency	*	Undetermined/comparative
Number of digital ulcers you think are related to calcinosis	Quantity/frequency	—	Undetermined
Stem to below items is: "In the past TWO WEEKS, what is the worst degree that…"			
Raynaud's interfered with daily activities?	Reference	*	0–10 for comparative reference
Digital ulcers interfered with daily activities?	Reference	*	0–10 for comparative reference
Experienced pain from calcinosis?	Pain/sensation	*	0–10 for scoring
You felt any areas of calcinosis getting tighter or having more pressure?	Pain/sensation	*100%	0–10 for scoring
You felt any areas of calcinosis GROWING under your skin?	Pain/sensation	*	0–10 for scoring
Your felt any areas of your calcinosis THROBBING?	Pain/sensation	*	0–10 for scoring
Your calcinosis has been TENDER to TOUCH?	Pain/sensation	*100%	0–10 for scoring
You felt the need to PROTECT areas of your calcinosis?	Psychological impact	*100%	0–10 for scoring
You have been FEARFUL or WORRIED that any of the calcinosis areas are infected?	Psychological impact	*	0–10 for scoring
You have been worried that a calcinosis wound might not heal?	Psychological impact	*100%	0–10 for scoring
Your calcinosis interfered with ability to care for self?	Physical function	*	0–10 for scoring
Your calcinosis interfered with your ability to use your hands?	Physical function	*	0–10 for scoring
Your calcinosis interfered with walking?	Physical function	(25%)	0–10 for scoring
Your calcinosis interfered with your ability to work (paid or unpaid)?	Physical function	*	0–10 for scoring
Your calcinosis made you feel down, depressed, or hopeless?	Psychological impact	—	0–10 for scoring

Your calcinosis interfered with your ability to enjoy and "be there" for your friends and family?	Psychological impact	—	0–10 for scoring
Your calcinosis interfered with your ability to enjoy recreational activities (hobbies, sports, and so forth)?	Psychological impact	—	0–10 for scoring

Item domains preferred by FT participants with majority ratings of ≥ 4 (very to extremely useful).

* = >80% of participants rated the item with greater or equal to 4 ('very useful' to 'extremely useful').

Mawdsley Calcinosis Questionnaire

Patient Name or Reference_____   Current geographical location _____

Hemisphere/season _____   Month/Day _____

Part A.

1. a. How many calcinosis lesions (open or closed) do you ACTUALLY have today? _____

1. b. How many calcinosis do you FEEL that you have today? _____

2. a. How many digital ulcers do you have today? _____

2. b. How many of these digital ulcers do you think are related to calcinosis? ____

Part B.

In the past TWO WEEKS, what is the worst degree that...

1. Your Raynaud's has interfered with daily activities?

| No Limitation | 0 1 2 3 4 5 6 7 8 9 10 | Maximum limitation/ Worst possible |

2. Your DIGITAL ULCERS interfered with daily activities?

| No Limitation | 0 1 2 3 4 5 6 7 8 9 10 | Maximum limitation/ Worst possible |

3. You experienced PAIN from your calcinosis?

| No Pain | 0 1 2 3 4 5 6 7 8 9 10 | Worst Possible Pain |

4. You felt any areas of your calcinosis getting TIGHTER or having more pressure?

| Not at all | 0 1 2 3 4 5 6 7 8 9 10 | Maximum |

5. You felt any areas of your calcinosis GROWING under your skin?

| Not at all | 0 1 2 3 4 5 6 7 8 9 10 | Maximum |

6. You felt any areas of your calcinosis THROBBING?

| Not at all | 0 1 2 3 4 5 6 7 8 9 10 | Maximum |

7. Your calcinosis has been TENDER to TOUCH?

| Not at all | 0 1 2 3 4 5 6 7 8 9 10 | Maximum |

8. You felt the need to PROTECT areas of your calcinosis?

| Not at all | 0 1 2 3 4 5 6 7 8 9 10 | Maximum |

9. You have been FEARFUL or WORRIED that any of your calcinosis areas are INFECTED?

| Not at all | 0 1 2 3 4 5 6 7 8 9 10 | Maximum |

10. You have been worried that a calcinosis wound MIGHT NOT HEAL?

| Not at all | 0 1 2 3 4 5 6 7 8 9 10 | Maximum |

11. Your calcinosis interfered with ability to CARE FOR SELF?

| No Limitation | 0 1 2 3 4 5 6 7 8 9 10 | Maximum limitation/ Worst possible |

12. Your calcinosis interfered with your ability to USE YOUR HANDS?

| No Limitation | 0 1 2 3 4 5 6 7 8 9 10 | Maximum limitation/ Worst possible |

13. Your calcinosis interfered with WALKING?

| No Limitation | 0 1 2 3 4 5 6 7 8 9 10 | Maximum limitation/ Worst possible |

Test question: Your calcinosis interfered with your ability to USE YOUR HANDS or to WALK?

14. Your calcinosis interfered with your ABILITY TO WORK (paid or unpaid)?

| No Limitation | 0 1 2 3 4 5 6 7 8 9 10 | Maximum limitation/ Worst possible |

15. Your calcinosis made you FEEL DOWN, DEPRESSED or HOPELESS?

| Not at all | 0 1 2 3 4 5 6 7 8 9 10 | Worst Possible |

16. Your calcinosis interfered with your ability to enjoy and 'be there' for your FRIENDS and FAMILY?

| No Limitation | 0 1 2 3 4 5 6 7 8 9 10 | Maximum limitation/ Worst possible |

17. Your calcinosis interfered with your ability to enjoy RECREATIONAL ACTIVITIES (hobbies, sports, etc)?

| No Limitation | 0 1 2 3 4 5 6 7 8 9 10 | Maximum limitation/ Worst possible |

Fig. 1. The current version of the MCQ. (*Courtesy of* LA Saketkoo MD, MPH, New Orleans, LA.)

Table 9
Selected Patient Quotes

"I think we all go through that with temperature changes—the air conditioning can set it off quickly"

"It's like intense—it racks your whole body"

"It's like I need a heated blanket—give me a heated blanket, an electric pad, heater, just to warm up"

"When I get home, I put the wristies on and get into bed and really cover up"

"Yes! Cover your whole body"

"Blankets! And you trap your own body heat underneath"

"I have a big calcinosis here on that finger and then I have it on the tips of my thumbs"

"I get them in my fingers and on my palms"

"I got those over my hands (pointing to her proximal interphalangeal joints)"

"Mine only that I had on the top of my elbow was when I was first diagnosed"

"Arms, elbows, toes, and the bottom of my spine"

"I have an elbow that kills me"

"I went to the doctor because my wrist really really hurt, it was just the beginning of this"

"I also get in my hair, little grainies, and in my ears and inside my ears"

"I also got one on my lip"

"And then I noticed these white spots on my face and chest"

"It was the other parts of my body that I get them, like my arms and my head"

"I get some on my chin...little sandy things"

"The most painful ones I get on the eyelid"

"I even got some on my head"

"On the scalp, I've had those several times"

"I got a few of them really bad actually on my earlobe and behind my ear"

"The only ones I get now are on the edge of my eyes"

"I started getting little calcium bumps like on my eyelid"

"On my feet...it's like right on the side"

"I've got a small group in my heels—and that really hurts"

"The tips of both of my big toes and the heel of my foot"

"If I soaked it in hot water a couple of times a day, it helps the skin to open and then eventually it drains by itself and the calcium will come out by itself"

"It seems like anytime temperature changes—if there's a breeze, it feels like someone is cutting my skin"

"It is really painful when you're really cold"

"You see this pinky? It really hurts when I write because it touches the paper, and it starts to burn"

"Just the tips, the tips or the knuckles, you brush it, you bang it, you touch it the wrong way. It hurts—right away—and you do it too hard it hurts a lot, and it will open up"

"Whenever you turn the wrong way at night"

"I would just touch the table and it would just shoot pain through my finger"

"It aches even if you don't touch it on anything—it aches till it opens and drains"

"The ones on the ear hurt if I scratch them by accident or hit them"

"I got these over my hands, they are hard, painful"

"The most painful ones I get on the eyelid"

(continued on next page)

Table 9
(continued)

"I've got a small group in my heels—and that really hurts"

"I got a few of them really bad actually on my earlobe and behind my ear. I did take the one in my earlobe out because it was really painful"

"They drain and then they're relieved"

"It is horribly painful"

"Paralyzing pain—you have to pause for a minute"

"It's still tender, even though it's completely healed"

"The less you use your hands the better"

"I still drive but am limited, and I do as much as I can, and I'm very careful with a knife—scissors, forget it"

"I'm sick of filling the pill boxes—because I can't do it easily"

"I try to avoid touching things…the car seat…I use my knuckles and try to use other ways—and the kid is sitting in the car seat for like 5 minutes before I can get him out"

"And I don't use my thumb anymore for the microwave. I'm very cognizant of what I'm doing with my thumb and my knuckles. I'm a manager and I do a lot of typing"

"Most of the time you learn to live with it—it's painful, and controlling the circulation is prominent"

"So, when you ask what is the most burdensome part of calcinosis, for me right now it's not knowing"

"Well, the ulcers from the calcinosis on the fingers are not just painful, it's debilitating and keeps you from doing what you are normally able to do. And when they are very active, it's a really painful part of life…really painful"

"I can't even thread a needle, I can't knit, I can't crochet …all of those things are kind of sad. I read now"

"I can't even hold her (child)"

"Her hair I can't brush well enough"

"And sometimes I just want to do something. Like trim the hedges—I haven't done that in years…but I'll hit it or irritate it"

"I'm sitting here in a wheelchair because…I had a calcinosis…on the bottom of my heel"

"This is one of the biggest challenges, how to relieve the pain so you can function"

"As an attorney, and using the computer a lot with my fingertips. That was very, very painful"

"I know winter's coming because these come up…become tight"

"I think there is a relationship between cold and calcinosis and ulcer development"

"As soon as the weather started changing these hurt much more"

"Say you open the freezer…you are there in the frozen food aisle feeling absolutely frozen and hands are cold…I think it's a combination of the cold and the Raynaud's and the calcium"

"The cold makes it worse especially when they're open"

"She went out and bought me gloves—helped with the calcinosis"

"By spring as it gets warmer, they'll be less"

"I think it (warmth) helps prevent calcinosis"

"Summer makes a difference—all get better in the summer"

"I've noticed that as the Raynaud's has progressed, I've gotten the calcinosis"

"If you bang it and you're going through Raynaud's, it's going to be a lot worse"

"When the Raynaud's attacks are worse, the calcinosis is more noticeable"

(continued on next page)

Table 9
(continued)

"The more severe the Raynaud's attacks are the more they push up to the surface of the skin"

"I see a connection between Raynaud's and...[the development of calcinosis]"

"I do think there is a relationship for me between Raynaud's and the development of calcinosis"

"I was thrown from a carriage...and did something to my pelvic area; and that seemed to trigger calcinosis throughout my pelvic area and hip area"

"I closed the step stool. I pinched here...that's how it started—it was an injury that started in the one"

"I did notice that if I bang my finger...the red will stay and the calcium will develop"

"But if I banged it somehow, it would open right up"

"It was building up at the incision site"

"The normal use of your hands can cause calcinosis by just bumping it in everyday activities"

"That was the worst one—I guess because I hit it and it took a long time to heal"

"Do you think the less you bang the calcinosis the more likely it is to heal? ..." "Yes I do." "I do." "I do."

"Mine [worsening of calcinosis] is absolutely stress. Emotional stress"

"Dr X did this thumb, did the same thing with the calcinosis. And I really have not had any more infections in that thumb"

"I don't have those anymore because he went in there and straightened them out and scraped it all out and put a little screw in"

"In terms of recurrence, most of the surgery has been successful"

"I haven't taken that kind of care I'm used to with my gloves on and everything...and now it's the first time again with this"

"I've always had peeling and leaking and whenever I peeled a scab...it is a relief"

"I actually always have a scab and when it's too thick—the scab—it's painful, relieving the scab helps"

"Oh yeah, you get relief from taking them out"

"I did take the one in my earlobe out because it was really painful"

"I made an elbow puff so I couldn't touch too much of the bed"

"I always wear gloves, I always wear padding"

"What about protective gloves? ... hard to put 'em on"

"I can't wear gloves—because of the pressure"

"Movement and circulation are helpful because it increases the circulation in my fingertips"

"And you know what helped me a lot? Washing the hands in the paraffin wax"

"Wrapping my fingers tight with the Band-aid will really help too"

"My hands start to sweat and that is like when my hands get wet...and they start to drain"

"The contact with water helps them to drain"

"I'll soak them in warm water, and sometimes they will just come to the surface"

"I soak it in hot salt water, warm salt water"

"When you soak them...it breaks itself and drains out and relieves a lot of pain that way"

"I think the biggest disadvantage of having scleroderma and calcinosis is...not enough people know about it, and not enough doctors and nurses" was perceived to prevent worsening occurrence and intensification of pain. There were some sporadic assertions regarding various systemic, vasodilatory, and other medications.

Of great interest, several described a disabling phenomenon involving a decrease of core temperature with a rapid physical decline and concomitant extreme fatigue, requiring prolonged recovery potentially lasting hours—"*it's like intense—it racks your whole body.*" The authors include this feature as described, as it may prove relevant and an investigation-worthy feature in patients with calcinosis and other vascular manifestations, such as ulcers and acro-osteolysis.

Theme 5: self-management
Participants reported diverse targeted strategies and general approaches to mitigating the routine diverse interference related to and potentially worsening of SSc-calcinosis. Most participants reported taking steps to protect against Raynaud and cold sensation to reduce the development and impact of SSc-calcinosis symptoms. When tactile tolerance allowed, many participants described applying cushioned coverings in the hopes of averting or lessening the occurrence of prolonged pain intensification of potential physical impact/trauma. Only a few participants knew of topical lidocaine products, and oral analgesics were infrequently discussed.

A majority of participants reported engaging in strategies to extrude calcinosis with either pressure, warm water ± salt soaking, or at-home surgical techniques, and often a combination of these. "*I actually have homemade surgical tools to get these out.*" Participants who engaged in extrusion concomitantly reported care in instrument cleanliness and the use of antibiotic ointment.

The majority of patients expressed needing more guidance and assistance in SSc-calcinosis care. A strong need was expressed by 65% of participants for a calcinosis self-management protocol or care book.

Theme 6: emotional impact
Experiences of SSc-calcinosis deliver an emotional impact on patients that reflect a range of degrees of frustration, embarrassment, irritation, anxiety, and distress. The impact of SSc-calcinosis as a multifaceted impediment interfering with family and self-care, remunerative work, social participation, and engagement in previously enjoyable leisure activities was a source of emotional discomfort, distress, isolation, and dysphoric self-identity or guilt, especially in roles revolving around family care.

Theme 7: uncertainty
Uncertainty is a recurring, and perhaps the most complex, theme across FG, a resultant impact for which the preceding themes converged. However, uncertainty is closely tied to anxiety and could be considered under the emotional impact theme. Both relate to worrying about future circumstances; uncertainty appears to be a strong, somewhat independent operative driver with diffuse and pervasive causes for fueling anxiety. Participants described continual negotiation in discrete situations and overarching projections of uncertainty in daily life and the long term. Uncertainty spans broadly to include how SSc-calcinosis may reflect overall SSc disease progression and worsening, the presence of underlying infection, whether recalcitrant or deep DUs will develop, the prospect of future and further disability or need for amputation, or the potential for worsening calcinosis recurrence. Treatment and self-management are laden with uncertainty, despite participants being seemingly "seasoned" in navigating calcinosis self-care, which sometimes resulted in self-punitive feelings of regret if insufficient measures to prevent occurrence and complications were suspected.

DISCUSSION

The authors report the first investigations dedicated to the patient experience of SSc-calcinosis that yielded both astonishing and confirmatory information on the natural history and management of SSc-calcinosis. Clear concepts were generated and subsequently confirmed by multichoice FT, that have implications for assessment, clinical care, and counseling for SSc-calcinosis. Concepts yielded PROM domains and question items that were relevant, meaningful, functional, and discriminating in detecting change over time in the experience of SSc-calcinosis.

The physical symptoms of SSc-calcinosis, of which the pervasive driver is complex pain sensations, leads to considerable emotional distress and impaired ability to use hands or be mobile, resulting in a significant impact on daily life. During instrument development, concepts such as cognitive slowing and fatigue were introduced, especially concerning the toll of SSc-calcinosis pain or impairment. However, participants voiced that these symptoms were difficult to distinguish and would not be valuable PROM elements as the source as SSc-calcinosis from other SSc features such as lung involvement.

Participant reports corroborate hypotheses of prior trauma. SSc-calcinosis arose in areas of antecedent trauma and recurred in the absence of repeated trauma. More common was SSc-calcinosis occurring and recurring in areas routinely exposed to pressure or repeated trauma. In the authors' analysis, cold exposure and cold prevention were perceived as influential in SSc-calcinosis. A strong correlation was voiced between Raynaud preventive care and the development of calcinosis and DUs, "*I learned early on, if you want to keep your fingers, you gotta keep your hands warm.*"

A recurrent and surprising discussion was that of "*core warmth*" and its impact on systemic and constitutional symptoms leading to short-term general function impairment. Debilitation related to loss of core warmth, although not specific to calcinosis and hence not included in the MCQ, has not yet been reported in the literature. The authors communicate this concept in publication, as they believe it is worth deeper consideration by SSc education and research communities.

Participants' self-management approaches were extraordinary and sometimes withheld from their treating physician's knowledge for fear of disapproval. Despite participants' ability to generate valuable insights for clinical care, participants' consistently expressed self-management was fraught with uncertainty (fear of infection, resultant nonhealing DUs, need for amputation), insufficient guidance from the medical community, and the need for self-management protocols.

Patients sought daily relief by taking substantial and diverse measures to avoid intensifying symptoms and complications of SSc-calcinosis. The most common was repetitive warm water soaking ($\pm$ salt compound) with self-extrusion, for which several patients reported self-assembled surgical kits to assist in extrusion. Patients conveyed being vigilant for signs of infection and other red flags possibly requiring clinician attention, and frequently using topical antibiotics during extrusion. This knowledge of "underground" self-management and self-care is pivotal to developing relevant patient-clinician alliances and anticipatory guidance for safe self-management.

The frequency of expressions of psychological impact and emotional impact was not discretely tabulated in the analyses. These impressive concepts were less often directly expressed in word units but rather imbued by the tone and context of the narrative. This was also true of "*living with uncertainty,*" which seems to erode one's perception of general well-being, ability to care for self and others, ability to enjoy family, and employment performance. Therefore, items of psychological impact were reported by usual qualitative standards without quantifying occurrence.

Not reported in the results, but a predominant participant preference was using non-possessive references and avoiding use of "your "or "my" when referring to SSc or SSc-calcinosis. This was expressed as an essential differentiation of true self from the health condition as overtaking their identity.

This study's strengths were multifold because of the research team, including SSc patient leaders as parallel experts and a study design robustly compliant with FDA guidance. Qualitative researchers with prior experience in PROM development and in-depth clinical knowledge of SSc led thematic analysis. The multicenter global design with inductive methodology strengthened the generalizable representation of the SSc-calcinosis patient experience described here. The design strove to achieve diversity in representation of age, gender, race, disease duration, SSc phenotype, and geographic, cultural, and ethnic participation. This appears to have been accomplished to a very reasonable degree and to an extent fairly unusual of studies in SSc.[19]

The stewardship and scientific engagement by PRPs with experience in peer leadership and SSc qualitative research were essential in facilitating a feasible, effective design. Patient expertise drove the efficient development of a PROM from analysis and interpretation to question item development.

The generalizability of the MCQ PROM is evident in the extremely high agreements across variable selections in the multichoice FT phase. Great care was taken to select simple language and words to clearly carry the intent of the question item and to reach a diversity of cultures and languages, and facilitate future translation efforts into other languages. Involving trainees interested in SSc and in qualitative research had bidirectional benefits for both the deeper humane understanding of SSc for the learner and the fresh perspective brought by the trainees to the project.

Study limitations are mostly related to selection bias by preferentially attracting sufficiently aware, educated, connected, and able-bodied patients to respond to the participation announcement. Although 5 participants attended with caregivers who enabled patient travel and supported their needs during the FG or interview, this degree of support may not be available to the majority with significant SSc-related disability. Along similar lines, higher levels of motivation or education may have influenced the insights into coping, self-management, and influential factors, that may not be reflective of all people struggling with SSc-calcinosis. Another potential selection bias is that all participants acquired the required rheumatologist SSc-calcinosis confirmation, whereas patients with less self-efficacy may have desired to participate but were discouraged by the requirements for participation.

The MCQ, although not yet fully validated, is currently being used in multicenter clinical studies. The MCQ is undergoing further validation steps, which are anticipated to finalize a scoring and weighting system. Translation of the MCQ is planned for in several languages via standardized translation protocols.

SUMMARY

The patient experience of SSc-calcinosis was explored iteratively in a diverse and representative international cohort, reaching concept saturation. Pervasive disability, frustration, symptom distress, and uncertainty created largely by complex, severe pain sensations are related to daily living with SSc-calcinosis. Patient observations and self-management behavior provide opportunities to educate clinicians and patients. Patients are eager for self-management guidance. This investigation informed the development of a novel PROM, the MCQ, developed according to FDA guidance[20,21] to assess the severity and impact of SSc-calcinosis for use in clinical studies and clinical practice. Further validation and translation studies of the MCQ are underway.

Significance and Innovations/Key Messages

- Patients provide novel insight into the cause, complex pain and sensation features, influencing factors, natural history, and management of calcinosis.
- SSc-calcinosis can result in high symptom distress with significant and pervasive disability in daily living with intense feelings of stress, frustration, and uncertainty about current and future living.
- This is the first study investigating the patient experience of SSc-calcinosis resulting in a novel PROM that is undergoing further validation steps and future translations.
- The MCQ is named in honor of Anne Mawdsley—an original research member of this team, founder of the Raynaud's & Scleroderma Association UK, and a person living with SSc who raised over £10 million for SSc research, education, and advocacy in her lifetime.

SOURCES OF SUPPORT

Rheumatology Research Foundation, Scleroderma and Raynaud's Society UK, The Scleroderma Foundation, Federation of European Scleroderma Associations, Scleroderma Clinical Trials Consortium, EUSTAR, Georgetown University, and the Hospital for Special Surgery.

CONFLICTS OF INTEREST

None of the authors report any conflicts of interest relevant to the content of this work.

DEDICATION

This research is dedicated to the memory, life, and work of A. Mawdsley, founder of the *Raynaud's & Scleroderma Association UK* (SRUK) and a tireless engine of patient education and advocacy, procuring more than £10 million of research funding.

CLINICS CARE POINTS

- Patients' observations from living with SSc-calcinosis and their descriptions of self-management behavior provide key learning opportunities for healthcare providers.
- Patients are eager for healthcare providers to educate on anticipatory and self-management guidance to manage and prevent complications of SSc-calcinosis.
- Patients engage in various methods of protecting vulnerable areas and extrusion of SSc-calcinosis. Open conversations with patients about their self-management strategies and anticipatory guidance on when to seek medical care may help prevent complications.

ACKNOWLEDGMENTS

The authors acknowledge the Rheumatology Research Foundation, Scleroderma Clinical Trials Consortium, The Scleroderma Foundation, and the Federation of European Scleroderma Associations. This work could not have been done without the knowledge and proactive expertise of Dr Tracy M. Frech at Vanderbilt University Scleroderma Center, whose editorship precludes her place in the author line. Her involvement in the project will be marked by her initials in the article where relevant.

REFERENCES

1. Muktabhant C, Thammaroj P, Chowchuen P, et al. Prevalence and clinical association with calcinosis cutis in early systemic sclerosis. Mod Rheumatol 2021; 31(6):1113–9.

2. Pai S, Hsu V. Are there risk factors for scleroderma-related calcinosis? Mod Rheumatol 2018;28(3):518–22.

3. Gauhar R, Wilkinson J, Harris J, et al. Calcinosis preferentially affects the thumb compared to other fingers in patients with systemic sclerosis. Scand J Rheumatol 2016;45:317–20.

4. Cruz-Dominguez MP, Garcia-Collinot G, Saavedra MA, et al. Clinical, biochemical, and radiological characterization of the calcinosis in a cohort of Mexican patients with systemic sclerosis. Clin Rheumatol 2017;36:111–7.

5. Morgan ND, Shah AA, Mayes MD, et al. Clinical and serological features of systemic sclerosis in a multicenter African American cohort: analysis of the genome research in African American scleroderma patients clinical database. Medicine 2017;96. e8980.

6. Christensen A, Khalique S, Cenac S, et al. Systemic sclerosis related calcinosis: patients provide what specialists want to learn. J La State Med Soc 2015;167(3): 158–9.

7. Avouac J, Lepri G, Smith V, et al. Sequential nailfold videocapillaroscopy examinations have responsiveness to detect organ progression in systemic sclerosis. Semin Arthritis Rheum 2017;47(1). 86e94.

8. Shah AA, Wigley FM, Hummers LK. Telangiectases in scleroderma: a potential clinical marker of pulmonary arterial hypertension. J Rheumatol 2010;37(1): 98–104.

9. Avouac J, Mogavero G, Guerini H, et al. Predictive factors of hand radiographic lesions in systemic sclerosis: a prospective study. Ann Rheum Dis 2011;70(4): 630–3.

10. Administration USDoHaHSFaD. Guidance for industry: patient-reported outcome measures: use in medical product development to support labeling claims 2009. Available from: http://www.fda.gov/downloads/Drugs/GuidanceCompliance RegulatoryInformation/Guidances/UCM193282.pdf. Accessed June 1, 2016.

11. Valenzuela A, Song P, Chung L. Calcinosis in scleroderma. Curr Opin Rheumatol 2018;30(6):554–61.

12. Krueger R, Casey M. Focus groups: a practical guide for applied research. 3rd edition. Thousand Oaks (CA): Sage; 2000.

13. Guest GB,A, Johnson L. How many interviews are enough? An experiment with data saturation and variability. Field Method 2006;18:59–82.

14. Patton MQ. Qualitative research and evaluation methods. 3rd edition. Thousand Oaks (CA): Sage; 2002.

15. van den Hoogen F, Khanna D, Fransen J, et al. 2013 Classification criteria for systemic sclerosis: an American College of Rheumatology/European League Against Rheumatism collaborative initiative. Ann Rheum Dis 2013;72(11): 1747–55.

16. Braun V, Clarke V. Using thematic analysis in psychology. Qual Res Psychol 2006; 3:77–101.

17. Saketkoo LA, Jensen K, Nikoletou D, et al. Sarcoidosis illuminations on living during covid-19: patient experiences of diagnosis, management, and survival before and during the pandemic. J Patient Exp 2022;9. 23743735221075556.

18. Steen VD, Medsger TA Jr. The value of the health assessment questionnaire and special patient-generated scales to demonstrate change in systemic sclerosis patients over time. Arthritis Rheum 1997;40(11):1984–91.
19. Dougherty DH, Kwakkenbos L, Carrier ME, et al. SPIN investigators. The scleroderma patient-centered intervention network cohort: baseline clinical features and comparison with other large scleroderma cohorts. Rheumatology (Oxford) 2018;57(9):1623–31.
20. U.S. Department of Health and Human Services FDA Center for Drug Evaluation and Research, U.S. Department of Health and Human Services FDA Center for Biologics Evaluation and Research, U.S. Department of Health and Human Services FDA Center for Devices and Radiological Health. Guidance for industry: patient-reported outcome measures: use in medical product development to support labeling claims: draft guidance. Health Qual Life Outcomes 2006;4:79.
21. Speight J, Barendse SM. FDA guidance on patient reported outcomes. BMJ 2010;340. c2921.

Primary Cardiac Involvement in Systemic Sclerosis

Best Approach to Diagnosis

Erin Chew, MD[a],*, Vineet Agrawal, MD, PhD[b], Tracy Frech, MD[a,c]

KEYWORDS

- Systemic sclerosis • Cardiac • Arrhythmia • Myocardial

KEY POINTS

- Primary cardiac involvement can be detected on routine cardiopulmonary screening and requires further diagnostics.
- Cardiovascular magnetic resonance is the gold standard for imaging cardiac anatomy, function, and advanced myocardial tissue characterization.
- Serum cardiac soluble biomarkers can help identify cardiac involvement but do not distinguish between primary and secondary causes.
- The role of algorithm-based cardiac evaluation both before and after therapeutic initiation is one of the many unmet needs for systemic sclerosis clinical care.

INTRODUCTION

Systemic sclerosis (SSc) is an autoimmune disease characterized by vasculopathy and fibrosis. Although monitoring patients with SSc for skin, pulmonary, and renal complications are defined by expert guidelines, evidence-based recommendations for the identification of primary cardiac involvement is less clear.[1] Primary cardiac involvement can include the pericardium, myocardium, conduction system, and, less commonly, valves. Primary cardiac involvement is recognized as being distinct from heart complications secondary to other disease manifestations, such as ischemic heart disease and right heart failure from pulmonary hypertension, but unfortunately lacks standard consensus definitions.[2] Nonetheless, autopsy studies suggest that primary cardiac involvement, especially myocardial lesions, are common in SSc, regardless of antemortem cardiac symptoms and are a major cause of mortality.[3–5] Therefore, understanding diagnostics that allow for early identification of primary cardiac involvement in patients with SSc is

[a] Division of Rheumatology and Immunology, Vanderbilt University Medical Center, VUMC 1161 21st Avenue South, MCN #3113, Nashville, TN 37232, USA; [b] Division of Cardiovascular Medicine, Vanderbilt University Medical Center, Nashville, TN, USA; [c] Division of Rheumatology, Tennessee Valley Healthcare System, Veterans Affair Medical Center, Nashville, TN, USA
* Corresponding author.
E-mail address: erin.chew@vumc.org

Rheum Dis Clin N Am 49 (2023) 483–488
https://doi.org/10.1016/j.rdc.2023.01.018
0889-857X/23/© 2023 Elsevier Inc. All rights reserved.

important for practicing rheumatologists. Classification of primary cardiac involvement in SSc is particularly critical to define because several immunomodulatory therapeutics have possible adverse cardiac effects.

ROUTINE CARDIOPULMONARY SCREENING IN SYSTEMIC SCLEROSIS

Interstitial lung disease (ILD), pulmonary arterial hypertension (PAH), and scleroderma renal crisis (SRC) are well-recognized causes of mortality in SSc.[6] As such, routine cardiopulmonary screening is the standard of care for all patients with SSc. Patients are educated to routinely monitor their blood pressure in order to screen for SRC. Experts recommend the routine use of pulmonary function testing for ILD monitoring and high-resolution chest computed tomography (CT) for high-risk patients.[7] Serum levels of myocardial natriuretic peptide N-terminal probrain natriuretic peptide (NT-proBNP) and electrocardiograms (ECGs) are incorporated into some composite PAH screening algorithms.[8] The regular use of noninvasive Doppler echocardiography with subsequent right heart catheterization to confirm the presence of precapillary pulmonary hypertension allows for an early detection and prompt initiation of therapy for PAH.[9] Echocardiography techniques including speckle-tracking echocardiography for the measurement of strain and strain rate can provide additional regional contractility information that detects early myocardial dysfunction.[10] As such, the routine use of cardiopulmonary screenings in patients with SSc can assist the rheumatologist in the early detection of primary cardiac involvement.

APPROACH TO PRIMARY CARDIAC INVOLVEMENT DIAGNOSTICS

Abnormal parameters of diastolic function and conduction abnormalities may be early indicators of primary cardiac involvement in SSc and require further diagnostics.[11] Cardiovascular magnetic resonance (CMR) is the gold standard for imaging cardiac anatomy, function, and advanced myocardial tissue characterization. Advances in parametric mapping enable direct, quantitative comparisons that can detect both focal and diffuse perfusion defects, myocardial fibrosis, and myocardial edema, without the need for contrast agents.[12] Although the clinical and prognostic significance of subclinical findings remains unclear, obtaining CMR to further evaluate structural abnormalities found on echocardiogram can identify patients who are at high risk of significant conduction and rhythm disturbances that may require therapeutic or prophylactic intervention.[11] Another noninvasive technique that is highly sensitive in the quantitative evaluation of inflammation is 18F-fluorodeoxyglucose-positron emission tomography/computed tomography (PET/CT). Although potentially promising in SSc, its use to guide diagnosis and therapeutics is not yet clear.[13,14] Nonetheless, CMR with parametric mapping and PET/CT reduces the need for invasive myocardial biopsy to diagnosis primary cardiac involvement due to SSc.[15] However, there is a role for myocardial biopsy if infective myocarditis or drug reaction is suspected.[11] The most common pathologic finding in SSc-associated cardiomyopathy is patchy interstitial or perivascular fibrosis[16] (**Fig. 1**). However, Hematoxylin & Eosin, Masson trichrome, and immunofluorescence stains may identify infective myocarditis in patients.[17] In patients with accompanying diastolic dysfunction, a common finding in cardiomyopathy associated with SSc, the combination of Congo Red and immunostains for immunoglobulin chains may be used to identify cardiac amyloidosis as a treatable cause of underlying diastolic dysfunction.[11,18] Finally, in patients with suspected drug-induced cardiomyopathy (eg, hydroxychloroquine), electron microscopic evaluation of myocardial biopsy samples may identify lamellar body inclusions suggestive of a drug-induced cardiomyopathy.[19]

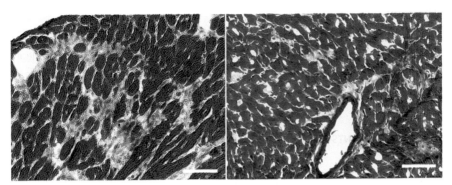

Fig. 1. Typical findings of interstitial (*left*) and perivascular (*right*) fibrosis that are found in patients with SSc with myocardial involvement (*bar* = 50 μm).

If there is a concern for conduction abnormalities and a 12-lead ECG is nondiagnostic, an ambulatory ECG monitoring (for 24 hours or longer) should be performed.[20] The implantable loop recorder (ILR), also known as insertable cardiac monitor, is a subcutaneous device that can stay in place subcutaneously for up to 3 years, and is used for diagnosing heart rhythm disorders without providing an intervention such as rate control.[21,22] CMR-extracellular volume (indicating diffuse fibrosis) and cardiac biomarkers may identify at-risk patients who would benefit from ILR screening for the initiation of antiarrhythmic therapy.[23] The importance of diagnosis is clear because automatic implantable cardioverter defibrillators have shown beneficial results in SSc.[24]

Cardiac soluble biomarkers can help identify cardiac involvement but do not distinguish between primary and secondary causes. Although, NT-proBNP has an established role in the screening and prognostication of SSc-associated PAH, troponin I is more specific to the myocardium than troponin T, and is helpful in cases where there is comorbid skeletal myopathy.[25] In one study, patients with both an elevated troponin T and NT-proBNP levels had higher risk of cardiac death.[26] However, elevated cardiac biomarkers have been more consistently reported when functional abnormalities are detectable by echocardiogram or clinical symptoms are present. There is a need for specific cardiac biomarkers that define primary cardiac involvement particularly in asymptomatic patients.

THERAPEUTIC CONSIDERATIONS REQUIRING PRIMARY CARDIAC INVOLVEMENT CHARACTERIZATION

Certain treatments for SSc require an understanding of primary cardiac involvement due to potential therapeutic adverse effects. Cyclophosphamide, which historically has been used to treat ILD and skin disease in SSc, is associated with dose-dependent cardiac toxicity.[27] Nintedanib is a tyrosine kinase inhibitor, which is FDA-approved for the treatment of SSc-ILD with ad hoc data for other indications concerning its proarrhythmic, hypertensive, and arterial thromboembolic events.[28] Janus kinase (JAK) inhibitors, a novel class of targeted synthetic disease-modifying antirheumatic drugs approved for the treatment of rheumatoid arthritis, are being investigated for SSc.[29] Progression of atherosclerosis, lipid profile disturbance, and risk of thromboembolic complications are a concern with this class of drug.[30] Of note, CMR is recommended as part of the preevaluation for hematopoietic stem cell transplantation for SSc.[31] The role of algorithm-based cardiac evaluation both before and after therapeutic initiation is one of the many unmet needs for SSc clinical care.[11]

SUMMARY

Patients with SSc regularly complete cardiopulmonary screening as a part of their rheumatology care. Abnormalities found on these routine screens require additional investigation. CMR, PET/CT, soluble biomarkers, ambulatory ECG, and ILR are options to further investigate primary cardiac involvement, which may be particularly useful before therapeutic initiation with concerning cardiovascular adverse event profiles.

CLINICS CARE POINTS

- Routine use of cardiopulmonary screenings such in patients with SSc such as high-resolution chest CT, NT-proBNP, ECGs, and doppler echocardiography can assist the rheumatologist in the early detection of primary cardiac involvement.

- Abnormal parameters of diastolic function and conduction abnormalities may be early indicators of primary cardiac involvement in SSc. Patients may benefit from further diagnostics including CMR, PET/CT, soluble biomarkers, ambulatory ECG, and ILR.

DISCLOSURES

Authors declare no conflicts of interests.

FUNDING

T. Frech is supported by VA Merit Award I01CX002111. V. Agrawal is supported by Veterans Affairs 1IK2BX005828 (VA) and NIH NHLBI 1K08HL153956 (VA).

REFERENCES

1. Smith V, Scirè CA, Talarico R, et al. Systemic sclerosis: state of the art on clinical practice guidelines, RMD Open 2018;4:e000782.
2. Ross L, Prior D, Proudman S, et al. Defining primary systemic sclerosis heart involvement: a scoping literature review, Semin Arthritis Rheum, 48, 2019, 874–887.
3. Bulkley BH, Ridolfi RL, Salyer WR, et al. Myocardial lesions of progressive systemic sclerosis. A cause of cardiac dysfunction. Circulation 1976;53:483–90.
4. D'Angelo WA, Fries JF, Masi AT, et al. Pathologic observations in systemic sclerosis (scleroderma). A study of fifty-eight autopsy cases and fifty-eight matched controls. Am J Med 1969;46:428–40.
5. Elhai M, Meune C, Boubaya M, et al. Mapping and predicting mortality from systemic sclerosis. Ann Rheum Dis 2017;76:1897–905.
6. Denton CP, Khanna D. Systemic sclerosis. Lancet 2017;390.1685–99.
7. Roofoh D, Khanna D. Management of systemic sclerosis: the first five years. Curr Opin Rheumatol 2020;32:228–37.
8. Weatherald J, Montani D, Jevnikar M, et al. Screening for pulmonary arterial hypertension in systemic sclerosis. Eur Respir Rev 2019;28. https://doi.org/10.1183/16000617.0023-2019.
9. Avouac J, Airò P, Meune C, et al. Prevalence of pulmonary hypertension in systemic sclerosis in European Caucasians and metaanalysis of 5 studies. J Rheumatol 2010;37:2290–8.

10. Schattke S, Knebel F, Grohmann A, et al. Early right ventricular systolic dysfunction in patients with systemic sclerosis without pulmonary hypertension: a Doppler Tissue and Speckle Tracking echocardiography study. Cardiovasc Ultrasound 2010;8:3.

11. Bruni C, Ross L. Cardiac involvement in systemic sclerosis: getting to the heart of the matter. Best Pract Res Clin Rheumatol 2021;35:101668.

12. Ferreira VM, Piechnik SK. CMR parametric mapping as a tool for myocardial tissue characterization. Korean Circ J 2020;50:658–76.

13. Besenyi Z., Ágoston G., Hemelein R., et al., Detection of myocardial inflammation by 18F-FDG-PET/CT in patients with systemic sclerosis without cardiac symptoms: a pilot study, Clin Exp Rheumatol, 37 (Suppl 119), 2019, 88–96.

14. Krumm P, Mueller KAL, Klingel K, et al. Cardiovascular magnetic resonance patterns of biopsy proven cardiac involvement in systemic sclerosis. J Cardiovasc Magn Reson 2017;18:70.

15. Liangos O, Neure L, Kühl U, et al. The possible role of myocardial biopsy in systemic sclerosis. Rheumatology 2000;39:674–9.

16. Mueller KA, Mueller II, Eppler D, et al. Clinical and histopathological features of patients with systemic sclerosis undergoing endomyocardial biopsy. PLoS One 2015;10:e0126707.

17. Cooper LT Jr. Myocarditis. N Engl J Med 2009;360:1526–38.

18. Pucci A, Aimo A, Musetti V, et al. Amyloid deposits and fibrosis on left ventricular endomyocardial biopsy correlate with extracellular volume in cardiac amyloidosis. J Am Heart Assoc 2021;10:e020358.

19. Soong TR, Barouch LA, Champion HC, et al. New clinical and ultrastructural findings in hydroxychloroquine-induced cardiomyopathy–a report of 2 cases. Hum Pathol 2007;38:1858–63.

20. Bissell LA, Anderson M, Burgess M, et al. Consensus best practice pathway of the UK Systemic Sclerosis Study group: management of cardiac disease in systemic sclerosis. Rheumatology 2017;56:912–21.

21. Bisignani A, De Bonis S, Mancuso L, et al. Implantable loop recorder in clinical practice. J Arrhythm 2019;35:25–32.

22. Hung G, Mercurio V, Hsu S, et al. Progress in understanding, diagnosing, and managing cardiac complications of systemic sclerosis. Curr Rheumatol Rep 2019;21:68.

23. Bissell LA, Dumitru RB, Erhayiem B, et al. Incidental significant arrhythmia in scleroderma associates with cardiac magnetic resonance measure of fibrosis and hs-TnI and NT-proBNP. Rheumatology 2019;58:1221–6.

24. Bernardo P, Conforti ML, Bellando-Randone S, et al. Implantable cardioverter defibrillator prevents sudden cardiac death in systemic sclerosis. J Rheumatol 2011;38:1617–21.

25. Allanore Y, Komocsi A, Vettori S, et al. N-terminal pro-brain natriuretic peptide is a strong predictor of mortality in systemic sclerosis. Int J Cardiol 2016;223:385–9.

26. Bosello S., De Luca G., Berardi G., et al., Cardiac troponin T and NT-proBNP as diagnostic and prognostic biomarkers of primary cardiac involvement and disease severity in systemic sclerosis: a prospective study, Eur J Intern Med, 60, 2019, 46–53.

27. Fraiser LH, Kanekal S, Kehrer JP. Cyclophosphamide toxicity. Characterising and avoiding the problem. Drugs 1991;42:781–95.

28. Shah RR, Morganroth J. Update on cardiovascular safety of tyrosine kinase inhibitors: with a special focus on QT interval, left ventricular dysfunction and overall risk/benefit. Drug Saf 2015;38:693–710.

29. Lescoat A, Lelong M, Jeljeli M, et al. Combined anti-fibrotic and anti-inflammatory properties of JAK-inhibitors on macrophages in vitro and in vivo: Perspectives for scleroderma-associated interstitial lung disease. Biochem Pharmacol 2020;178: 114103.

30. Kotyla PJ, Islam MA, Engelmann M. Clinical Aspects of Janus Kinase (JAK) Inhibitors in the Cardiovascular System in Patients with Rheumatoid Arthritis. Int J Mol Sci 2020;21. https://doi.org/10.3390/ijms21197390.

31. Farge D, Burt RK, Oliveira MC, et al. Cardiopulmonary assessment of patients with systemic sclerosis for hematopoietic stem cell transplantation: recommendations from the European Society for Blood and Marrow Transplantation Autoimmune Diseases Working Party and collaborating partners. Bone Marrow Transplant 2017;52:1495–503.

State-of-the-art, balanced coverage of all aspects of rheumatology

Rheumatology, 8th Edition

Edited by Marc C. Hochberg, Ellen M. Gravallese, Josef S. Smolen, Desiree van der Heijde, Michael E. Weinblatt, and Michael H. Weisman

Covering both the scientific basis of rheumatology and practical, clinical information for rheumatologists and trainees, Rheumatology, 8th Edition, remains a leading text in this fast-changing field. Fully updated from cover to cover, this two-volume text is designed to meet the needs of all practicing and academic rheumatologists as well as arthritis-related health care professionals and scientists interested in rheumatic and musculoskeletal diseases.

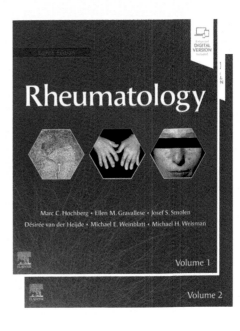

www.elsevierhealth.com

Moving?

Make sure your subscription moves with you!

To notify us of your new address, find your **Clinics Account Number** (located on your mailing label above your name), and contact customer service at:

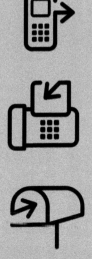

Email: journalscustomerservice-usa@elsevier.com

800-654-2452 (subscribers in the U.S. & Canada)
314-447-8871 (subscribers outside of the U.S. & Canada)

Fax number: 314-447-8029

Elsevier Health Sciences Division
Subscription Customer Service
3251 Riverport Lane
Maryland Heights, MO 63043

*To ensure uninterrupted delivery of your subscription, please notify us at least 4 weeks in advance of move.

9780323960793